CANCER CLINICAL TRIALS:

PROACTIVE STRATEGIES

Cancer Treatment and Research
Steven T. Rosen, M.D., *Series Editor*

Sugarbaker, P. (ed): *Peritoneal Carcinomatosis: Principles of Management.* 1995. ISBN 0-7923-3727-1.
Dickson, R.B., Lippman, M.E. (eds): *Mammary Tumor Cell Cycle, Differentiation and Metastasis.* 1995. ISBN 0-7923-3905-3.
Freireich, E.J, Kantarjian, H. (eds): *Molecular Genetics and Therapy of Leukemia.* 1995. ISBN 0-7923-3912-6.
Cabanillas, F., Rodriguez, M.A. (eds): *Advances in Lymphoma Research.* 1996. ISBN 0-7923-3929-0.
Miller, A.B. (ed.): *Advances in Cancer Screening.* 1996. ISBN 0-7923-4019-1.
Hait, W.N. (ed.): *Drug Resistance.* 1996. ISBN 0-7923-4022-1.
Pienta, K.J. (ed.): *Diagnosis and Treatment of Genitourinary Malignancies.* 1996. ISBN 0-7923-4164-3.
Arnold, A.J. (ed.): *Endocrine Neoplasms.* 1997. ISBN 0-7923-4354-9.
Pollock, R.E. (ed.): *Surgical Oncology.* 1997. ISBN 0-7923-9900-5.
Verweij, J., Pinedo, H.M., Suit, H.D. (eds): *Soft Tissue Sarcomas: Present Achievements and Future Prospects.* 1997. ISBN 0-7923-9913-7.
Walterhouse, D.O., Cohn, S. L. (eds): *Diagnostic and Therapeutic Advances in Pediatric Oncology.* 1997. ISBN 0-7923-9978-1.
Mittal, B.B., Purdy, J.A., Ang, K.K. (eds): *Radiation Therapy.* 1998. ISBN 0-7923-9981-1.
Foon, K.A., Muss, H.B. (eds): *Biological and Hormonal Therapies of Cancer.* 1998. ISBN 0-7923-9997-8.
Ozols, R.F. (ed.): *Gynecologic Oncology.* 1998. ISBN 0-7923-8070-3.
Noskin, G. A. (ed.): *Management of Infectious Complications in Cancer Patients.* 1998. ISBN 0-7923-8150-5.
Bennett, C. L. (ed.): *Cancer Policy.* 1998. ISBN 0-7923-8203-X.
Benson, A. B. (ed.): *Gastrointestinal Oncology.* 1998. ISBN 0-7923-8205-6.
Tallman, M.S., Gordon, L.I. (eds): *Diagnostic and Therapeutic Advances in Hematologic Malignancies.* 1998. ISBN 0-7923-8206-4.
von Gunten, C.F. (ed.): *Palliative Care and Rehabilitation of Cancer Patients.* 1999. ISBN 0-7923-8525-X
Burt, R.K., Brush, M.M. (eds): *Advances in Allogeneic Hematopoietic Stem Cell Transplantation.* 1999. ISBN 0-7923-7714-1.
Angelos, P. (ed.): *Ethical Issues in Cancer Patient Care* 2000. ISBN 0-7923-7726-5.
Gradishar, W.J, Wood, W.C. (eds): *Advances in Breast Cancer Management.* 2000. ISBN 0-7923-7890-3.
Sparano, J. A. (ed.): *HIV & HTLV-I Associated Malignancies.* 2001. ISBN 0-7923-7220-4.
Ettinger, D. S. (ed.): *Thoracic Oncology.* 2001. ISBN 0-7923-7248-4.
Bergan, R. C. (ed.): *Cancer Chemoprevention.* 2001. ISBN 0-7923-7259-X.
Raza, A., Mundle, S.D. (eds): *Myelodysplastic Syndromes & Secondary Acute Myelogenous Leukemia* 2001. ISBN: 0-7923-7396.
Talamonti, M. S. (ed.): *Liver Directed Therapy for Primary and Metastatic Liver Tumors.* 2001. ISBN 0-7923-7523-8.
Stack, M.S., Fishman, D.A. (eds): *Ovarian Cancer.* 2001. ISBN 0-7923-7530-0.
Bashey, A., Ball, E.D. (eds): *Non-Myeloablative Allogeneic Transplantation.* 2002. ISBN 0-7923-7646-3.
Leong, S. P.L. (ed.): *Atlas of Selective Sentinel Lymphadenectomy for Melanoma, Breast Cancer and Colon Cancer.* 2002. ISBN 1-4020-7013-6.
Andersson , B., Murray D. (eds): *Clinically Relevant Resistance in Cancer Chemotherapy.* 2002. ISBN 1-4020-7200-7.
Beam, C. (ed.): *Biostatistical Applications in Cancer Research.* 2002. ISBN 1-4020-7226-0.
Brockstein, B., Masters, G. (eds): *Head and Neck Cancer.* 2003. ISBN 1-4020-7336-4.
Frank, D.A. (ed.): *Signal Transduction in Cancer.* 2003. ISBN 1-4020-7340-2.
Figlin, R. A. (ed.): *Kidney Cancer.* 2003. ISBN 1-4020-7457-3.
Kirsch, M.; Black, P. McL. (ed.): *Angiogenesis in Brain Tumors.* 2003. ISBN 1-4020-7704-1.
Keller, E.T., Chung, L.W.K. (eds): *The Biology of Skeletal Metastases.* 2004. ISBN 1-4020-7749-1.
Kumar, R. (ed.): *Molecular Targeting and Signal Transduction.* 2004. ISBN 1-4020-7822-6.
Verweij, J., Pinedo, H.M. (eds): *Targeting Treatment of Soft Tissue Sarcomas.* 2004. ISBN 1-4020-7808-0.
Finn, W.G., Peterson, L.C. (eds.): *Hematopathology in Oncology.* 2004. ISBN 1-4020-7919-2.
Farid, N. (ed.): *Molecular Basis of Thyroid Cancer.* 2004. ISBN 1-4020-8106-5.
Khleif, S. (ed.): *Tumor Immunology and Cancer* Vaccines. 2004. ISBN 1-4020-8119-7.
Balducci, L., Extermann, M. (eds): *Biological Basis of Geriatric Oncology.* 2004. ISBN
Abrey, L.E., Chamberlain, M.C., Engelhard, H.H. (eds): *Leptomeningeal Metastases.* 2005. ISBN 0-387-24198-1
Platanias, L.C. (ed.): *Cytokines and Cancer.* 2005. ISBN 0-387-24360-7.
Leong, S. P.L., Kitagawa, Y., Kitajima, M. (eds): *Selective Sentinel Lymphadenectomy for Human Solid Cancer.* 2005. ISBN 0-387-23603-1.
Small, Jr. W., Woloschak, G. (eds): *Radiation Toxicity: A Practical Guide.* 2005. ISBN 1-4020-8053-0.
Haefner, B., Dalgleish, A. (eds): *The Link Between Inflammation and Cancer.* 2006. ISBN 0-387-26282-2.
Leonard, J.P., Coleman, M. (eds): *Hodgkin's and Non-Hodgkin's Lymphoma.* 2006. ISBN 0-387-29345.
Leong, S. P.L. (ed:) *Cancer Clinical Trials: Proactive Strategies.* 2006. ISBN 0-387-33224-3.

CANCER CLINICAL TRIALS:

PROACTIVE STRATEGIES

edited by

STANLEY P. L. LEONG, MD, FACS
Professor and Director of Sentinel Lymph Node Program
University of California San Francisco Medical Center
at Mount Zion
San Francisco, CA, USA

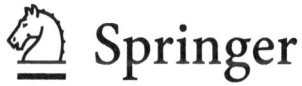

Stanley P. L. Leong
Department of Surgery
University of California
Medical Center at Mount Zion
1600 Divisadero Street
San Francisco, CA 94143
leongs@surgery.ucsf.edu

CANCER CLINICAL TRIALS: PROACTIVE STRATEGIES

Library of Congress Control Number: 2006927192

ISBN-10: 0-387-33224-3 e-ISBN-10: 0-387-33225-1
ISBN-13: 978-0387-33224-6 e-ISBN-13: 978-0387-33225-3

Printed on acid-free paper.

© 2007 Springer Science+Business Media, LLC
All rights reserved. This work may not be translated or copied in whole or in part without the written permission of the publisher (Springer Science+Business Media, LLC, 233 Spring Street, New York, NY 10013, USA), except for brief excerpts in connection with reviews or scholarly analysis. Use in connection with any form of information storage and retrieval, electronic adaptation, computer software, or by similar or dissimilar methodology now known or hereafter developed is forbidden.
The use in this publication of trade names, trademarks, service marks and similar terms, even if they are not identified as such, is not to be taken as an expression of opinion as to whether or not they are subject to proprietary rights.
While the advice and information in this book are believed to be true and accurate at the date of going to press, neither the authors nor the editors nor the publisher can accept any legal responsibility for any errors or omissions that may be made. The publisher makes no warranty, express or implied, with respect to the material contained herein.

Printed in the United States of America.

9 8 7 6 5 4 3 2 1

springer.com

Cover figure modified and printed with permission © 2002 Coalition of Cancer Cooperative Groups.

CONTENTS

Contributors		vii
Foreword		xiii
Preface		xvii
Acknowledgement		xix

1. **Historical Perspective and Evolving Concerns for Human Research** — 1
   Bernard Lo and Nesrin Garan

2. **Cancer Trials and the Institutional Review Board (IRB)** — 11
   Scott Kurtzman and Zita Lazzarini

3. **NCI's Cancer Therapy Evaluation Program: A Commitment to Treatment Trials** — 31
   Jeffrey S. Abrams, Anthony Murgo and Michaele C. Christian

4. **Practical Guide for Cancer Clinical Investigators** — 51
   Steven Hirschfeld

5. **The Role of Cooperative Groups in Cancer Clinical Trials** — 111
   Ann M. Mauer, Elizabeth S. Rich and Richard L. Schilsky

6. **The Advocate Role in Clinical Study Development and Partnering with Patient Advocates in Your Local Institution** — 131
   Barbara Parker

7. **The National Breast Cancer Coalition: Setting the Standard for Advocate Collaboration in Clinical Trials** — 143
   Fran Visco

8. **The Role of the Principal Investigator in Cancer Clinical Trials** — 157
   Stanley P. L. Leong

9.	**The Audit Process and How to Ensure a Successful Audit** Y. Nancy You, Lisa Jacobs, Elizabeth Martinez and David M. Ota	179
10.	**The Privacy Rule (HIPAA) As It Relates To Clinical Research** John M. Harrelson and John M. Falletta	199
11.	**The Commission on Cancer, American College of Surgeons' Response to HIPAA** E. Greer Gay	209
12.	**Ethical and Legal Issues in the Conduct of Cancer Clinical Trials** Gerianne J. Sands and Peggy A. Means	219
13.	**The Role of the Office of Research Integrity in Cancer Clinical Trials** Peter Abbrecht, Nancy Davidian, Samuel Merrill and Alan R. Price	231
14.	**Strategies for the Administration of a Clinical Trial Infrastructure: Lessons from a Comprehensive Cancer Center** Leonard A. Zwelling and Carleen A. Brunelli	241
15.	**The Clinical Research Process: Building a System in Harmony with Its Users** Greg Koski	275
16.	**Cancer Research and Clinical Trial in Action: An Important Exercise Before You Embark on Your Study** Stanley P.L. Leong, Larry Carbone and Scott Kurtzman	291
	Index	311

CONTRIBUTORS

Peter Abbrecht, MD, PhD
Medical Expert
Office of Research Integrity
Department of Health and Human Services
Rockville, Maryland

Jeffrey S. Abrams, MD
NCI Project Officer
Cancer Therapy Evaluation Program
Division of Cancer Treatment and Diagnosis
National Cancer Institute
Bethesda, Maryland

Carleen A. Brunelli, PhD, MBA
Chief Research and Regulatory Affairs Officer
Office of Research Administration
The University of Texas M.D. Anderson Cancer Center
Houston, Texas

Larry Carbone, DVM, PhD
Clinical Veterinarian
Department of Veterinary Medicine
University of California San Francisco Medical Center
San Francisco, California

Michaele C. Christian, MD
Associate Director
Cancer Therapy Evaluation Program
Division of Cancer Treatment and Diagnosis
National Cancer Institute
Bethesda, Maryland

Nancy Davidian, PhD
Clinical Case Expert
Office of Research Integrity
Department of Health and Human Services
Rockville, Maryland

John M. Falletta, MD
IRB Chairman Institutional Review Board
Professor of Pediatrics
Duke University Health System
Durham, North Carolina

Nesrin Garan
Program in Medical Ethics
Department of Medicine
University of California San Francisco
San Francisco, California

Greer Gay, RN, PhD, MPH
Manager, Research Unit National Cancer Data Base
Division of Research and Optimal Care
American College of Surgeons
Chicago, Illinois

John M. Harrelson, MD
Associate Professor Pathology/Orthopedic Surgery
Director Musculoskeletal Oncology Division
Director Diabetic Foot Clinic
Duke University Health System
Durham, North Carolina

Steven Hirschfeld, MD, PhD
CAPT USPHS
Office of Cellular, Tissue and Gene Therapy
Center for Biologics Evaluation and Research
Food and Drug Administration
Rockville, Maryland

Lisa Jacobs, MD
Assistant Professor of Surgery
Department of Surgery
Johns Hopkins University
Baltimore, Maryland

Greg Koski, MD, PhD
Associate Professor of Anesthesia
Senior Scientist
Institute for Health Policy
Massachusetts General Hospital
Harvard Medical School
Boston, Massachusetts

Scott Kurtzman, MD, FACS
Director of Surgery
Waterbury Hospital
Waterbury, Connecticut
Department of Surgery
University of Connecticut School of Medicine
Farmington, Connecticut

Zita Lazzarini, JD
Division Director and Associate Professor
Department of Surgery
University of Connecticut School of Medicine
Farmington, Connecticut

Stanley P. L. Leong, MD, FACS
Professor and Director, Sentinel Lymph Node Program
Department of Surgery
University of California San Francisco Medical Center at Mount Zion
Member, UCSF Comprehensive Cancer Center, San Francisco, California

Bernard Lo, MD
Professor
Program in Medical Ethics
Department of Medicine
University of California San Francisco
San Francisco, California

Elizabeth Martinez, LPN, BS
Lead Auditor
American College of Surgeons Oncology Group
Durham, North Carolina

Ann M. Mauer, MD
Assistant Professor of Medicine
Cancer and Leukemia Group B
Central Office of the Chairman
Chicago, Illinois

Peggy A. Means
Consultant
Fred Hutchinson Cancer Research Center
Seattle, Washington

Samuel Merrill, PhD
Scientist-Investigator
Office of Research Integrity
Department of Health and Human Services
Rockville, Maryland

Anthony Murgo, MD
Acting Chief Investigational Drug Branch
Associate Chief for Developmental Chemotherapy Evaluation Program
Cancer Therapy Evaluation Program
Division of Cancer Treatment and Diagnosis
National Cancer Institute
Bethesda, Maryland

David M. Ota, MD
Department of Surgery
Duke University Medical Center
Durham, North Carolina
American College of Surgeons Oncology Group
Durham, North Carolina

Barbara Parker
Breast Cancer SPORE and
American College of Surgeons Oncology Group
Duke University Medical Center
Durham, North Carolina

Alan R. Price, PhD
Associate Director for Investigative Oversight
Office of Research Integrity
Rockville, Maryland

Elizabeth S. Rich, MD, PhD
Assistant Professor of Medicine
Cancer and Leukemia Group B
Central Office of the Chairman
Chicago, Illinois

Gerianne J. Sands
Associate General Counsel
Fred Hutchinson Cancer Research Center
Seattle, Washington

Richard L. Schilsky, MD
Professor of Medicine
Cancer and Leukemia Group B
Central Office of the Chairman
Chicago, Illinois

Fran Visco
President
National Breast Cancer Coalition
Washington, DC

Y. Nancy You, MD
Surgical Research Fellow
American College of Surgeons Oncology Group
Durham, North Carolina

Leonard A. Zwelling, MD, MBA
Vice President for Research Administration
Office of Research Administration
The University of Texas M.D. Anderson Cancer Center
Houston, Texas

FOREWORD

Samuel A. Wells, Jr., MD
Professor of Surgery
Duke University Medical Center
Durham, North Carolina

The formal organization of a clinical trial program for the treatment of patients with malignant diseases began in this country over 50 years ago and resulted in a large part from the availability of promising therapeutic agents for the treatment of leukemia, and subsequently solid tumors. The National Cancer Institute (NCI) initiated this effort, which has gradually expanded to include twelve cooperative clinical trial groups involving 1700 institutions in Canada, Europe and the United States. The cooperative groups, administered by the Cancer Therapy Evaluation Program of the NCI, enter over 22,000 patients on clinical studies each year. The groups are large and complex organizations that include a number of specialists, such as: clinical oncologists, statisticians, other medical specialists, basic scientists, nurses, epidemiologists, health services researchers, data managers, information technologists, auditors, data and safety monitoring committee members, and patient advocates. Additional cancer clinical trials are supported by investigator-initiated grants or by the N01 contract mechanism. The individual groups have conducted highly important clinical trials, which have substantially improved the treatment of patients with cancer. To appreciate the contributions of the cooperative group program, one need only review the accomplishments of the National Surgical Adjuvant Breast Project, which greatly improved the management of patients with carcinoma of the breast, or the role of the Children's Cancer Group and the Pediatric Oncology Group (now combined as the Children's Oncology Group), which reduced the mortality of childhood cancer (Figure 1A) despite an increasing incidence (Figure 1B). The pediatric clinical trial groups have had a remarkable impact on the survival of children with cancer, due in a large part to their ability to accrue over half of children with cancer in the U.S. and Canada to their clinical trials, a rate more than ten times that achieved by the adult cooperative groups.

Dr. Leong has edited and authored an important book on *Cancer Clinical Trials: Proactive Strategies.* There are contributions from a series of international experts on clinical trials. This book provides an important historical context and thoroughly addresses the broad operational aspects of cancer clinical trials. Substantial personal effort and resources are required to develop a cancer clinical research program, whether in the academic or the private practice setting. The institutional review board, regulatory personnel, and ethicists are essential to the efficient and safe performance of clinical research. Furthermore, the role of a dedicated principal investigator, skilled in the theory and practice of clinical research, is critical to a successful clinical trial program. Above all the patients are the key element of successful clinical trials, as it is they who serve as both the participants and the direct beneficiaries of the clinical research process.

This book is especially timely, as we are entering one of the most important eras of cancer research and treatment, characterized by the development of targeted therapeutics. These novel compounds, a direct result of the human genomic project, have already shown great promise in the treatment of patients with leukemia and malignant solid tumors. We are also into an era of financial constraint in the government-supported clinical research. A well-organized, economically efficient, clinical research infrastructure, in part supported by the federal government, is essential for the critical evaluation of these new compounds, either alone or in combination with existing therapies. It is important that there be a close communication and interaction among the NCI, the Food and Drug Administration, the pharmaceutical and biotechnology industries, basic scientists, and clinical investigators with their institutions if these new therapeutics are to be evaluated in a timely manner.

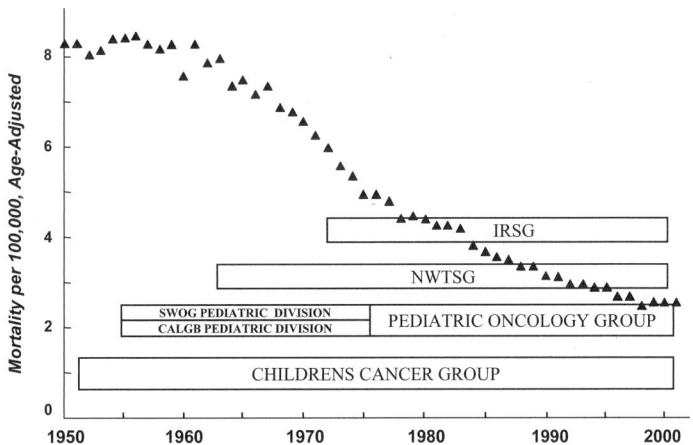

Figure 1A: Decrease in the mortality rate of thyroid cancer in children less than 15 years of age (denoted by closed triangles), since the 1950s when the National Cancer Institute (NCI) began the Cooperative Group Clinical Trials Program. The NCI Cooperative Clinical Trial Groups are shown as horizontal bars: CALGB (Cancer and Leukemia Group B), IRSG (Intergroup Rhabdomyosarcoma Study Group), NWTSG (National Wilms' Tumor Study Group), and SWOG (Southwest Oncology Group). U.S. SEER (United States Surveillance Epidemiology and End Results).

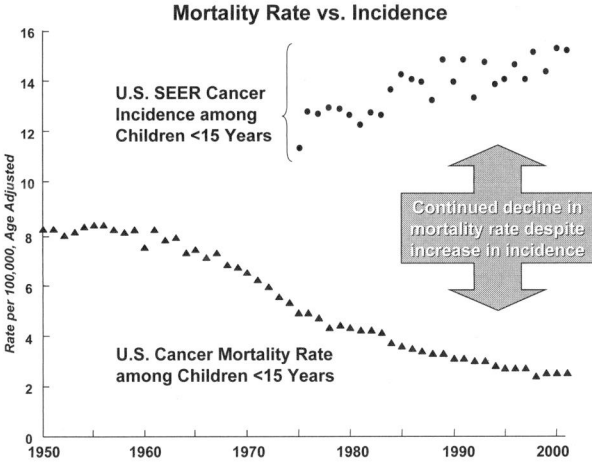

Figure 1B: Decrease in the mortality rate of thyroid cancer in children less than 15 years of age (denoted by closed triangles) as a function of time in decades, beginning in 1950. The decrease has occurred despite an increasing incidence of childhood cancer (denoted by closed circles) in children of the same age group beginning in 1975. U.S. SEER (United States Surveillance Epidemiology and End Results).

PREFACE

According to the American Cancer Society, about 1 million persons in the United States will be diagnosed with solid cancer every year. About 50% of them will be potentially cured by surgery. The other half of the population may develop metastatic cancer. To date, there is no systemic treatment available to cure metastatic cancer. Therefore, cancer clinical trials are critical to evaluate reliable treatment modalities against metastatic cancer. Likewise, adjuvant trials are needed to prevent high risk patients from developing recurrence following definitive surgical resection of their cancer. Only about 3-5% of the cancer patients are enrolled in clinical trials. Multiple barriers exist to block patients from entering into clinical protocols. The ever-changing regulations for clinical trials and the ethical dilemma of treating cancer patients as subjects have made it ever so difficult for the principal investigators to conduct clinical research, especially when they are often ill-informed of the complex nature of the regulations. Therefore, cancer clinical trials are at a critical junction. The objective of this book is to bring the issues of cancer clinical trials into focus so that proactive strategies may be developed to make such trials more user-friendly. Ultimately, the cancer patients will be benefited.

Stanley P. L. Leong, M.D.
Professor of Surgery
UCSF

ACKNOWLEDGEMENT

We would like to thank Jorge Arteaga and Regina Hopkins of the Department of Surgery, UCSF for the preparation of this book.

We are grateful to Laura Walsh and Maureen Tobin of Springer for their advice and expertise in making this book a reality.

Chapter 1

HISTORICAL PERSPECTIVE AND EVOLVING CONCERNS FOR HUMAN RESEARCH

Bernard Lo, MD and Nesrin Garan

*Program in Medical Ethics, Department of Medicine, University of California San Francisco
San Francisco, California, USA*

1. INTRODUCTION

Clinical trials have identified effective new cancer therapies and screening strategies. Additional clinical trials are needed for further progress in cancer prevention, screening, and treatment. However, clinical trials raise ethical concerns because volunteers take on risk for the primary goal of advancing scientific knowledge and helping future patients. Moreover, the risks and benefits of interventions studied in clinical trials are not yet fully known. If a research question has already been answered and the efficacy and safety of the intervention have already been established, there would be no point in carrying out the study. Indeed, it would be unethical to assign participants in a clinical trial to an intervention that was known to be less effective or less safe than the intervention in another arm of the trial. Furthermore, in several historical and recent cases, participants in clinical research suffered serious harm due to ethical lapses in research conduct. In response to such tragic cases, government regulations have been enacted. However, the current regulatory system is flawed: it is burdensome on researchers and institutions, yet does not cover all clinical research and may not be effective in achieving its goals.

2. HISTORICAL BACKGROUND

Research studies that involved serious ethical lapses have led to federal regulations and professional guidelines regarding the ethical conduct of research with human participants. During World War II, Nazi "experiments" intentionally inflicted serious harms on prisoners who gave no consent. In response to these atrocities, the Declaration of Helsinki of 1964 required consent from research subjects and established the need to balance the risks and benefits of the study.[1] In 1972, news reports revealed egregious misconduct in the Tuskegee study, which was conducted by the U.S. government. Researchers deceived impoverished, poorly educated, African-American men into believing they were receiving treatment for syphilis and later withheld antibiotics after they became available.[2] Revelations about the Tuskegee study led to the promulgation of federal regulations on the ethical conduct of human subjects research, the requirement of informed consent from subjects, and the creation of Institutional Review Boards (IRBs) to review federally sponsored human research. These federal regulations form the basis for oversight of clinical trials today.

More recently, 18-year-old Jesse Gelsinger died in 1999 from liver failure during a gene transfer trial at the University of Pennsylvania.[2,3] In retrospect, investigators did not pay sufficient heed to animal data indicating the possibility of adenovirus-induced liver failure and overlooked abnormalities in Gelsinger's liver function tests. The principal investigator was also the founder of the biotechnology company that produced that adenovirus vector used in the study and thus had a significant financial interest in the success of the clinical trial. The researchers in this study also failed to use the consent form approved by the IRB and failed to report as adverse events instances of mild liver toxicity in previous participants. The tragic outcome in this highly publicized case led to additional federal regulations regarding conflicts of interest, training investigators in human participant's protection, and reporting adverse events.

Public outrage at such egregious cases is understandable. All clinical research raises ethical concerns. In clinical care, patients who accept the risk of treatments are the same individuals who will benefit from the treatments. In research, however, participants assume risk primarily for the benefit of future patients and for the advancement of scientific knowledge. The effectiveness of interventions in clinical trials is not known until the study is completed. Also, the risks of new therapies are identified only after data from the clinical trial are analyzed. Participants in research do not have as much knowledge about the risks and potential benefits of a clinical trial as do investigators, peer reviewers, and IRBs. Participants depend on them to assure that the risks of the study are reasonable and minimal. Thus, if there is excessive risk or misrepresentation during the consent process, participants, as well as the public, feel betrayed. This sense of betrayal and mistrust is particularly strong when research is publicly sponsored. Taxpayers may feel complicit if participants in federally funded research are seriously harmed. One response to egregious cases is a demand for greater oversight, which usually means greater government regulation.

The Gelsinger case and other recent cases in which research volunteers died or suffered grave harm indicate serious problems with the current system of human subjects protection.[2,4] IRBs have come under strong criticism because they are underfunded and understaffed.[2,5] In some highly publicized cases, IRBs failed to follow federal regulations and keep adequate records. In these incidents, IRBs reviewed protocols when no member with relevant clinical expertise was present, or when the university official charged with promoting research in the institution was present.[5] Hence research volunteers may not be adequately protected by the current system. However, stricter enforcement of existing regulations or promulgation of additional regulations may not be beneficial. Many IRBs and researchers complain that administrative burdens of compliance with federal regulations are increasing, while doing little to protect research participants.

Changes in the organization of clinical trials raise additional concerns. Traditionally, the bulk of clinical research was funded by the federal government and carried out at academic health centers. However, the majority of clinical research is now funded privately or carried out at contract research organizations (CROs). Federally sponsored research undergoes rigorous peer review and must comply with federal regulations for the protection of human subjects. Most academic health centers agree to apply these regulations to all research at their institution. In contrast, research funded by for-profit sponsors may not receive external peer review. Moreover, federal regulations apply to privately funded research only if the study will be submitted to the Food and Drug Administration (FDA) as part of a new drug application or if the research is carried out in an institution that has agreed to apply the federal human subjects regulations to all research. Many private sponsors follow the Guideline for Good Clinical Practice of the International Conference of Harmonization, which require informed consent and review by an IRB. However, these international guidelines have no provisions regarding conflicts of interest or on training investigators in human subjects protection.

In response to these problems, several broad suggestions have been made to improve human participant's protection. First, accreditation of IRBs may be a less burdensome and more effective and flexible alternative to increased government regulation.[2] Moreover, it may provide more assurance that appropriate guidelines and procedures to protect research participants are actually being followed at the institution. Second, a quality improvement approach would focus attention on improving outcomes of the oversight system rather than on compliance with regulations for its own sake.[2] The challenge is to devise outcomes measures that capture the goal of human subjects protection and that can be readily measured. Third, greater representation of nonscientists and community members on IRBs may help assure that the perspective and concerns of research participants and vulnerable communities are appropriately considered.[6] Lay and noninstitutional IRB members may identify unappreciated risks in the study and problems with the consent process, as well as suggest how to ameliorate them.

3. EVOLVING ETHICAL CONCERNS: OVERSIGHT OF MULTICENTER CLINICAL TRIALS

Conducting research at multiple institutions is desirable because it results in shorter and more efficient trials and more generalizable findings. Also if pivotal trials are conducted in several countries simultaneously, the sponsor can apply for licensing a new drug in those countries at the same time. However, multicenter trials also present many challenges in oversight. Local IRBs differ widely on their assessment of risk and benefit in clinical research.[7] Inconsistent reviews by IRBs at different sites lead to delays in finalizing a common protocol.[7] Moreover, full review by multiple local IRBs requires considerable duplication of effort for busy IRBs, leads to few substantive changes, and places unnecessary burden on sites that enroll few participants.[8]

The National Cancer Institute (NCI) is currently experimenting with a centralized review process for Phase 3 multicenter clinical trials,[8] with the goal of improving the quality and efficiency of IRB review. A national IRB whose members have appropriate ethical, legal, and scientific expertise carries out in-depth review. The local IRBs maintain a role in determining whether local context requires restrictions or minor changes in the protocol or consent form and in assuring that the local researchers are qualified to carry out the research and receive adequate training in human subjects protection. The local IRB may choose to make the central IRB responsible for annual reviews and reviews of adverse events. This central NCI review board will need to work out how it interacts with the NCI scientific review committees and data and safety monitoring boards. In addition, the national IRB needs to determine the extent to which its review of the ethical aspects of a protocol also requires consideration of the scientific aspects of the study. A similar centralized IRB system introduced in the U.K. faced procedural difficulties, mostly because local research ethics committees were unwilling to defer to a centralized authority.[9]

3.1 Conflicts of interest

Industry sponsorship of clinical research has increased dramatically, now exceeding federal support for clinical research. Federal policies promote technology transfer to the private sector, in order to better translate publicly funded discoveries into clinical therapies. These policies have resulted in universities' and their researchers' developing close relationships with for-profit companies, through founding companies, holding stock and options, and forming long-term consulting arrangements.[10] These closer ties between industry and academic institutions, while having the promise of bringing discoveries to the bedside more efficiently, raise concerns about conflicts of interest. University-based researchers play an important public role as impartial and independent agents, distinct from the role of partisan employees of for-profit companies who are manufacturing a drug.[11] This distinction may be particularly important in clinical trials, whose results will influence clinical care of patients.

Studies show that industry-sponsored clinical trials and studies conducted by investigators with ties to industry are more likely to report positive findings for the investigational intervention.[12,13] While this may represent more careful selection of drugs under study, it may also be due to an unwillingness to report negative findings or bias in the design of trials and interpretation of findings.[14-18] In several cases, sponsors refused to allow investigators to publish negative findings about the study drug,[19-21] even though such publication is essential to establish a rigorous evidence base for clinical practice and ultimately to provide the best care to patients. Moreover, typical contracts between academic researchers and industry sponsors do not provide access to data and freedom to publish all findings.[22] To address concerns about academic freedom to publish findings, many leading medical journals now require investigators in clinical trials to disclose conflicts of interest when they submit manuscripts for publication and to certify that they had full access to data, had responsibility for data analysis and interpretation, and controlled the decision to publish.[23]

Under the current system, researchers at an institution receiving federal funding must disclose financial conflicts of interest to the institution, which then has considerable discretion in managing conflicts and implementing conflict of interest policies.[10] Federal regulations do not require researchers to disclose conflicts of interest to the IRB or to research participants.

However, such disclosure should be carried out as a matter of sound ethical practice. Recent voluntary guidelines establish a presumption that academic researchers in a clinical trial should not hold stock or stock options in the manufacturer of the therapies under study, nor be officers in the company.[24] Instead, researchers should be compensated only for their time, effort, and expenses; their remuneration should not increase if the trial shows that the investigational therapy is effective and safe.

3.2 Informed consent

Informed consent from research participants is essential for the ethical conduct of clinical trials. However, it is difficult to achieve. The so-called "therapeutic misconception" is common[25] among research participants, indicating a fundamental misunderstanding about clinical trials. Many participants believe that clinical trials provide individualized treatment and direct benefit to subjects, whereas research by definition has the goal of generalized knowledge and involves unproven interventions. The popular press reinforces this misconception by portraying research too optimistically.

A recent study assessed the quality of informed consent in cancer therapy trials. Researchers found that 48% of subjects believed that all treatments and procedures in the clinical trial were standard therapy for their type of cancer.[26] Thirty-eight percent believed that the clinical trial did not carry any additional risks or discomforts compared with standard treatments, while 29% believed that the treatment being studied was proven to be the best treatment for their type of cancer.[26] In fact, clinical trials generally involve nonstandard treatment, potentially increased risks, and unproven benefits.

Moreover, cancer researchers frequently have misunderstandings about the purpose of clinical trials. One study found that 43% of medical oncologists enrolled patients in clinical trials to assure they got the most state-of-the-art treatment, while 41% enrolled them to improve the treatment of future cancer patients.[27] However, there is no rigorous evidence that patients who enroll in clinical trials have better outcomes than comparable patients who do not participate in clinical trials.[28] Thus the claim that "the best cancer care is in a clinical trial" is not substantiated by convincing evidence.

Researchers often fail to distinguish between different types of benefit that participants may experience in clinical trials. Direct benefits result from the intervention being studied, which may turn out to be more effective or safer than standard care. However, at the onset of a clinical trial it is unknown which arm is superior. Thus it is more accurate to speak about the "prospect" of direct benefit. Several dimensions of direct benefit need to be distinguished. Cancer clinical trials commonly evaluate whether the size of the tumor decreased – a so-called "objective response." An objective response may be partial or complete, long-lasting or short-lived. A short-term partial response in a Phase 1 clinical trial may be sufficient evidence to justify further studies. However, a temporary decrease in the size of the tumor is unlikely to lead to any clinically meaningful outcome.

Collateral benefits of participating in a clinical trial might include closer follow-up, more personal attention, or greater attention to the timing and dosage of therapies, which in turn might lead to improved outcomes, even if the intervention being studied is no more effective than standard care.[25,29] Finally, a clinical trial may provide hope, particularly to patients for whom no effective therapy is available. Hope is always desirable, but unrealistic hope can lead to uninformed decisions to participate in clinical trials. A participant may realize that the probability of a meaningful response to an experimental intervention is low, yet still hope, despite long odds, that he will gain such a response. Such hope is completely consistent with informed consent.

Recent empirical studies highlight the difficulties in attaining informed consent. For example, cancer patients commonly decide to enter a clinical trial before they meet the researchers and hear about the potential benefits and risks. Despite researchers' efforts to explain the experimental nature of clinical trials, there may be difficulties in effectively communicating this information to patients. A recent study found that 50% of parents who enrolled their children in clinical leukemia trials did not understand the concept of randomization, a key factor distinguishing these trials from standard treatment in which the choice of therapy is an individualized decision based on what is best for the patient.[30] In addition, some consent forms may reinforce the therapeutic misconception. Vague wording, such as "you may or may not benefit" or "we cannot guarantee that you will benefit," may imply that benefit is in fact likely.[31] Another study found that in NCI-sponsored clinical trials, consent forms are generally clear in explaining potential risks, harms, and benefits to subjects in Phase I trials.[32] Hence improving consent forms per se is unlikely to solve all problems with informed consent. Other studies found that innovative means of providing information, such as videotapes or CDs, did not consistently enhance participants' understanding of key features of clinical trials.[33] Taken together, these studies underscore that informed consent must be viewed as a process or an ongoing dialogue between researcher and participant, rather than a lengthy legal form that patients must sign before they enroll in clinical research.[34]

4. CONCLUSION

Historically, scandals that shook public trust in research have led to new government regulations. These regulations, however, may be burdensome yet ineffective in protecting research participants. In a systems approach to research oversight, multiple parties have responsibility for protecting participants – sponsors, research institutions, IRBs, and investigators.[34] Investigators have particular responsibilities because they have power over what happens to research subjects and because their decisions and actions during the course of a project cannot be effectively monitored. Thus the ethical integrity and judgment of the investigators are crucial protections for research participants, particularly in situations where the regulations are silent, ambiguous, or controversial. It is essential that researchers fulfill their ethical obligations when designing and carrying out clinical trials. Failure to do so might lead to additional government regulations, thus further complicating the current system rather than facilitating further progress in cancer research.

REFERENCES

1. World Medical Association, World Medical Association Declaration of Helsinki: Ethical Principles for Medical Research Involving Human Subjects.
2. Committee on Assessing the System for Protecting Human Research Subjects. Preserving Public Trust: Accreditation and Human Research Participant Protection Programs. Washington, DC: National Academy Press, 2001.
3. Lo B, Wolf LE. Ethical issues in clinical research: an issue for all internists. Am J Med 2000;109:82-85.
4. Steinbrook R. Protecting research subjects--the crisis at Johns Hopkins. N Engl J Med 2002;346:716-20.
5. Steinbrook R. Improving protection for research subjects. N Engl J Med 2002;346:1425-30.
6. National Bioethics Advisory Commission. Ethical and Policy Issues in Research Involving Human Participants. Bethesda, MD: National Bioethics Advisory Commission, 2001.
7. McWilliams R, Hoover-Fong J, Hamosh A, Beck S, Beaty T, Cutting G. Problematic variation in local institutional review of a multicenter genetic epidemiology study. JAMA 2003;290:360-366.
8. Christian MC, Goldberg JL, Killen J, et al. A central institutional review board for multi-institutional trials. N Engl J Med 2002;346:1405-1408.
9. Tully S. The Party's Over. Fortune June 26, 2000: 156.

10. Committee on Assessing the System for Protecting Human Research Subjects. Responsible Research: A Systems Approach to Protecting Research Participants. Washington, DC: National Academies Press, 2002.
11. Moses H, Martin JB. Academic relationships with industry: a new model for biomedical research. JAMA 2001;285:933-935.
12. Friedman LS, Richter ED. Relationship between conflicts of interest and research results. J Gen Intern Med 2004;19:51-56.
13. Bekelman JE, Li Y, Gross CP. Scope and impact of financial conflicts of interest in biomedical research: a systematic review. JAMA 2003;289:454-465.
14. Van Kolfschooten F. Can you believe what you read? Nature 2002;416:360-363.
15. Rennie D, Flanagin A. Publication bias; the triumph of hope over experience. JAMA 1991;267:411-412.
16. Rennie D, Flanagin A. Conflicts of interest in the publication of science. JAMA 1991;266:266-267.
17. Rennie D, Flanagin A. Thyroid storm. JAMA 1997;277:1238-1243.
18. Rennie D, Flanagin A, Yank V. The contributions of authors. Jama 2000;284:89-91.
19. Chopra SS. Industry Funding of Clinical Trials: Benefit or Bias? JAMA 2003;290:113-114.
20. Dong BJ, W.W. H, Gambertoglio JG, et al. Bioequivalence of generic and brand-name levothyroxine products in the treatment of hypothyroidism. JAMA 1997;277:1205-1213.
21. Kahn JO, Cherng DW, Mayer K, Murray H, S. L. Evaluation of HIV-immunogen, an immunologic modifier, administered to patients infected with HIV having 300 to 549 x 10^6/L CD4 cell counts. JAMA 2000;284:2193-2202.
22. Schulman KA, Seils DM, Timbie JW, et al. A national survey of provisions in clinical-trial agreements between medical schools and industry sponsors. N Engl J Med 2002;347:1335-1341.
23. DeAngelis CD, Fontanarosa PB, Flanagin A. Reporting financial conflicts of interest and relationships between investigators and research sponsors. JAMA 2001;286:89-91.
24. Association of American Medical Colleges, Protecting subjects, preserving trust, promoting progress: policy and guidelines for the oversight of individual financial interests in human subjects research.
25. King NMP. Defining and Describing Benefit Appropriately in Clinical Trials. Journal of Law, Medicine, and Ethics 2000;28:332-343.
26. Joffe S, Cook EF, Cleary PD, Clark JW, Weeks JC. Quality of informed consent in cancer clinical trials: a cross-sectional survey. Lancet 2001;358:1772-7.
27. Joffe S, Weeks JC. Views of American clinical oncologists about the purpose of clinical trials. J Natl Cancer Inst 2002;94:1847-53.
28. Peppercorn JM, Weeks JC, Cook EF, Joffe S. Comparison of outcomes in cancer patients treated within and outside clinical trials: conceptual framework and structured review. Lancet 2004;363:263-270.

29. Churchill LR, Nelson DK, Henderson GE, et al. Assessing benefits in clinical research: why diversity in benefit assessment can be risk. IRB 2003;3:1-8.
30. Kodish E, M. E, Noll RB, et al. Communication of randomization in childhood leukemia trials. JAMA 2004;291:494-496.
31. RAC Informed Consent Working Group. NIH Guidance on Informed Consent For Gene Transfer Research. NIH Office of Biotechnological Activities. Updated Accessed March 2004,
32. Horng S, Emanuel E, Wilfond B, Rackoff J, Martz K, Grady C. Descriptions of benefits and risks in consent forms for phase 1 oncology trials. N Engl J Med 2002;347:2134-2140.
33. Agre P, Campbell FA, Goldman BD, et al. Improving informed consent: the medium is not the message. IRB 2003;25:11-19.
34. Federman DD, Hanna KE, Rodriguez LL, ed. Responsible Research: A Systems Approach to Protecting Research Participants. Washington, D.D.: National Academies Press, 2002.

Chapter 2

CANCER TRIALS AND THE INSTITUTIONAL REVIEW BOARD (IRB)

Scott Kurtzman, MD[1,2] and Zita Lazzarini, JD[1]
[1]*University of Connecticut School of Medicine, Farmington, Connecticut, USA*
[2]*Waterbury Hospital, Waterbury, Connecticut, USA*

Key words: human subjects, Institutional Review Boards, ethics, regulatory issues, and clinical research

1. INTRODUCTION

The issues involved in clinical trials involving cancer patients are often unique. IRBs may be unfamiliar with aspects of such trials that differ from studies involving other types of patients such as healthy subjects and patients with infectious or chronic diseases. Often for cancer patients, there may be no effective treatment for example when metastases have occurred. Experimental treatments might be based on chemotherapeutic regimens that have been used in other cancers or in patients in the adjuvant setting but not in that particular cancer patient population.

Cancer patients are often willing to accept risks of treatment that other patients would not, even in the adjuvant setting. In a recent study, women with breast cancer who had completed adjuvant chemotherapy were asked knowing the discomforts and expenses that they had experienced, how much benefit would be necessary for them to be willing to take the chemotherapy if they had it to do over again. Roughly three quarters of the women said that they would be willing to take chemotherapy again for what might be considered modest gains, e.g. an increase in survival from 15 to 17 years.[1]

As oncologists, we are comfortable offering very toxic treatment to patients who we know might or might not even need the treatment. We knowingly accept the fact that as many as 70% of patients with early stage breast cancer are cured by the operation and radiation therapy that they receive and don't actually harbor occult metastases. Nevertheless, we offer Stage II breast cancer patients adjuvant chemotherapy because we don't yet have the tools to determine which patients harbor metastatic cells. IRB members who come from a variety of non-oncological backgrounds don't necessarily share our view on this problem. In this chapter we will describe the issues that the IRB considers in reviewing cancer clinical trials and give some practical suggestions for improving the study and hopefully ensuring passage of the trial.

2. HISTORY OF CLINICAL RESEARCH

In 1966 Henry Beecher published a landmark article identifying at least 22 studies recently published in the medical literature that suggested serious ethical problems in the treatment of human subjects[2] Beecher's, as well as other scientists' and journalists' revelations about the risks of research that emerged during the 1960s and early 1970s led to increasing calls for government regulation of research. In 1974 Congress passed the National Research Act. Title II of the Act created the National Commission for the Protection of Subjects of Biomedical and Behavioral Research (National Commission). The National Commission worked from 1974 to 1978 and issued 17 reports. Perhaps the most well-known and influential of these reports, published April 8, 1979, was the Belmont Report, described below, which identified key ethical principles that should guide human subjects' research and which formed the basis for regulations issued by the Department of Health Education and Welfare (DEHW, now HHS) and the Food and Drug Administration (FDA). These regulations, originally published January 19, 1981, as "DHHS Regulations for the Protection of Human Subjects and FDA Regulations for Clinical Research and Informed Consent" and issued as 45 CFR part 46 and 21 CFR parts 50 and 56, were more consistent than earlier regulatory efforts and had a tremendous impact on biomedical research. Ten years later efforts to bring all government sponsored research under similar rules was finally realized with publication of the Common Rule in 1991, covering all research using human subjects sponsored by 16 federal agencies. The Common Rule retained most of the provisions of the 1981 regulations, including the requirement for prior ethical review of all studies and the establishment of Institutional Review Boards (IRBs) for this purpose with specific responsibilities.

The remainder of this chapter deals with the requirements of the CFR in regulating research and particularly role of the IRB in relation to cancer trials, but necessarily much of the information is generalizable to other types of studies as well.

As with most significant bodies of federal regulation, a government body exists to implement and enforce the regulations. Originally established in 1972, this entity was called the Office for Protection from Research Risks (OPRR); it was part of NIH and reported directly to the director. In 2000 that office was renamed the Office of Human Research Protections (OHRP). OHRP has continued the activities of OPRR and has issued guidance for research in specific settings.

3. BOUNDARIES BETWEEN PRACTICE AND RESEARCH

3.1 Basic ethical principles

The Belmont Report, issued in 1979, described fundamental ethical principles that should guide research involving human subjects. The Commission was charged specifically with providing guidance on: (1) the boundaries between clinical practice and research; (2) assessing risk and benefits as part of the process of reviewing human subject research; (3) fair selection of subjects; and (4) informed consent for research. Researchers and clinicians often have difficulty defining what constitutes research and what is clinical practice. One simple definition is that research is the collection of data from live human subjects for the purpose of producing generalizable knowledge. Thus, testing new medications or treatments for cancer patients with the intention to present the results to peers would certainly qualify as research. An example of a project that would not be considered research would be a quality assurance program such as a survey of infections in the hospital where the purpose is to improve the care at that particular institution without influencing other hospitals. Sometimes such quality assurance projects yield such interesting information that publication or presentation is valuable. In those cases, the IRB will need to review the project and create the parameters for the use of the data so that the rights of the participants are adequately protected. It is often wise to seek IRB approval for projects that might carry such promise.

The Commission identified what it considered three basic ethical principles, although it acknowledged that other principles could also be important. These principles, respect for persons, beneficence, and justice are familiar from the realm of clinical ethics, but when applied to research additional safeguards and rules need to be considered.

3.2 Respect for persons

The principle of respect for persons requires that scientists recognize the individual worth and dignity of all potential human subjects and it encompasses two important concepts. First, respect for persons requires that scientists and caregivers honor the right of self-determination, or "autonomy", for persons in relation to both medical care and participation in research. That means that individuals who are competent to make medical decisions generally have the right to freely choose whether or not to participate in biomedical or behavioral research. Second, those individuals who are not able to make decisions for themselves, are non-autonomous, deserve additional protection.

In practice, respect for persons has its most direct applications to research in that it requires that autonomous subjects of biomedical or behavioral research be fully informed of the nature, risks, benefits and alternatives to research, and that they consent voluntarily to participate. Respect for persons also requires that individuals or groups with diminished autonomy be protected in the research setting, usually by designating special steps to be taken to limit risk and by designating a process for obtaining consent for research from parents, guardians, or legal representatives.

3.3 Beneficence

The principle of beneficence requires that those conducting biomedical and behavioral research maintain as their primary focus "securing the well-being" of human subjects. This means both that subjects should be protected from harm and that, where possible, the likelihood of benefit be maximized. Beneficence requires that the clinical researcher remain a clinician first. Where the roles of clinician and researcher conflict, the researcher should resolve the conflict in favor of promoting the well being of the patient.

Applying the principle of beneficence to research requires that investigators, IRBs and institutions always minimize risks to human subjects throughout the study process, maximize the possible benefits in relation to risks, and ensure that no study proceeds where the risks remain disproportionate to the potential benefits. It requires the researcher, in relation to individual subjects, to withdraw a subject from a study or trial if the researcher believes continued participation would be particularly dangerous to that subject. IRBs can and will require criteria in most protocols to determine when and if subjects should be withdrawn.

3.4 Justice

The principle of justice requires that the researcher consider whether the risks and benefits of his or her proposed research are equitably distributed. True justice or fairness does not mean purely "equal" treatment. In medicine, public health and research there are well-accepted criteria for treating different individuals differently (e.g., only those with cancer ought to be considered candidates for chemotherapy, or only pregnant women need prenatal care), however it can often be difficult to determine what exactly is "equitable" distribution of the risk and benefits of research.

In practice the principle of justice is most clearly applied to subject selection. Researchers and IRBs must ask, "is the choice of subjects fair?" are any group of subjects being exploited or unjustifiably excluded from the research? This requires consideration of several sub-questions: 1) are the proposed subjects roughly representative of the population affected by this disease or condition? 2) Does the research address a significant health need of the study population? 3) Are any groups excluded from the study without clear medical justification, and if so, why? 4) Is any group chosen purely for convenience? And 5) will the groups chosen as potential subjects be able to benefit from the results of research if they are positive?

These and other applications of the three fundamental ethical principles will be examined further below.

4. APPLICATION OF THE PRINCIPLES

4.1 Informed Consent

The Belmont report, the Helsinki agreement and other similar documents have helped raise the general awareness of the critical nature of informed consent in human subject research. Beyond safety this is the most important issue that the IRB will consider in deciding whether or not to approve the research.

Many have wondered what really constitutes informed consent in this context. Although it is tempting to try and make the subjects understand the scientific basis of the protocol, this is not a practical or reasonable goal. Subjects need to be told in clear language the overall purpose of the study, the potential benefits and risks of their participation, and alternatives to participation. The informed consent form (ICF) must also be written in a language understandable to the patient. If subjects' primary language is not English, the IRB is likely to insist that the ICF be translated into the primary language of the subjects. The ideal way to accomplish this is to have the ICF translated into the second language and then translated back into English by another interpreter (called "back-translation") to ensure accuracy. It is reasonable for the IRB to require the investigators to translate the ICF into some of the major languages in the vicinity of the study site, but the PI should not be expected to translate the ICF for one or two patients who speak a very obscure language.

The upper limit for the language of the consent form should be a 10th grade reading level. Often, even simpler language should be used. If the subjects are likely to have lower levels of education, the language level should be adjusted accordingly. Consent forms that are overly complex or technical are likely to be rejected by the IRB and neither read nor understood by the potential subjects. If the investigators desire to try and convey complex topics such as the molecular biology of the new agent, this can easily be presented in additional documents supplementary to the ICF.

Researchers must also be aware that modern IRBs consider informed consent a process, not just a document. Leaving a patient encounter with a signed trophy will not satisfy this important requirement. In examining the validity of the informed consent process, the IRB will consider broadly two major factors: are the patients *adequately informed* about the study and is their choice *fully voluntary*. In addition to ensuring that the ICF is written in a level suitable for the reading level and education of the potential subjects, the IRB will check that all the requisite information discussed below is included in the ICF (and thus should be discussed in the process). To ensure that patients who enter the study do so voluntarily, the IRB will consider whether the study and the process of informed consent are designed to minimize potential coercive influences on the potential subjects. Specifically, the informed consent should include the overall purpose of the study, the nature and duration of the subjects' involvement, the risks of the study, and an explanation of what will be done to minimize those risks, and alternatives to study participation. Benefits of the participation, if any, and incentives should also be listed, but should not be overstated. IRBs will scrutinize benefits and incentives to determine both if the ICF paints too rosy a picture of the actual clinical benefits that are possible and to ensure that neither the benefits nor the incentives (payments or other gifts to research subjects) are so valuable as to be coercive.

In determining whether the informed consent process is likely to result in subjects who are "fully informed," an IRB will first consider the type of study. There are clearly different standards for non-therapeutic trials, where the purpose of the research is simply to find out about the biology of the cancer, compared to a Phase I trial using an untested investigational agent, compared to Phase II and III trials evaluating safety and efficacy of new agents, or to trials comparing previously approved agents.

4.2 Non-therapeutic trials

There is a great deal to be learned about the biology of cancer. Patients who have clinically apparent disease are a potential rich source of biological information. Demographic, diet, and genetic information can provide important clues as to the etiology of tumors. Blood, urine and other biological specimens can provide material for protein, genetic and other studies. Fresh or preserved tumor and normal tissue specimens not needed for diagnosis or staging are also invaluable clues in the fight against cancer. Sometimes studies such as these are independent of treatment trials other times they are imbedded in therapeutic trials. The ICF must clearly state whether or not participation in the therapeutic portion of the study is contingent on participation on the non-therapeutic part. If this is the case, then participation in this portion of the study might be viewed as coercive, and must be dealt with carefully by the investigators.

The risks of participation in the information, specimen and tissue portions must be fully described. Often researchers focus on the actual physical risks associated with this portion of the study. Sometimes this is important. For example, if bone marrow samples are being taken or if an invasive procedure needs to be carried out that would not occur during the normal course of treatment. If the collection is relatively risk free, such as blood drawing of small samples (i.e., less than 450 ml from healthy adults), then the consent should focus on the implications of the sampling. It is not necessary to spend many paragraphs on bruising and infection, but rather on the significance of the information that might be obtained and potential uses of the information within the study or by others. If the information is not clinically useful, then the explanation might be simple. If for example, however, genetic information is the focus of the study, then the consent process should focus on what the risk to the patient and their family might be with respect to learning about the fundamental building blocks of their inherited genetic information. If the test is examining markers of tumor status or progression, then issues regarding disclosure of experimental information might be relevant. The researcher must inform the patient as to whether or not the information will be available to the patient or the healthcare team. Will the information become part of the medical record? Might knowledge of the information change the planned clinical care?

4.3 Phase I studies

Phase I studies are designed to gather information about safety and answer biological questions. They are not designed to result in benefit to the subjects although occasionally there might be some therapeutic gain. Therefore, research subjects are true volunteers, allowing the research team to learn about the effects of drugs or biologic agents. For that reason, the IRB expects several additional items. First, the research protocol must make abundantly clear what steps are taken to minimize risks to the subjects in a more comprehensive manner than in trials with therapeutic potential. If the investigators manufacture the drug or biologic agent tested, then the protocol must present safety data with respect to good laboratory practices. Usually, if a pharmaceutical company manufactures the agent, the IRB will accept that the manufacturing process meets standards. Similarly, the ICF must be more explicit, and often more detailed. Subjects need to be told in simple language that there is no expectation that their participation in the research will help them in any way. The ICF must state that there are known and unknown hazards associated with the agent.

Some studies raise questions of ownership interest in a valuable product developed using subjects' tissues (blood, tumor cells, etc). Subjects, researchers, institutions and funders may all make plausible ownership claims to products developed using such tissues and ICFs must describe whether or not the researchers intend to reimburse or otherwise compensate the volunteer if the study is successful and results in financial profit. This issue is often confusing for investigators as well as IRB members. CFR Section 46.116 regulations prohibit asking subjects to waive their rights in any way in a consent form "No informed consent, whether oral or written, may include any exculpatory language through which the subject or the representative is made to waive or appear to waive any of the subject's legal rights, or releases or appears to release the investigator, the sponsor, the institution or its agents from liability for negligence." Investigators and research facilities are usually unwilling to share in the profit if the research results in a profitable product. In this situation, research subjects who provide such material cannot be asked to waive their rights to seek financial compensation. In this case however, the researcher can inform the subject as part of the consent process that there is no intention to compensate the patient under any circumstance. It is then up to the patient to seek compensation through the legal system. Whether or not they are successful is up to the courts, not the researcher or the hospital.

4.4   Phase II and III studies

In Phase II and III clinical trial, there is an expectation that there might be some clinical benefit to the subjects as a result of their participation. The protocol and ICF should reflect this. In many cases, the test therapy will be compared to treatment that is considered the standard of care for the disease. The research design must describe the rationale for withholding effective standard treatment for those subjects who will receive the experimental arm. Decisions regarding study design with respect to the issue of parity or superiority studies must also be fully explained and justified in the power analysis.

The ICF must clearly state why the subjects are being asked to participate. The subjects must be told what standard treatment would be if they elect not to participate in the research and how likely that treatment would be to succeed. The document and informed consent process should then contain enough lay language information to allow the potential participant to understand why they should accept potential assignment to an unproven treatment arm. The ICF need not go into technical details, but should convey the rationale in a clear and succinct manner.

The second task of the IRB in evaluating the informed consent process is to ensure that subjects who participate do so voluntarily and free from undue coercion, and that they know they can withdraw from the study at any time. Cancer patients are often more vulnerable than non-cancer patients for several reasons and therefore susceptible to the influence of others. The diagnosis of cancer is extraordinarily stressful. No matter what we as clinicians know about the natural history of the disease, patients almost always view cancer as a threat to their existence in a very current and imminent manner. Additionally, because of the non-optional nature of treatment for most cancers, the patients have a need to please their caregivers and may mistakenly feel that entry into a clinical trial is their only option. Therefore, they might be willing to accept risks or recommendations in order to please the clinician or the staff that they would not otherwise accept. Cancer treatment is also very expensive. Often participation in a clinical trial will lower the cost of treatment to the patients who are underinsured or have high deductibles. This factor might also influence patients to accept risks that they would not otherwise. The significant financial benefit of participation (through lowered costs) is similar to the issue of payment to subjects. The IRB will consider whether the financial implications of participation, like payment, will unduly influence the patient's ability to make an informed and non-coerced decision.

The ICF must also contain a number of procedural and administrative details. Subjects should be reminded that their participation is voluntary and that they can withdraw permission at any time. Withdrawal from the study might subject the patients to unexpected risks, e.g., if subjects withdraw during the nadir count portion of chemotherapy special protective measure might be required. Until data have actually been published, subjects should have the right to withdraw permission to use their data, to contact them in the future, or to bank their tissues, if these remain identifiable. The ICF should also contain accurate information on who is in charge of the study, who can be contacted with questions, where a subject should go with concerns about side effects of drugs or adverse events that occur during the study, and who to call if they have general questions about their rights as human subjects. Most institutions have developed language that can be used in ICFs to convey this type of information, but it is the responsibility of the investigators to ensure that the names and contact information are accurate.

5. ASSESSMENT OF RISK AND BENEFITS

Some degree of risk is inherent in almost all research on human subjects. Cancer trials are no exception. When an IRB reviews such clinical trials, their role is not to eliminate all risk but rather to ascertain that all foreseeable risks have been minimized and that the potential for benefit is maximized. The risks of the research must then be balanced and put into context of the clinical scenario. Once this is done, it is assumed that a competent adult can decide whether or not they are willing to accept the risks of the trial and elect to participate. For example, a greater degree of risk would be permitted for clinical trials involving patients who have no standard clinical option. Research using subjects with otherwise incurable malignancy would fall under this heading. On the other end of the spectrum would be basic science studies for which there is no foreseeable benefit to the patient. Under those circumstances, there would be little tolerance for risk.

Cancer clinical trials often involve the use of chemotherapeutic or biologic agents. These drugs might be standard combinations of approved drugs, new dosages or formulations, the use of non-accepted regimens, or the use of investigational agents. From a human subject point of view, the safety requirements would necessarily vary. If the agent being used is not a standard drug manufactured by an established company, then the IRB will need to monitor not only the application of the material and the ethical nature of the study, but also the manufacturing process. Investigators need to satisfy the IRB that a safety system is in place to ensure that good laboratory practices will prevent chemical and biologic contamination. Additionally, they need to establish quality assurance programs to ensure that: 1) the material that is manufactured is the product intended; 2) the concentrations and doses are reliable and match those listed in the protocol; and 3) the product is sterile and non-pyrogenic. Biologic agents manufactured from living tissue or cell lines raise other concerns. Specifically, the IRB will be expecting to hear how molecular material and viral contamination or transmission will be tested for and prevented.

5.1 Selection of subjects

Historically, clinical researchers often chose subjects based on groups who were immediately available (ward or clinic patients), easy to follow for periods of time (incarcerated or institutionalized adults and children), or unlikely to question the type of care they received (uneducated, poor or minorities). As a result, the burden of research fell disproportionately on the poor, minorities, and those with limited autonomy. Such patients might have been easy to enroll and follow, but they often also had less capacity to understand the potential risks and benefits of participation in trials and may have not have freely chosen to participate. Although it could be argued that for some patients, participating in trials was the only way to access care, this cannot justify exposing only needy patients to the risks of research and may, in fact, interfere with the voluntariness of their choice.

In many ways the Tuskegee Syphilis study provides a classic example of a study which enrolled poor, uneducated subjects who were denied real choice in entering or continuing in the study and suffered various harms as a result of their participation. In that study, poor black men with a diagnosis of syphilis were observed without treatment over a period of decades. When inexpensive and highly effective antibiotic treatment for syphilis became available, the men were denied treatment. In addition they were never clearly informed of the purpose of the study or the nature of their disease. As a result, most subjects experienced the long-term complications of syphilis and some transmitted the disease to their spouses, partners, and children. The subjects in Tuskegee were African-American, poor, unable at the outset to obtain treatment outside the study, largely uneducated, and unlikely to question the "treatment" they received.

Recruitment of subjects in developing countries is a more current example where the benefit of treatment argument can be made but is often surpassed by other considerations of equity in risk sharing. This is discussed more fully below.

In order to avoid exploitation of subjects, investigators' protocols must justify their selection of subjects as equitable, based on the particular condition studied and the risks and benefits of treatment. The investigator must make it clear to the IRB that no particular population or class of subjects will bear an undue burden of the risks. Unless the study involves a disease or condition that is unique to a patient population such as homeless people or patients of a particular race or ethnicity, the methods section must include a plan to offer participation in a fair and equitable manner.

Subject selection also raises another issue. While some studies have unfairly singled out specific groups to bear the risks of research other studies have unjustifiably excluded groups of potential subjects. Besides depriving these potential subjects as individuals of the advantages of participation such as access to free medications or drugs that have clinical promise otherwise not available to them, exclusion can pose larger societal problems. If a group of subjects, such as fertile women, is systematically excluded from research, then information regarding the benefits and risks of the drugs tested are not available to those patients. For example, if a drug is only tested in post-menopausal women, even if it is found to be effective, it might not be used in pre-menopausal women because of the lack of data on safety and efficacy. Similarly, drugs for diseases such as hypertension have been shown to have differing efficacy depending on the race of the patient. If the clinical trial does not include enough subjects of different racial backgrounds, then those patients are deprived of the benefits of the research. Until recently there were very few clinical trails on the safety and efficacy of numerous drugs in children. Consequently, physicians treating children often had little empirical data to guide safety, efficacy, and dosing for children.

The research plan submitted to the IRB must take these factors into consideration. Some funding agencies will require a plan to recruit a percentage of patients from particular racial or ethnic groups. In multi-institutional trials this can be accomplished by including hospitals and clinics in a variety of settings. In single institution studies the plan may be more complex. If subject selection for a particular trial cannot be sufficiently diverse to broadly reflect the population that could benefit from the drug, the researcher must explain and justify the less diverse plan. For pilot studies with limited funding, recruiting patients that don't exist in that community might not be practical. This too should be carefully described and justified.

6. SPECIAL SITUATIONS

An important assumption of the modern approach to research on human subjects is that a competent patient has the capacity to understand the implications of participating in the study. Furthermore, there is an expectation of a lack of coercion. There are clearly circumstances, however, when potential subjects might not have the capabilities to understand the research or have the same ability to make voluntary choices regarding participation. The implications for the IRB are considered below.

6.1 Prisoners

Prisoners were used as research subjects millennia ago by Persian kings. Researchers in the U.S. used prisoners in pellagra studies in the late 1800s and malaria studies in the early 20th century. During World War II, U.S. prisoners participated in numerous medical experiments and received public praise for their "contribution to the war effort."[3] As pharmaceutical research expanded dramatically after WWII, many prisoners became research subjects. Some prisons even had special units dedicated to drug company research.[3] By the end of the 1960s an estimated 85% of new pharmaceuticals were tested on prisoners.[4,5] There were many potential advantages to researchers and pharmaceutical companies for using this captive population. Prisoners were stably housed and easy to follow throughout the study period. Conducting studies in prisons could be less expensive than among the non-incarcerated.

Participation often provided tangible benefits to prisoners also. Participation was rewarded with early parole or better treatment and privileges. Better food, housing, health care, and safety were also often available to prisoners in drug trials. The material benefits of participation often made for easy recruiting, even for studies that involved treatments or procedures that the non-incarcerated population would not accept. Prisoners, however, also faced risks from inclusion in trials including: the risks of unproven drugs, the possibility that the drugs would be less effective than those already approved, harms to healthy prisoners from drugs taken in non-therapeutic trials, or procedures associated with therapeutic or non-therapeutic trials.

Even when prisoners were not directly harmed in studies, however, their participation could rarely be described as fully voluntary. Prisoners are subject to coercion on many levels. They are deprived of freedom of movement, assembly, employment, and communication with the outside world. The health care provided to them has historically been poor to nonexistent and they are prevented, by their confinement, from choosing alternative health care providers. In recognition of their greatly reduced autonomy, and the potential coercive nature of both therapeutic and non-therapeutic trials in prisons, a subchapter of the Code of Federal Regulations[6] specifically addresses the additional protections necessary for prisoners as a "vulnerable group." The IRB is legally bound to only approve research that meets the strict requirements of Subpart C.

Briefly, with respect to cancer trials, prisoners can only participate in clinical research if there is a reasonable expectation of personal benefit to them as a patient with a disease. They may participate in non-therapeutic trials only if the study is investigating questions about being a prisoner or about a select population that is incarcerated. These rules therefore narrow the scope of research that prisoners may be enrolled in. They may not be included in any clinical trials that do not contain a therapeutic arm. This would include studies regarding the biology of tumors, markers, etc. However, if the study is a comparison of potentially therapeutic treatment arms and there is also a tissue collection portion of the study that will likely be approved unless the specimen collection is deemed to carry an excess risk. A good barometer is whether a competent non-prisoner would be willing to contribute tissue under the same circumstances.

A critically important interpretation of the rule is that prisoners cannot participate in a therapeutic trial that has a placebo arm. The reason is that they might be randomized to the non-therapeutic arm and therefore not receive the same treatment that they would ordinarily be offered. Although researchers might argue that for some cancers no treatment might be best or that no proven, effective treatment exists, this argument is unlikely to succeed under the current narrow interpretations of this rule.

IRBs reviewing studies that include prisoner subjects must also meet certain requirements themselves, including having a member with expertise in prisoner issues[6] who is not affiliated with the prison system **46.304 (b)** "At least one member of the Board shall be a prisoner, or a prisoner representative with appropriate background and experience to serve in that capacity, except that where a particular research project is reviewed by more than one Board only one Board need satisfy this requirement.". If researchers are considering prisoners as research subjects for a cancer trial, they also need to comply with any administrative and other requirements of the correctional system itself. Often these requirements can be far more time consuming than standard IRB approval and must be factored into the proposed timeline for a clinical trial. Although the requirements for enrolling prisoners as research subjects add a measure of complexity to conducting a clinical trial, they are critically important to ensuring protection of prisoners as a class and as individuals. Such requirements were established to protect against repetition of abuses in the past. Researchers or IRBs that violate these rules have faced sanctions in the recent past.

7. INTERNATIONAL STUDIES

Given the ease of communication and travel in our modern times, multi-national studies have become quite common, especially in Europe. Many trials now include patients in both Europe and North America. When the study population includes subjects of similar socio-economic backgrounds, then the experimental design is generally simpler to construct.

The issues are different when scientists from industrialized countries conduct clinical trials that will primarily involve subjects in developing countries. IRBs are accustomed to assessing clinical trials within the framework of the Belmont Report. Studies in poor nations raise issues of beneficence, respect for persons (informed consent), and justice in ways that differ from studies conducted solely among patient populations in industrialized countries.

Investigators may consider many reasons to consider the option of conducting clinical trials in poor countries. The costs of conducting studies may be far less, the numbers of subjects with a particular disease may be higher, or recruitment might be expected to be easier. One rationale for permitting such trials is that without the clinical trial, the population in that country would likely not have access to the medications or treatments that would be available with participation. Similarly, some researchers (and funding agencies) have argued for inclusion of non-treatment (placebo) control arms in international studies, even where an effective treatment is available in the industrialized home country of the researchers[7-9] because the "standard of care" in the developing country might be no treatment at all. Both sides in these debates have claimed to be acting out of beneficence. In favor of these studies, researchers argue that some of the subjects may benefit directly from the study's active regimen that would not otherwise be available, while the entire population will benefit if research identifies inexpensive, effective alternatives to regimens used in industrialized countries. Those opposing such studies argue that it is unethical to give a placebo to subjects where a known, effective regimen exists, because the researchers will knowingly be exposing some subjects to worsening of their condition or even death. They argue that poor subjects should never be used as a "means" to discovering less expensive treatments where their participation will definitely harm them.

Therefore, in the absence of extraordinary circumstances most IRBs will find a protocol using a placebo or non-treatment control arm that could not be conducted in US unacceptable in a developing country.[7-9] Although it might be true that without the trial there might be no treatment, it is generally considered an injustice to treat certain subjects in a way that would be viewed as below the standard of care in this country.

For international studies to meet the standard of respect for persons, the issue of informed consent will be critical to the IRB. Keeping in mind the concept of informed consent as a process, not a document, careful attention must be paid to regional, cultural and religious considerations. At the very least, the informed consent process must be conducted in a language familiar to the subjects. A beautifully constructed ICF in English will not be acceptable in a non-English speaking country. In order to pass this test, the ICF must be translated into the native language and then translated back into English to ensure accuracy. Cultural, religious and idiomatic sensitivities are critical. Additionally, investigators in international research face a daunting task of explaining the concept of research and uncertainty in simple lay language to potential subjects whose education and literacy levels may be very low and the local understanding of biology and the scientific method may be very limited. In some cases oral consent might be needed and so a mechanism for accomplishing this will be expected by the IRB.

The lack of access to care makes subjects in developing countries especially vulnerable to coercion. In order to get treatment for their cancer, such patients might be willing to accept risks that patients in this country would not. A study that includes payment to subjects for their participation will be a red flag for the IRB.

The issue of justice is particularly important in relation to selection of subjects, including the choice to conduct studies in a developing country. Fundamentally, research in developing countries should address health problems that are important to the local population and provide potential benefit for that population in the future. If adequate numbers of patients with the target disease could be found easily in the researchers' home country, then his or her choice to use subjects in a developing country should be subject to closer scrutiny. An IRB will ask, are these subjects being chosen merely to lower research costs or to recruit subjects for dangerous or unpalatable studies? If the answer to either question is "yes," then the study should not be allowed to proceed. Additionally, according to international standards (WMA Declaration of Helsinki, paragraph 30 and clarification) "every patient entered into the study should be assured of access to the best proven prophylactic, diagnostic and therapeutic methods identified by the study." Furthermore, Helsinki requires that the plan for ensuring access must be included in the study protocol so that review committees can consider its adequacy. In practice this could mean, at a minimum, that if a new therapy is found safe and efficacious, all subjects who can still benefit from it should have immediate access to it at the conclusion of the trial. Where such access is impossible, as where subjects have died or recovered, researchers should consider offering the new treatment at an affordable cost to community in which the research is conducted. For similar reasons, non-therapeutic trials will be subject to close scrutiny because subjects ordinarily do not benefit directly.

In summary, international studies can be done, but important issues need to be addressed carefully with the IRB. Issues of safety of the subjects treated in local settings need attention as well.

7.1   Terminal patients

Despite our best efforts, our treatments will fail some patients. As experienced oncologists we recognize that at some point patients will have exhausted all therapy with curative intent. Such patients might become the subject of clinical investigations. For this group, Phase I drug studies, tumor sampling, and end of life research might be contemplated. While there is a great deal to be learned from these patients, there is also the risk that their inclusion in non-therapeutic research might diminish the quality of the remainder of their lives. There is, however, an opportunity to conduct studies that could not otherwise be done.

The IRB members who are not oncologists might not have the same appreciation for the condition of these patients that a seasoned oncologist would. The IRB should frame decision making in the context of the Belmont Report principles, respect for persons, beneficence and justice. Dying patients clearly must be afforded the same rights and dignities that apply to patients who have therapeutic options available to them. Their willingness to accept risks however might be higher. The distinction between experimentation and treatment with therapeutic intent is more critical for them than for any other group. While these patients may be motivated by altruism, their desperate situation makes them susceptible to misunderstanding regarding the boundaries between clinical care and experimentation. IRBs ought to ensure that non-therapeutic, or Phase I trials with little likely benefit are accurately described to terminal patients to ensure that entry into a 'trial' is not confused with effective treatment.

7.2   Tissue and gene banking

Remarkable progress has been made in the understanding of the biochemical and metabolic nature of cancer. Advances in molecular biology and protein chemistry have resulted in extraordinary opportunities to gain information. These advances almost always require the acquisition of biologic material from humans with cancer. While this material is especially valuable, the rights of the patients submitting this material must be respected.

Cancer studies might involve collection of a variety of different tissues, including blood or serum, fresh tissue, or archived tissue. Such samples might be obtained prospectively (i.e., the investigator might be looking for fresh tissue or blood from patients diagnosed with a particular cancer) or might want tissue already collected. The samples might be removed as part of a therapeutic procedure or might only be collected for the purpose of non-therapeutic research. Some of these issues have been covered in the section on non-therapeutic research.

Federal regulations govern some aspects of collection of such materials. Section **46.110** of the Code of Federal Regulations provides guidance for exempt studies that use tissue that already exist. Such studies must use tissues that have been stripped of all personal identifiers. For this research, it is not possible to collect any further information on the patients. Information stripped of identifiers can be stored in a properly secured tumor bank. The use of these specimens must not jeopardize the rights of the subject in any way. It is up to the IRB, not the investigator, to determine whether or not the research is considered exempt.

If the samples do not already exist (i.e., they are to be collected), then the research might approved through the expedited process if the tissues will be collected as part of routine care, or are obtained through non-invasive methods. Section **46.110** of the CFR includes a list that describes the types of samples that are appropriate to this regulation. The investigator must bear in mind that the ability to obtain tissue through an expedited protocol is a separate question from the need for informed consent from the patient. As a general rule, if any information might be obtained that could affect the patient or the patient's family, then specific consent will need to be obtained.

The investigator must also ensure that the study meets the requirements of current federal privacy and security regulations, promulgated as part of HIPAA. Researchers who are not part of the patient care team may not review patient charts looking for subjects. The IRB application must describe the method of recruitment. Separate HIPAA regulations will apply to this process. HIPAA permits waiver of some requirements for appropriate circumstances. Clinicians who are treating the patient must recruit these patients not researchers who are not entitled to review protected health information (PHI). Individual patients may contact the researchers without going through their own physicians if there are IRB approved advertisements. If it will be important to collect additional tissue samples or to gather follow-up information from the subjects, then specific consent and HIPAA-specific authorization must be obtained.

Many hospitals have established tumor and tissue banks. These serve as an invaluable resource to researchers looking to study cancer. Some institutions have constructed their surgical consent form to allow for the storage of excess tissues that are not needed for the purpose of making a diagnosis or other pathologic assessment. Such resources need to be approved by the IRB. They must be carefully managed and the identity of the subjects protected.

When research involves stored samples the important issue is whether or not the patients need to give permission to use the tissues. As stated above, some research will qualify as "exempt" under federal rules, and the patients do not need to be contacted. An example of such research would be a study looking for tumor markers in archived tissue. The tumor bank can supply samples from patients with a particular disease, but cannot disclose personal identifiers. However, as a general rule, if information on genetic material is being investigated, then the IRB will expect that permission from the patient will be sought due to the sensitive nature of the study, and the possible implications for the patient's family. For example, if the research is to find genes that result in susceptibility to cancer, then it would be highly relevant to the family. If the research is looking at genes (or other factors) that would predict the response to a particular therapy such as chemotherapy, then the patient would have an interest in knowing that their tissue (or blood cells) was being examined. A separate issue is the potential financial aspects of the research. This has been covered above.

8. CONCLUSION

Decades of quality research has led to improved patient survival and quality of life. It is our hope and society's expectation that continued research will result in even more successes. Unfortunately it is our failures and poor outcomes that often dictate policy. As Mark Antony stated regarding the slain Caesar "The evil that men do lives after them; The good is oft interred with their bones".[10] Our obligation to our patients is to conduct safe and ethical research. It is the duty and responsibility of the IRB to ensure this. While the rules might seem onerous, a clear understanding of the ethical underpinnings and a pot of hot coffee are the tools needed to reach the goal.

REFERENCES

1. Simes, R.J. and A.S. Coates, *Patient preferences for adjuvant chemotherapy of early breast cancer: how much benefit is needed?* Journal of the National Cancer Institute. Monographs, 2001(30): p. 146-52.
2. Beecher, H., *Ethics and Clinical Research.* N Engl J Med, 1966. **274**: p. 1354-1360.
3. Lazzarini, Z. and F.L. Altice, *A review of the legal and ethical issues for the conduct of HIV-related research in prisons.* AIDS & Public Policy Journal, 2000. **15**(3-4): p. 105-35.
4. *Survey-Use of Prisoners in Drug testing,* in *Report to the National Commission.* 1976, Pharmaceutical Manufacturers Association.
5. *Prison Drug Test: Choice or Coercion,* in *Los Angeles Times.* 1981: Los Angeles. p. 27.
6. in *Code of Federal Regulations.* 2001.
7. Steinbrook, R., *Testing medications in children.[see comment].* New England Journal of Medicine, 2002. **347**(18): p. 1462-70.
8. Gurwitz, J.H., *Testing medications in children.[comment].* New England Journal of Medicine, 2003. **348**(8): p. 763-4; author reply 763-4.
9. Crawley, F.P., R. Kurz, and H. Nakamura, *Testing medications in children.[comment].* New England Journal of Medicine, 2003. **348**(8): p. 763-4; author reply 763-4.
10. Shakespeare, W, *Julius Caesar.* Act 3, scene 2.

Chapter 3

NCI'S CANCER THERAPY EVALUATION PROGRAM: A COMMITMENT TO TREATMENT TRIALS

Jeffrey S. Abrams, MD, Anthony Murgo, MD, Michaele C. Christian, MD
Cancer Therapy Evaluation Program, Division of Cancer Treatment and Diagnosis, National Cancer Institute, Bethesda, Maryland, USA

1. INTRODUCTION

As the lead federal agency for cancer research, the National Cancer Institute supports a broad array of interventional clinical trials, using medical, surgical and/or radiation therapies to treat, prevent and control symptoms of cancer.[1] The trials are coordinated or conducted by different Divisions/Programs within the NCI, including the Division of Cancer Treatment and Diagnosis (DCTD), the Division of Cancer Prevention, the Cancer Centers Program, the Specialized Programs of Research Excellence (SPOREs) and the Center for Cancer Research. This chapter will focus on the cancer treatment trials sponsored by the Cancer Therapy Evaluation Program (CTEP) located in the DCTD, the largest program sponsoring cancer treatment trials at NCI. CTEP is organized into distinct branches (Figure 1) that work closely together, in many ways similar to the functioning of a large pharmaceutical firm, with the important difference that the primary stakeholders are the American public. Because development of effective therapies in the public interest is CTEP's prime mission, achieving this goal requires multiple collaborations with pharmaceutical firms, public and private academic institutions and physicians in oncology practices in the

U.S. and abroad. This myriad of public-private partnerships has made CTEP one of the largest sponsors of oncology trials in the world.

Development of new therapies traditionally occurs through a logical sequence of trials, moving from the first trials in humans (phase 1) to disease-specific efficacy trials (phase 2), and finally, to definitive trials comparing the new therapy to a standard control (phase 3). CTEP is organized to support and evaluate all phases of these trials. Staff in the Regulatory Affairs Branch submit and manage the investigational new drug (applications), termed INDs, and coordinate interactions with the Food and Drug Administration (FDA). As an example, their efforts have resulted in contractual language acceptable to different companies, thereby allowing two or more targeted, investigational agents to be co-developed in a single trial (Figure 2). The Pharmaceutical Management Branch monitors distribution and dispensation of investigational agents, and forecasts drug supply needs. Quality assurance for CTEP-sponsored trials is managed by the Clinical Trials Monitoring Branch, and its staff oversees an extensive on-site auditing program. Medical and statistical input into the planning and evaluation of new trials is supplied by the Investigational Drug Branch, the Clinical Investigations Branch, and the Biometrics Research Branch. This multidisciplinary structure allows CTEP to provide broad expertise and experience regarding the conduct and evaluation of clinical trials.

With its primary focus being the accumulation of useful knowledge to treat cancer, CTEP-sponsored trials are not exclusively directed towards drug approvals. The goal is not to find a niche for the agent, but rather to find an effective treatment for the disease. Thus, a hallmark of CTEP-sponsored trials is the inclusion of translational science and other correlative studies. Knowledge gained in this way is shared with all investigators whether or not it is supportive of the agents in the actual study. Review of these scientific efforts is accomplished by including experts from other NCI programs (quality of life, prevention, imaging, biomarkers, and preclinical models) in the CTEP review processes. Non-NCI reviewers provide valuable input in the solicitation process for new agents in the phase 1-2 program and disease experts and patient advocates serve as reviewers for concepts for phase 3 trials.

In view of its broad scope and interactive components, the CTEP review process is complex. The schema in Figure 3 provides an explanation of both the NCI-supported studies that are subject to review and the types of reviews conducted for each. Full review involves contributions from the entire CTEP program, and includes relevant internal and external non-CTEP reviewers. Development strategy reviews and/or safety reviews are limited to select CTEP reviewers whose recommendations are usually non-binding, whereas "file only" studies are listed in CTEP's Protocol and Information Office database for reference but the studies are not reviewed formally. Why audit?

Clinical trials have played pivotal roles in the care of cancer patients. Randomized comparisons of therapies have defined the optimal treatment strategy; early-phase investigations involving novel agents have stimulated and advanced cancer care; and multi-institutional trial participation has propagated promising new treatments to many patients. As scientists and care providers, clinical trialists must assure and protect the integrity of clinical trials. A *quality assurance audit* is a formal process by which the quality and completeness of the reported trial data are independently appraised in relation to the raw clinical data and the actual conduct of the trial. Detecting both systematic errors as well as deliberate falsifications of data is important for ensuring that trial outcomes are valid. Indeed, quality control represents both an ethical obligation to the human subjects who voluntarily participate in the clinical trials, as well as a scientific obligation to the trial investigators who contribute to the collective results of the trial.

The NCI has defined several goals for the quality assurance program of cooperative groups.[2]

Auditing aims to *prevent* problems, by fostering the development of a responsible research team. Investigators who understand the importance of faithful adherence to the trial protocol will likely recruit and train support staff who are careful and honest in data collection and reporting.[3] Building such a research team guards against noncompliance with the protocol or the regulatory requirements.

The audit program aims to *detect* problems through periodic monitors and checks. Random errors and systemic errors may result in data that are missing, incorrect or variable beyond expected ranges. These errors may be detected by statistical methods. Auditing, as defined above, is a process where reported data are checked against the original medical records or source documents, constitutes a more detailed and rigorous method of error detection.[1]

The third goal of the audit process is to ensure timely and effective *correction* of detected errors. Indeed, deficiencies identified in an audit require responses from enrolling institutions within a pre-defined time frame.

Finally, the quality assurance audit has been increasingly recognized as a valuable *educational* opportunity. Through on-site visits, the audit staff not only evaluates the trial support structure at individual institutions, but also compares and shares sound research practices from other member institutions. Additionally, as identified deficiencies are communicated and plans for corrective action are developed, the investigators and the institution have the opportunity to learn and improve their research practices in the future.

2. CTEP'S EARLY PHASE DRUG DEVELOPMENT PROGRAM

CTEP's early phase investigational drug development program is managed primarily by the Investigational Drug Branch (IDB). IDB directs the clinical development of a large number of investigational new drugs and biologics and makes them available for trials conducted by a vast, national network of investigators and Cooperative Clinical Trials Groups (hereafter referred to as the "Cooperative Groups").

IDB is staffed by physicians, all of whom have extensive experience in medical and pediatric oncology and in the development and conduct of cancer clinical trials. During pre-clinical testing, IDB works in close collaboration with scientists in the NCI's Developmental Therapeutics Program (DTP), providing medical input into the assessment and prioritization of agents considered for future or further pre-clinical development. Through each phase of clinical development, IDB works jointly with disease experts in CIB and in the extramural community to establish cancer treatment strategies that are grounded in the latest available knowledge of tumor targets and novel therapeutics.

CTEP's early drug development program involves a large number and variety of agents and the sponsorship of about 150 active INDs for drugs and biologics. These agents come from a variety of sources (Figure 4). Most are obtained through collaborations with biotechnology and pharmaceutical companies. NCI-CTEP has approximately 80 collaborative research and development agreements with over 60 different companies. The purpose of these agreements is to provide a regulatory and legal foundation for the exchange of funds, materials and information between NCI, industry, and academia, while addressing issues such as human safety, good clinical practice guidelines, data sharing, and intellectual property. The three agreement types - Collaborative Research and Development Agreements (CRADAs), Clinical Trials Agreements (CTAs) and Clinical Supply Agreements (CSAs) – are utilized, respectively, according to whether the research plan for an agent is broad (multiple phase 1-2 trial), targeted (just a few focused trials) or only involves distribution of the investigational agent for a multicenter trial. Some of the agents are "home grown" at the NCI. Others come from scientists at universities or other academic or research institutions, often produced with the support of NCI grants or NCI-funding agreements, such as RAID (Rapid Access to Intervention Development). The RAID program is designed to accelerate the transition to the clinic of novel anticancer therapeutic interventions, either synthetic, natural product, or biologic, arising in the academic community. Information about RAID can be obtained on the NCI DTP website.[2]

Before NCI can file an IND or expend significant resources on the development of an agent, approval must be obtained from NCI's multidisciplinary Drug Development Group (DDG).[3] The DDG is advisory to the NCI-DCTD Director, with membership that includes senior staff from DTP and CTEP and other relevant NCI programs. DDG meetings are confidential since proprietary information is reviewed (Figure 5). For each application discussed, there are usually two ad hoc external reviewers who are selected based on their expertise with the particular drug, target or indication. Agents can enter the DDG review process in various stages of preclinical (DDG I-II) or clinical (DDG III) development. Upon completion of the review, the DDG assigns priority scores (ranked 1-5; Outstanding=1.0, Excellent=1.5, Very Good=2.0, Good=3.0, Fair=4.0, Acceptable=5.0) which are weighted as follows: Strength of Proposal's Credentials (40%); Novelty (30%); Cost and Benefits (20%); Need for NCI Involvement (10%). A score of 2.5 or less is usually required for approval.

For agents considered for DDG III, CTEP commences clinical development upon DDG approval. In addition to involvement of industry collaborators, CTEP seeks input from extramural scientists in establishing drug development plans. The usual next step is the solicitation process whereby CTEP solicits for proposals to conduct clinical trials. These solicitations, which provide background information on the agent and the types of studies sought, are distributed to cancer centers, principal investigators of cooperative agreements (termed UO1s), contract holders (termed NO1s), SPORES and Cooperative Groups. Letters of Intent (LOIs) to conduct clinical trials are usually due within about 45 days from the solicitation date. Templates for preparation of the LOIs are provided on the CTEP website.[4] The LOIs are reviewed and prioritized by CTEP and selections are usually made within 4-6 weeks. CTEP also accepts unsolicited LOI's, recognizing the value of investigator initiated proposals. Priority scores are assigned for each proposal based on a variety of characteristics (Figure 6). The rating system is similar to that described for the DDG review and scores lower than 2.5 are usually successful. Even some very good proposals may not be approved if they are duplicative with ongoing studies or with other proposals with better priority scores. To improve a particular study's overall quality and accrual potential, CTEP may request that investigators with similar proposals collaborate and conduct the study as a multicenter trial to take advantage of the merits of both proposals. The approximate number of LOIs received and approved in 2004 is shown in Figure 7.

Investigators with approved LOI's are asked to submit protocols within 30-60 days. To assist in the preparation of the protocols and to standardize across all CTEP-sponsored studies, CTEP provides protocol templates specific for the phase of study. These protocol templates are available for down-loading from the CTEP website.[3] In addition, investigators with approved LOI's are provided with clinical brochures and often with agent-specific protocol templates to lessen the time and burden of document preparation.

There are a variety of ways to obtain funding to support the research costs of clinical trials. In addition to funding the Cooperative Groups, CTEP also provides funding for clinical trials through several other mechanisms, including about 16 U01 cooperative agreements to conduct early phase trials, with a focus on phase 1. In addition to support to conduct clinical trials, the U01 funds pharmacokinetic studies. CTEP also funds 7-8 N01 contracts to support the costs of conducting phase 2 trials with investigational agents. These contracts involve more than 18 cancer centers within the US and Canada. Unlike grants, these contracts provide funding on a fee for service basis. Patient accrual to U01-funded studies is shown in Figure 8. The accrual to N01-funded studies has steadily increased since the inception of the current structure in 2001 (Figure 9).

Support for the laboratory correlatives must be obtained from other sources such as R01 or R21 grants. Recognizing these research grants are often difficult to coordinate with the start date of a trial without requiring significant delays, CTEP provides support for these early correlative studies in these critical early development trials through its Translational Research Initiative (TRI). TRI is a contract mechanism to provide supplemental funding for correlatives studies that are part of an NCI-sponsored, early drug development trial. Only correlative studies that are considered to be relevant to the further development of the investigational agent are eligible for TRI support. Information about TRI funding can be obtained on the CTEP website.[3]

In addition to clinical trials, CTEP manages programs for "compassionate" and expanded use. If a CTEP-sponsored investigational agent has been found to have reproducible clinical efficacy, such as objective responses in the setting of a phase 2 trial, CTEP may provide the agent for "compassionate" use under its Special Exception program. These are single-patient protocols for individuals with the appropriate cancer type who have no other treatment options and are not eligible for an appropriate clinical trial. On average, about 8-12 investigational agents are available under this mechanism. Other CTEP-sponsored expanded access programs include Group C/Treatment IND and Treatment Referral Center (TRC) protocols. Further information about these programs can be found on the CTEP website.[5]

Investigators conducting CTEP sponsored clinical trials are required to follow certain requirements for data reporting. To manage and monitor the enormous amount of data from approximately 1000 active protocols, CTEP has in place several electronic submission systems. Many of the protocols involve investigational agents and, as such, must be monitored very closely. Investigators are required to submit serious adverse events through the Adverse Event Expedited Reporting System (AdEERS) according to timelines stipulated in the CTEP Guidelines for Adverse Event Reporting Requirements.[6] Investigators are also required to utilize CTEP electronic systems for routine reporting of data.[7] Data from Phase 1 trials are to be submitted via the Clinical Trials Monitoring System (CTMS) every two weeks whereas Phase 2 data are to be submitted quarterly using the Clinical Data Update System (CDUS). Compliance with data submission requirements is essential to allow CTEP to fulfill its regulatory responsibilities to the Food and Drug Administration (FDA) as an IND sponsor and its obligations to pharmaceutical company collaborators.

3. LATER PHASE CLINICAL TRIALS

Controlled, randomized phase 3 trials represent the gold standard in oncology and are required by the FDA for final approval of most new anti-cancer agents. To accomplish such trials, CTEP has sponsored a Cooperative Group program for the past 50 years that performs phase 3 trials utilizing new medical, surgical and radiation therapies, either alone or in combination. Multi-modality and specialty Groups (Figure 10) provide a unique, highly qualified, standing apparatus that permits the rapid testing of new agents and/or surgical and radiation techniques, and their integration into standard treatment. Cooperative Group trials have accounted for over 60% of plenary session presentations at the American Society of Clinical Oncology (ASCO) in the past 5 years, and these trials have often set the standard of care for the treatment of cancer patients world-wide.

The Groups are funded via cooperative agreements, a funding mechanism used when a collaborative relationship between extramural investigators and NCI staff is thought to be optimal to achieve the research goals. CTEP staff in the Clinical Investigations Branch (CIB), primarily physicians and nurses specializing in oncology, coordinate the overall Group research effort by emphasizing opportunities for collaboration, and by helping to integrate expertise in imaging, diagnostic, and correlative sciences from other NCI programs into Group trials. Because of their broad access to and knowledge of diverse research portfolios, CTEP staff can assist the Groups in identifying important research opportunities and questions. They also provide leadership in formulating a consensus review for all Group phase 3 trial concepts that go through the NCI review process. Investigators submit concepts for review utilizing the Concept Review Template[4]. Evaluation of concepts focuses on the scientific underpinnings of the clinical question, and spares investigators the time and effort required to prepare a protocol until a commitment to fund the trial is assured. Because approval of a concept implies that a large and costly study will be performed, effective concept evaluation requires that the investigators provide a strong preclinical/clinical rationale as well as the study design with treatment regimens, toxicities, and statistical plan in sufficient detail to allow an in-depth review. In addition to these factors, concepts are evaluated for the overall impact of the scientific question and its feasibility relative to the planned sample size. The scoring system is based upon a 5-point scale, similar to LOIs. Concepts scoring less than 2.5 are usually successful.

Over the past 5 years, CTEP has reviewed 219 concepts and has approved 154. Based upon these studies, enrollment into Group trials has consistently averaged approximately 20,000 patients annually for phase 3 studies with approximately 140 phase 3 studies open at any single time (Figure 11). Further details regarding the Cooperative Group research agenda are reviewed in Chapter 5.

Once a concept is approved, CTEP and Cooperative Group staff now work rapidly in tandem to develop the final protocol. Utilizing this new approach, several recent trials have gone from concept approval to approved protocol in under 100 days. This is a major improvement compared to the 9-18 month development periods that were required previously. To further facilitate joint protocol assembly, a new, web-based protocol authoring/review tool called Docu-Mart has been developed that permits on-line editing by multiple authors/reviewers. This new approach, due to be implemented in selected Groups in late 2005, should further speed protocol development since it avoids the sequential, paper-based processes used previously. To address an additional, oft-cited, barrier to clinical trials, CTEP has worked with the Cooperative Groups to build standardized case report forms for all diseases in which phase 3 trials occur. The approach is based upon a standard vocabulary, housed on-line by NCI in the Cancer Data Standards Repository (CaDSR)[8]. Data collection items with their respective valid values are stored on the website along with template case report forms for each disease. Utilization of common definitions and similar case report forms is a major benefit since it lowers staff training costs for intergroup trials by reducing confusion and inconsistencies, facilitating standardized data collection and rendering data sharing more feasible.

4. CANCER TRIALS SUPPORT UNIT (CTSU)

In an attempt to improve the rate of accrual to phase 3 trials, and to leverage advances in technology and communications, NCI created the Cancer Trials Support Unit. Its primary goals are to centralize regulatory support for Cooperative Group trials, previously maintained separately by the eight adult Cooperative Groups, and to establish a national network of physicians who can participate in NCI sponsored phase 3 adult cancer treatment trials, without regard for their individual Group affiliation.

The CTSU has increased physician and patient access to Phase 3 adult cancer treatment trials, the majority of which are led by the Cooperative Groups. Cooperative Group members are able to enroll eligible patients for any trial on the CTSU menu that is not available through their own Cooperative Group. For example, if a SWOG member is interested in a study on the CTSU menu that is being conducted by GOG, the SWOG member can open the study at their site through the CTSU.

This system appears to have broad appeal, as the number of accruals through the CTSU has steadily increased (Figure 12). During the past twelve months, the cumulative accrual through the CTSU since its inception in 1999 has nearly doubled, from 5000 to almost 10,000 patients. Additionally, using the CTSU as a readily available mechanism for collaboration, many more Group-led studies have been "endorsed" by other Groups such that most phase 3 studies are now Intergroup efforts both in terms of scientific leadership and accrual.

The steady increase in accruals is, in part, a function of the large variety of studies available on the CTSU menu (Figure 13). Initially, the CTSU protocol menu included protocols from 5 disease areas – gastrointestinal, genitourinary, lung, breast, and adult leukemia; however, the CTSU has expanded to include other diseases such as melanoma, head & neck, multiple myeloma, and some rare cancers. There are currently 58 trials on the CTSU menu, with 28 more in development. In addition to Group-led studies, the menu now also contains phase 3 trials led by International study groups, CCOP research bases, and some phase 2 studies in uncommon cancers. It is anticipated that eventually all phase 3 CTEP-sponsored studies will be available through the CTSU.

A unique aspect of the CTSU is its extensive use of the Internet. It has both a public web site[9] and a limited access, password protected members' web site[10]. All CTSU members have access to protocols, protocol-specific forms (e.g., case report forms, materials ordering forms) and patient educational materials on the members' web site. Protocol-specific materials that are provided on-line include the following: completed IRB submission applications, audit worksheets, protocol-specific time and events schedules, and pocket-sized protocol cards that outline protocol-specific eligibility requirements and treatment plans.

To assure that investigators would not be overly burdened by the requirements of participating in clinical trials led by different organizations, the CTSU consolidated regulatory processes (site and investigator credentialing, specific protocol requirements and IRB approvals). All adult Cooperative Group regulatory submissions, with the exception of some of the major phase 3 prevention trials, are now submitted to a single CTSU regulatory office. The CTSU and the Adult Cooperative Groups have collaborated to develop a web-based Regulatory Support System (RSS), capable of housing all Adult Cooperative Groups' regulatory documents in centralized repository. This consolidation has streamlined the regulatory process for investigators at local sites who can now submit their credentials once each year including a 1572 form for investigational drugs and a supplemental group membership form that are made available to all relevant Groups via RSS.

Cooperative Group trials supported by the CTSU are steadily migrating to electronic data capture from local sites, rather than the traditional paper- or fax- based approaches that have predominated previously. The CTSU is helping to standardize web-based data entry by utilizing an Oracle toolset that is potentially scalable across the country. Currently, a large pilot effort is underway to utilize this electronic data capture tool. Lessons learned during this pilot experience should enable NCI to rapidly move towards offering a national system for electronic data capture on multi-center studies. A single electronic data capture system will streamline training of research personnel and should further facilitate cross-group enrollments.

5. TOWARDS THE FUTURE

CTEP's commitment to the development of new drugs and better multi-modality treatments is evidenced by a solid track record of past accomplishments (Figure 14) and by novel approaches that address new challenges. The ability to combine multiple targeted agents early in their development, the inclusion of correlative science endpoints in the majority of phase 2 and 3 trials, and the integration of functional imaging approaches in early trials exemplify some of these innovations. In the phase 3 arena, the CTSU has proven to be a useful addition to NCI's longstanding Cooperative Group system. As the CTSU matures, cost savings should be realized as redundant activities conducted by individual Groups are eliminated. These efficiencies should permit Groups to focus their resources on study design and analysis thereby speeding the processes of protocol development and reporting. The CTSU's accomplishments – a unified menu of Group trials linked to a national system of qualified investigators managed in a consolidated regulatory database – indicates that the Cooperative Group system is evolving to meet new challenges. The formation of the CTSU has positioned NCI's Cooperative Groups to be more nimble partners for pharmaceutical companies seeking assistance with new drug development and to be more capable of addressing the most compelling cancer treatment research questions in a rapid and reliable manner.

The future evolution of NCI's approach to clinical trials has recently been charted. In June 2005, the NCI Clinical Trials Working Group (CTWG) presented their report to NCI's National Cancer Advisory Board[11]. Commissioned by NCI's Director to review all of NCI's clinical trials programs, the Working Group's report called for important changes in the development, prioritization, review and conduct of treatment, imaging, cancer control and prevention trials. It noted that even greater consolidation of standards across trials, with increased utilization of common data elements, uniform templates for protocols and legal contracts was essential. Consistent reporting tools were required so that a common database with trial information from all NCI-sponsored trials could be made available to the research community. Such a database was felt essential if treatment strategies were to be optimized and unnecessary redundancy was to be reduced.

Ultimately, the Working Group's vision calls for a more tightly integrated matrix of NCI-sponsored trials that, when realized, could more effectively synergize their efforts in moving anti-cancer strategies from early phase studies to definitive trials. The SPORE and Cancer Centers Program, CTEP, the Division of Cancer Prevention, the Cancer Imaging Program and NCI's intramural program have all committed to participating in this new framework for clinical trials. The plan also requires the extramural community to work closely with NCI staff to prioritize utilization of the Institute's finite, clinical trials resources. Towards this aim, tools for better communication and collaboration will be critical for success, and this effort is ongoing through NCI's Center for Bioinformatics, the leader of the CaBIG (Cancer Bioinformatics Grid) initiative[12].

6. CONCLUSION

In summary, the NCI's commitment to clinical trials remains strong. Collaborative by design and evolving with the times, the infra-structure is ready to confront the challenges posed by exciting, new, molecularly-based discoveries. NCI recognizes, however, that clinical trials could not be carried out without committed physicians and courageous patients. As we move forward, ensuring input from these key stakeholders is critical if we are to develop therapies that improve the lives of people with cancer in the communities where they are treated.

Figure 1. Cancer Therapy Evaluation Program (CTEP)

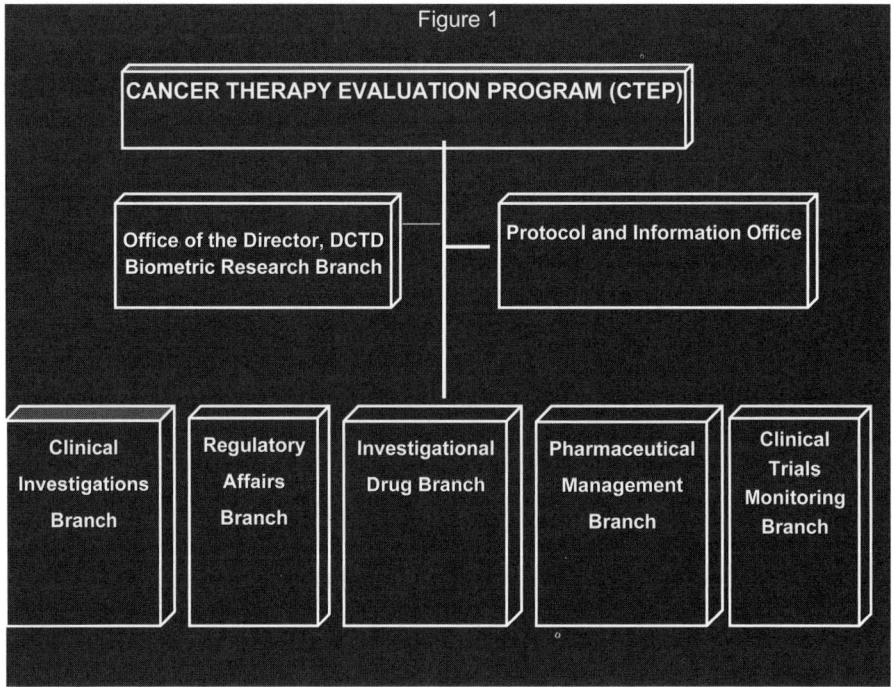

Figure 2. Investigational Drug Combinations Supported by CTEP

EGFR Inhibitor Combinations:
    Gefitinib +CCI-779   + mTor inhibitor
    Gefitinib +Bay43-9006   + raf inhibitor
    Erlotinib +bevacizumab   + angiogenesis inhibitor
    Erlotinib +cetuximab +bevacizumab   + angiogenesis inhibitor
    Cetuximab +bevacizumab + chemo   + angiogenesis inhibitor
    Erlotinib +R115776   + farneslytransferase inhibitor
    EKB-569 + CCI-779   + mTor inhibitor

Raf Kinase Inhibitors
    Bay43-9006 +bevacizumab   + angiogenesis inhibitor
    Bay43-9006 +R115776   + farneslytransferase inhibitor

mTor inhibitors
    CCI-779 + bevacizumab   + angiogenesis inhibitor
    CCI-779 + erlotinib   + EGFR inhibitor
    CCI-779 + imatinib   + kinase inhibitor

Trials conducted in multiple tumor types: renal, melanoma, glioblastoma, lung, ovary, pancreas, head & neck, colon, breast

Multiple companies involved: Sanofi, OSI, Novartis, AZ, Millennium, JJRD, Supergen, Genta Celgene, Fujisawa

Figure 3. CTEP Review Types Diagram

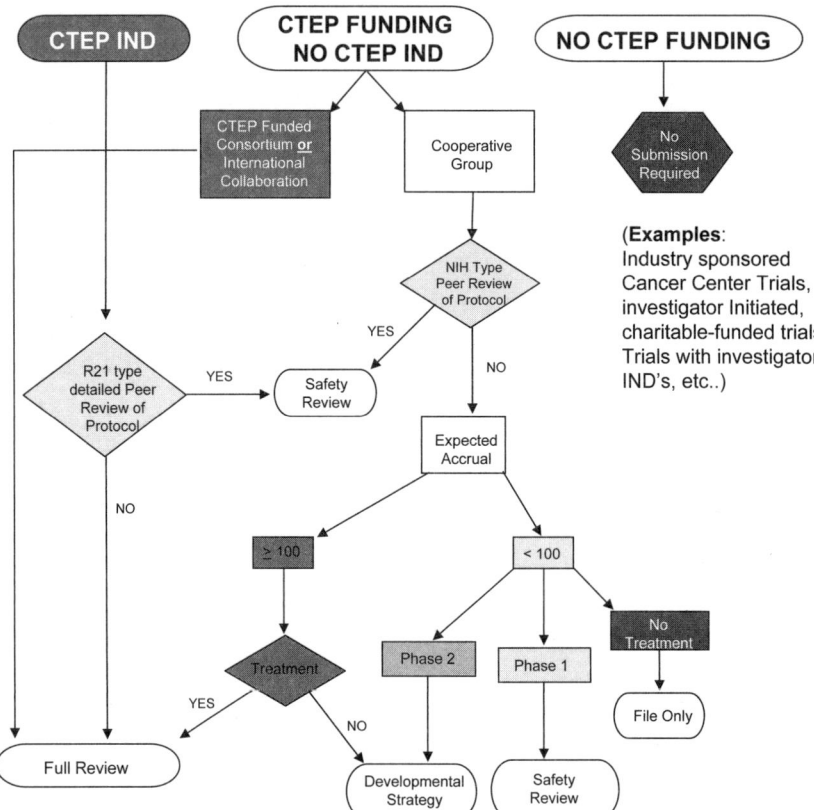

Figure 4. Source of Agents for CTEP

- Agents developed at NCI
- Agents developed under NCI-funding agreements (including RAID)*
- Agents developed independently by universities or other academic or research institutions
- Agents developed by biotech and pharmaceutical companies

Figure 5. Drug Development Group (DDG)

- DDG approval needed to expend NCI resources on development, IND filing, and sponsorship of clinical trials
- DDG is advisory to the Director, DCTD
- Preclinical
    - DDG I (Screening)
    - DDG 1B (Non-GMP drug synthesis, PK/PD, efficacy, schedule, molecular target clarification, pre-range finding toxicology)
    - DDG IIA (Range-finding toxicology, GMP synthesis, formulation)
    - DDG IIB (IND-directed toxicology, clinical lot manufacture)
- Clinical
    - DDG III (Clinical Trials, phase 1-3)
- DDG meetings closed to all but interested DCTD staff; ≈ every 6-8 weeks
- Membership
    - Representatives from NCI DTP & CTEP
    - External ad hoc reviewers (2)
- Priority Scores
    - Strength of proposals credentials (40%)
    - Novelty (30%)
    - Cost and benefits (20%)
    - Need for NCI involvement (10%)

Figure 6. Letter of Intent (LOI) CTEP Review

- Priority Scoring of Clinical and Laboratory Components:

    - Strength of scientific rationale
    - Consistency with CTEP development plan
    - Ability to accrue and complete study in timely manner
    - Appropriateness of patient population
    - Adequacy of study design
    - Quality and relevance of laboratory correlatives

Figure 7. Letters of Intent (LOI's) Received and Approved 2004

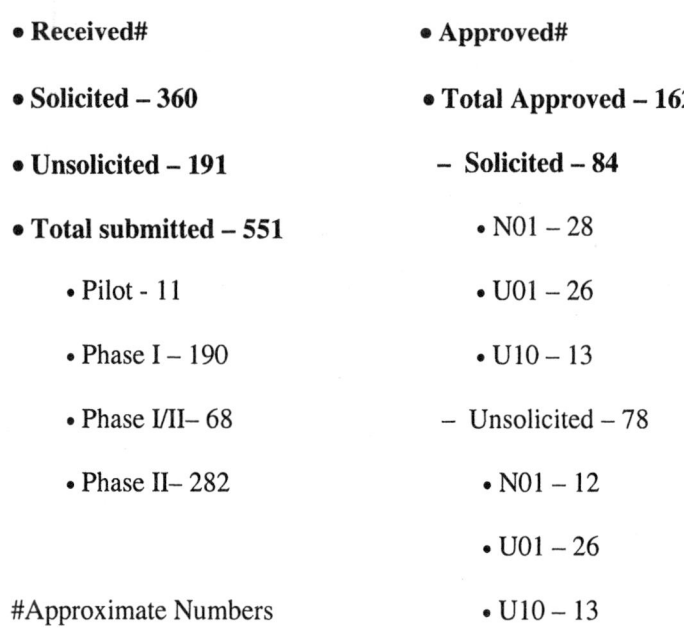

- **Received#**
- **Solicited – 360**
- **Unsolicited – 191**
- **Total submitted – 551**
  - Pilot - 11
  - Phase I – 190
  - Phase I/II– 68
  - Phase II– 282

#Approximate Numbers

- **Approved#**
- **Total Approved – 162**
  – Solicited – 84
  - N01 – 28
  - U01 – 26
  - U10 – 13
  – Unsolicited – 78
  - N01 – 12
  - U01 – 26
  - U10 – 13

Figure 8. U01 Annual Accrual (1998-2004)

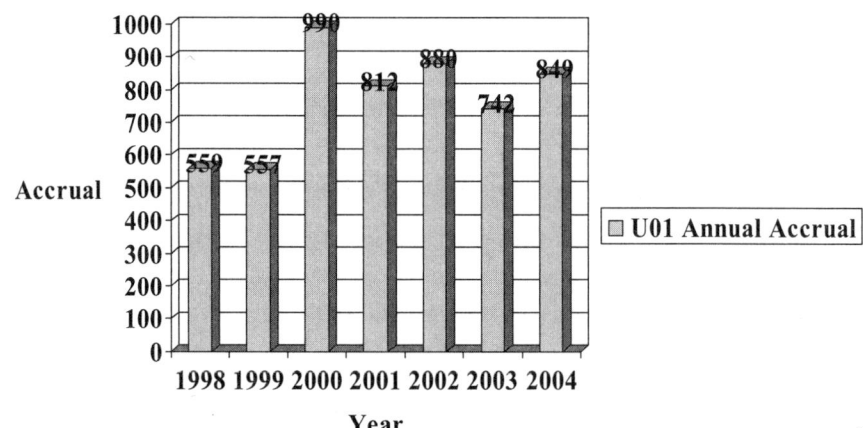

Figure 9. N01 Accrual by Year (2001-2004)

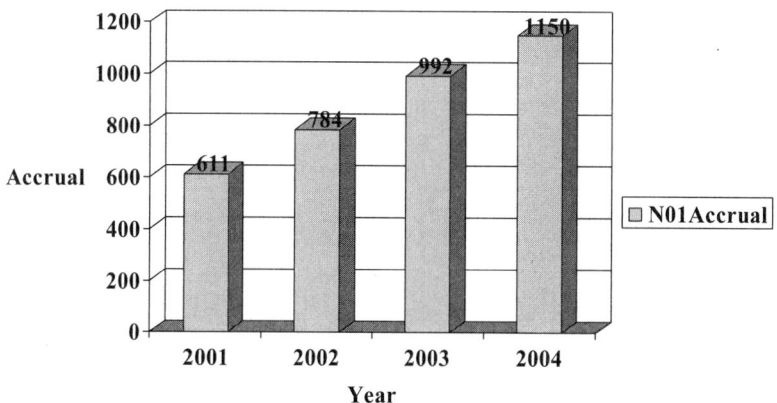

Figure 10. Late Clinical Trials – Cooperative Group Program*

10 Groups: 9 adult and 1 pediatric

Multimodality:
Cancer and Acute Leukemia Group B (CALGB)
Eastern Cooperative Oncology Group (ECOG)
North Central Cancer Treatment Group (NCCTG)
Southwest Oncology Group (SWOG)
National Cancer Institute of Canada – Clinical Trials Group
  (NCIC-CTG)**

Specialty:
American College of Surgeons Oncology Group (ACOSOG)
National Surgical Adjuvant Breast & Bowel Project (NSABP)
Gynecologic Oncology Group (GOG)
Radiation Therapy Oncology Group (RTOG)

Children's Oncology Group (COG)

- *includes CCOP participation
- ** NCIC-CTG funding limited to participation in Intergroup trials

Figure 11. Phase 3 Data for FY 2000 – 2004 for CTEP Treatment Trials

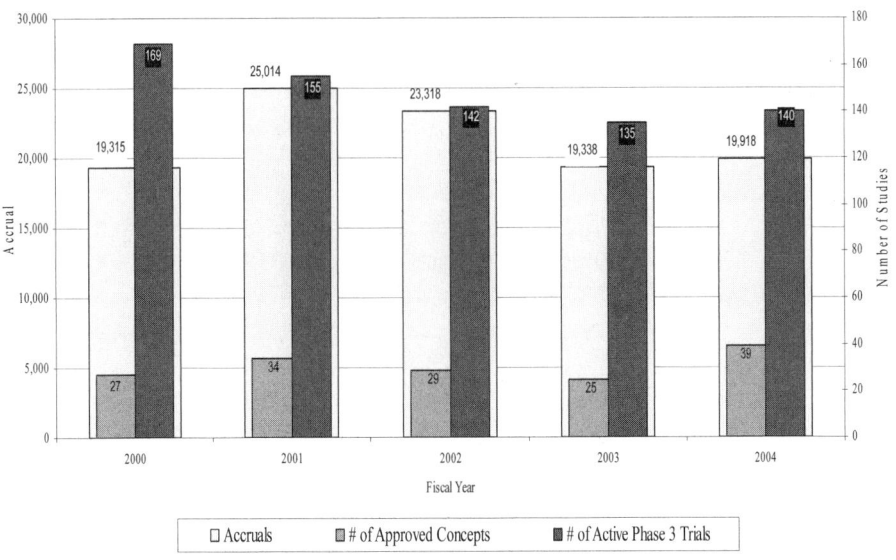

Figure 12. CTSU Accrual Summary May 31, 2005

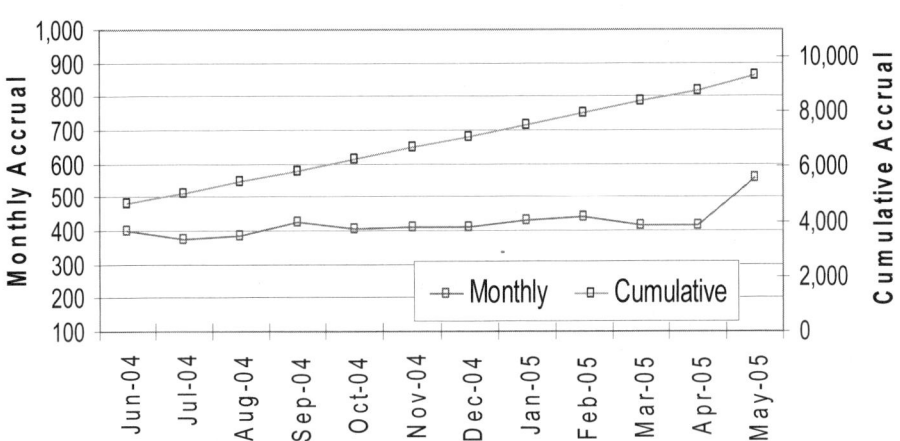

Figure 13. CTSU Protocol History as of May 31, 2005

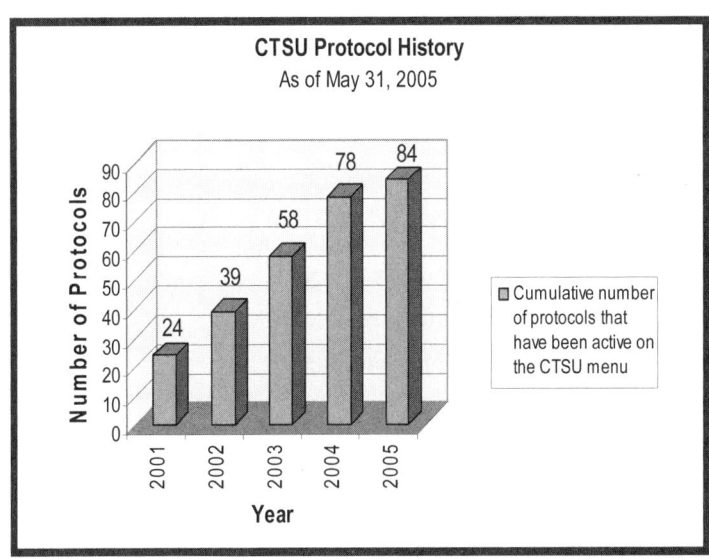

Figure 14. CTEP-sponsored Group trials contributing to FDA-approved/pending primary or secondary indications for new agents

    1991
        Fludarabine phosphate (SWOG)
        Pentostatin (CALGB, SWOG)

    1992
        Paclitaxel (GOG, CALGB, ECOG, NCCTG, SWOG)

    1993
        Melphalan IV (CALGB)

    1994
        Pegasparaginase (POG)

    2001
        Imatinib mesylate (COG, SWOG)

    2004
        Letrozole (NCIC, Intergroup)
        Taxotere (SWOG)

    2005
        Herceptin (NSABP, NCCTG, Intergroup) – pending
        Bevacizumab (ECOG, Intergroup) – pending

REFERENCES

1. World Wide Web: http://www.cancer.gov
2. World Wide Web: http://dtp.nci.nih.gov/docs/raid/raid_pp.html
3. World Wide Web: http://dtp.nci.nih.gov/docs/ddg/ddg_descript.html
4. World Wide Web: http://ctep.info.nih.gov
5. World Wide Web: http://ctep.info.nih.gov/requisition/compassion.html
6. World Wide Web: http://ctep.info.nih.gov/reporting/adeers.html
7. World Wide Web: http://ctep.info.nih.gov/reporting
8. World Wide Web: http://ncicb.nci.nih.gov/core/caDSR
9. World Wide Web: http://www.ctsu.org
10. World Wide Web: http://members.ctsu.org
11. World Wide Web: http://integratedtrials.nci.nih.gov/ict/
12. World Wide Web: https://cabig.nci.nih.gov/

Chapter 4

THE ROLE OF THE FDA IN CANCER CLINICAL TRIALS

Steven Hirschfeld, MD, PhD

Center for Biologics Evaluation and Response, Food and Drug Administration
Rockville, MD, USA

> -"The views and conclusions in this article have not been formally disseminated by the Food and Drug Administration and should not be construed to represent any agency determination or policy."

1. SCOPE OF THIS CHAPTER

This chapter is intended to assist the clinical investigator in developing products, with an emphasis on biological cellular and gene therapy products, due to their complexity, that may be used for cancer therapeutics. It is not intended as a guide for general product development or general clinical trial design and analysis nor as a guide to protective vaccine development, drugs, or devices except as those products have overlapping regulations and procedures.

2. DESCRIPTION OF THE FDA

The Food and Drug Administration (FDA) is a Federal agency in the Department of Health and Human Services with scientific, regulatory and public health responsibilities. The FDA mission statement notes that the FDA is responsible for protecting the public health by assuring the safety, efficacy, and security of human and veterinary drugs, biological products, medical devices, the nation's food supply, cosmetics, and products that emit radiation (http://www.fda.gov/opacom/hpview.html). The FDA is also responsible for advancing the public health by helping to speed innovations that make medicines and foods more effective, safer, and more affordable; and helping the public get the accurate, science-based information they need to use medicines and foods to improve their health.

There are about 10,000 FDA employees and the budget is derived from a combination of Congressional allocations and user fees.

3. BASIS OF FDA AUTHORITY AND SCOPE OF RESPONSIBILITY

The structure of the United States government apportions responsibilities among three major branches- the legislative branch that makes laws, the executive branch that enforces and implements laws, and the judicial branch that interprets and determines the validity of laws.

Development of a new law begins when a bill is proposed in Congress. . After the bill is passed by both Houses as an Act, it is signed by the President into law. The law, also known as a statute, is subsequently published in the United States Code (USC). Laws remain in effect until they are changed or in some cases, have an expiration date for some or all of the provisions.

In general, laws provide authority and responsibilities. The implementation of these responsibilities rests with the Executive Branch which includes the various Departments and Agencies. The detailed implementation of law is through the issuance of regulations developed by the Departments and Agencies. Typically, a regulation is first published in draft form in the Federal Register with a comment period, the comments are collated and addressed at the expiration of the period, and the regulation is issued as a Final Rule. Rule is a synonym for regulation. The Federal Register (FR) is a daily publication for rules, proposed rules, and notices of Federal agencies, executive orders, and other federal documents. All Final Rules are published in the Code of Federal Regulations (CFR) with citations to the relevant laws. Regulations, like laws, are binding and effective until revised or withdrawn. The authority for the FDA to issue regulations is contained in section 701 and other additional sections of the Food Drug and Cosmetic Act as amended.

The authority and responsibilities of the FDA are contained in many laws, and usually originate from the power given to Congress in Section 8 of the US Constitution to "regulate Commerce with foreign Nations, and among the several States..." (U.S. Const. art. I, sect. 8, cl. 3). Some of the laws are listed in Table 1.

Table 1. Examples of Laws Enforced by the Food and Drug Administration

Federal Food, Drug, and Cosmetic Act	Fair Packaging and Labeling Act
1997 Food and Drug Administration Modernization Act	Federal Advisory Committee Act
Public Health Service Act	Federal Advisory Committee Amendments
Congressional Reports Elimination Act of 1982	Federal Anti-Tampering Act
Controlled Substances Act	Orphan Drug Act
Controlled Substances Import and Export Act	Federal Fines and Sentencing Laws
Delegations of Authority to the Commissioner of Food and Drugs	Federal Import Milk Act
Prescription Drug User Fee Act	Federal Meat Inspections Act
Egg Products Inspection Act	Federal Trade Commission Act
Administrative Procedures Act	Fair Packaging and Labeling Act

An additional type of document, termed a Guidance Document, is published by the FDA to represent current thinking on a particular topic. In contrast to laws and regulations, Guidance Documents are not binding. A Guidance Document represents a position on a topic and represents expectations for FDA policy. Alternative approaches to the topic may be feasible and should be discussed with the FDA on a case by case basis. Within a Guidance Document, the FDA will distinguish between requirements, found in laws and regulations, which will be characterized by use of the word *must* and recommendations characterized by the word *should*. Examples of the products that the FDA regulates are listed in Table 2.

Table 2. Products regulated by the Food and Drug Administration

Biologics
Cosmetics
Drugs
Foods
Medical Devices
Radiation-Emitting Electronic Products

4. ORGANIZATION OF THE FDA

The FDA is organized into Centers based on the various regulated products. The FDA Centers are:

- Center for Biologics Evaluation and Research (CBER)
- Center for Drug Evaluation and Research (CDER)
- Center for Devices and Radiologic Health (CDRH)
- Center for Food Safety and Nutrition (CFSAN)
- Center for Veterinary Medicine (CVM)
- National Center for Toxicologic Research (NCTR)

Each product type has applicable laws and regulations.

Overall FDA Operations and Policy are coordinated in the Office of the Commissioner. The Office of the Commissioner also has special programs within its organizational structure that are not limited to one product type such as the Office for Orphan Product Development, the Office for Special Health Issues, and the Office for Combination Products. The Office of Combination Products assists in the coordination of regulatory responsibility for products that have components that would fall under the jurisdiction of more than one FDA Center.

5. HISTORY OF EVOLUTION OF FDA PRINCIPLES THAT APPLY TO BIOLOGICS

Government protection of the public health in the United States dates back to the 18th century. In 1785 the State of Massachusetts passed a law prohibiting the sale of diseased, corrupted, contagious or unwholesome provisions if known to the seller, but not the buyer, with the punishment to be inflicted according to the degree and aggravation of the offence. Punishments included fines, imprisonment or use of the pillory. In 1813 the United States Federal government passed the Vaccine Act which was signed by President James Madison. The law limited imports of certain foods and medicines, but it was one of the first national measures intended to protect consumers.

As the chemical industry matured during the 19th century and microbiology emerged as a science, means to detect contamination and adulteration became available. As better understanding of communicable diseases and immunology emerged, efforts were directed at combating infections and in 1894 a method for the production of diphtheria antitoxin by injection into horses and collection of the antiserum was developed. Subsequently production of antiserum was widespread, unregulated, and without standards.

Public health crises involving children were frequently the catalysts for Federal regulation of interstate commerce in health care products. The major principles were developed and legislation went into effect during the first two-thirds of the 20th century. These regulatory principles were adequate labeling, safety and efficacy.

In 1901 in St. Louis, Missouri a five year old girl died in a city hospital of tetanus following administration of tetanus antitoxin. The antitoxin serum was traced to a retired milk horse named Jim, who had been a prolific producer of antiserum, but who had been destroyed because of infection with tetanus. Unfortunately several lots of antiserum from this horse were not retrieved and destroyed as intended, so another 12 children died. When nine children in New Jersey died of contaminated small pox vaccine, the District of Columbia medical society initiated a bill that established federal control, including standards of manufacture and inspection for viruses, serums, toxins and antitoxins. The bill became law on July 1, 1902 as the Biologics Control Act, was signed into law by President Theodore Roosevelt, and the era of federal public health regulation began. The Surgeon Generals of the Marine Hospital Service, the Army and the Navy were named to a board with responsibility for developing regulations.

Similar legislation for drugs, the Pure Food and Drug Act, was signed into law in 1906, again by President Theodore Roosevelt. The unifying principle between the two laws was that products intended for interstate commerce must be labeled with regard to contents, must not be adulterated, and must conform to standards of purity.

Enforcement for the new laws was vested in the court system. In 1911 the US Supreme Court ruled in the US v. Johnson that federal authority was limited to false and misleading statements about the ingredients or identity of a product. This led to the 1912 Sherley Amendment to the Pure Food and Drug Act, that targeted false therapeutic claims for prosecution if intent to defraud could be proven. In 1927 the Food Drug and Insecticide Administration was established as an enforcement agency. In 1930 the name was shortened to the Food and Drug Administration.

In 1937 the Samuel Massengill Pharmaceutical Company in St. Louis, Missouri developed a liquid preparation of the antibiotic sulfanilamide that used diethylene glycol as the solvent and marketed the solution as an elixir. More than 100 people, including many children, died of glycol induced renal failure. Because the product was labeled as an elixir and did not include a full list of ingredients, the company could be charged with misbranding, but there was no law that made them responsible for the patient deaths.

In 1938 President Franklin Roosevelt signed the Food Drug and Cosmetic Act (FD&CA) into law, giving the FDA the authority to require that products establish safety prior to marketing. The FD&CA had additional provisions such as disclosure of all active ingredients, required directions for use, incorporation of warnings about misuse, provisions for facility inspections, prohibition of false claims, and extending authority to the regulation of cosmetics and devices.

In 1944 Congress passed the Public Health Service Act (PHS Act) which codified the regulation of biological products, control of communicable diseases, and additional topics such as certification of clinical laboratories.

The principle of establishing efficacy became law with the Kefauver Harris Amendment to the FD&CA in 1962. The catalyst was the submission for licensing for interstate commerce of a product generically known as thalidomide for use as a sedative. While the product was under FDA review data emerged that malformations in children were likely related to maternal thalidomide use during pregnancy. The product subsequently was not licensed for use in the United States and the FDA reviewer, Dr. Frances Kelsey, was awarded the Presidential Medal of Freedom by President John F. Kennedy.

In addition to requiring adequate and well controlled investigations, the Kefauver Harris Amendment required filing with the FDA an Investigational New Drug (IND) application prior to clinical testing.

The requirements to demonstrate efficacy and to file for initiating clinical investigations resulted in new regulations. The resulting regulations still form the basis for current clinical development.

Subsequent Federal regulations developed over the last quarter of the 20th century addressed the requirements for protection of participants in clinical research in two domains- investigations that receive Federal funding and investigations that utilize FDA regulated products. The two sets of regulations, 45 CFR 46 and 21 CFR 50 are similar and intended to be complementary but are not identical.

In the early 1980's the FDA took on a new, more proactive role by providing incentives and research support for products intended for underserved clinical populations with enactment of the Orphan Drug Act of 1983.

In addition to Federal regulations, the FDA has been a co-party to the efforts of the International Conference on Harmonization (ICH). The ICH is a global effort to coordinate medicinal product regulatory policy among three regions- the United States, Europe and Japan. Other regions and countries are incorporated into the process in an observer status. In the 1990's the ICH began to address topics related to product production, non-clinical studies, toxicology, clinical studies and other additional topics. The

ICH process and documents are detailed at www.ich.org. The document known as E-6 is devoted to standards for the conduct of clinical studies, known collectively as Good Clinical Practice (GCP). The principles and practices elaborated in GCP are emerging as an international standard. The FDA publishes the ICH documents as Guidance Documents, meaning that their content represents FDA policy and expectations, but that alternatives may be acceptable and should be discussed on a case by case basis.

To summarize, the three principles of regulation- adequate labeling, safety, and efficacy- were formalized during the first two-thirds of the twentieth century. Formal guidelines for the protection of participants in research, particularly children, are a product of the last third of the twentieth century. While the FDA regulates products that are shipped and marketed for interstate commerce, it does not regulate the practice of medicine, which is regulated through a licensing procedure by individual States.

6. BASIS OF AUTHORITY FOR REGULATING BIOLOGICS

The term biological product is defined by the PHS Act at 42 USC Section 262 as:

In this section, the term "biological product" means a virus, therapeutic serum, toxin, antitoxin, vaccine, blood, blood component or derivative, allergenic product, or analogous product, or arsphenamine or derivative of arsphenamine (or any other trivalent organic arsenic compound), applicable to the prevention, treatment, or cure of a disease or condition of human beings

For clinical development and licensure, biological products must meet criteria for safety, sterility, purity, and potency. These are defined in the applicable regulations (21 CFR Chapter I Part 600 Section 600.3) and are excerpted:

- *The word **safety** means the relative freedom from harmful effect to persons affected, directly or indirectly, by a product when prudently administered, taking into consideration the character of the product in relation to the condition of the recipient at the time.*
- *The word **sterility** is interpreted to mean freedom from viable contaminating microorganisms, as*

> determined by the tests prescribed in Sec. 610.12 of this chapter.
> - ***Purity*** *means relative freedom from extraneous matter in the finished product, whether or not harmful to the recipient or deleterious to the product. Purity includes but is not limited to relative freedom from residual moisture or other volatile substances and pyrogenic substances.*
> - *The word **potency** is interpreted to mean the specific ability or capacity of the product, as indicated by appropriate laboratory tests or by adequately controlled clinical data obtained through the administration of the product in the manner intended, to effect a given result.*

In 1993 the FDA published a Federal Register (FR) notice (58 FR 53248 October 14, 1993) outlining FDA authority to regulate somatic cell and gene therapy products, thereby requiring filing of an IND to conduct clinical investigations. The FR notice defines somatic cell therapy as the prevention, treatment, cure, diagnosis, or mitigation of disease or injuries in humans by the administration of autologous, allogeneic or xenogenic cells. The manufacture of products for somatic cell therapy involves the *ex vivo* propagation, expansion or other alteration of their biological characteristics.

The same 1993 Federal Register notice also articulated FDA authority to regulate gene transfer products as biologics. Operationally the FR notice defined gene therapy as the administration of genetic material in order to modify or manipulate the expression of a gene product or to alter the biological properties of living cells for therapeutic use. Thus whether the product is a gene transfer vector itself or cells modified by a gene transfer vector it is considered by the FDA to be a gene therapy.

In 2004 the FDA issued regulations under the communicable disease provisions of the Public Health Service Act (42 USC 264) that apply to all human cellular and tissue based products. The regulations can be found at 21 CFR Parts 1270 and 1271. While some products are regulated only under these regulations, other human cellular and tissue based products, meeting certain criteria, are in addition regulated as drugs, devices, or biological drugs.

If human cells, tissues and cellular and tissue based products (abbreviated as HCT/P) meet the following criteria:

(1) The HCT/P is minimally manipulated;

(2) The HCT/P is intended for homologous use only, as reflected by the labeling, advertising, or other indications of the manufacturer's objective intent;

(3) The manufacture of the HCT/P does not involve the combination of the cell or tissue component with a drug or a device, except for a sterilizing, preserving, or storage agent, and if the addition of the agent does not raise new clinical safety concerns with respect to the HCT/P; and

(4) Either:

(i) The HCT/P does not have a systemic effect and is not dependent upon the metabolic activity of living cells for its primary function; or

(ii) The HCT/P has a systemic effect or is dependent upon the metabolic activity of living cells for its primary function, and:

(*a*) Is for autologous use;

(*b*) Is for allogeneic use in a first-degree or second-degree blood relative; or

(*c*) Is for reproductive use.

and the establishment that would process the HCT/P qualifies for any of the exceptions listed in the applicable regulations, then the product is regulated only under section 361 of the Public Health Service Act (codified as 42 USC 264) to–

- Prevent the use of contaminated tissues that could spread infectious disease
- Prevent the improper handling or processing that might contaminate or damage tissues prevention of transmission of communicable diseases.

If any of the above conditions are not met or the establishment that would process the HCT/P does not qualify for any of the exceptions listed in the applicable regulations, then the product is regulated by both Section 351 of the PHSA (codified as 42 USC 262) and Section 361. This means that in addition to the communicable disease criteria, an IND is required for investigational use to demonstrate safety and efficacy for a marketing license.

CBER has responsibility for blood and blood products, cellular therapeutics, tissues, tissue engineered products, xenografts, and gene therapies. CDER has responsibilities for monoclonal antibodies for in-vivo use; cytokines, growth factors, enzymes, immunomodulators, thrombolytics, proteins intended for therapeutic use that are extracted from animals or microorganisms, including recombinant versions of these products (except clotting factors) and other non-vaccine therapeutic immunotherapies. The Health Resource Services Administration, a separate Federal Agency, has responsibility for bone marrow transplantation through operation of a national registry and for organ transplantation through the development of policies to ensure the fair distribution of organs (National Bone Marrow Donor Registry Reauthorization Act Public Law 105-196 July 16, 1998).

7. SCOPE OF INTERACTIONS BETWEEN THE FDA AND SPONSORS

An overview of the product development process along a time line is shown in Figure 1. The upper part of the time line notes the responsibilities of the product sponsor and the lower part of the time line notes the opportunities for interaction with and the responsibilities of the FDA that occur in parallel. Hash marks represent regulatory landmarks. The time line is hypothetical and follows a product through a 3 stage product development program with a marketing authorization granted and a post marketing commitment underway. The time between IND filing and licensing of the first use claim can be termed the clinical development time.

Figure 1. Overview of Therapeutic Development

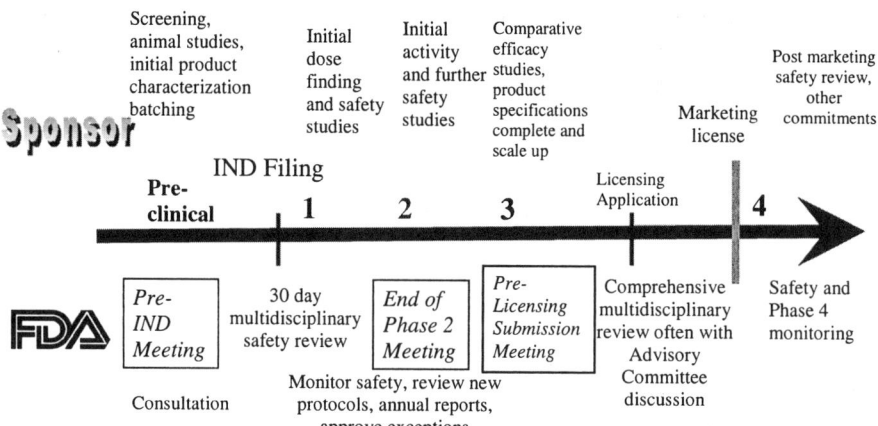

The role of the FDA in cancer clinical trials 61

8. THE IND PROCESS

8.1 Legal Basis for IND Process

Clinical investigations are conducted under Investigational New Drug (IND) applications and are described at 21 CFR 312. The IND regulations provide a mechanism to support the safe use of unlicensed investigational products (drugs and biologicals) in human clinical investigations and provide a mechanism to allow interstate shipment of products not approved for marketing

The authority citation for 21 CFR part 312 is cited in 312.1- "Scope", which states that the authority is derived from the following sections of the United States Code (USC): 21 U.S.C. 321, 331, 351, 352, 353, 355, 371; 42 U.S.C. 262.

The first 7 citations are from the Food, Drug and Cosmetic Act (FD&CA) and the last citation (42 USC 262) is from the Public Health Service Act (PHSA). FD&CA sections 321 (General Definitions), 331 (Prohibited Acts), 351 (Adulterated Drugs & Devices), 352 (Misbranded Drugs & Devices), 353 (Labeling Exemptions & Prescriptions), and 371 (Regulations & Hearings) are general in nature. The applicable section of the PHSA (42 U.S.C. 262) that addresses biological products states:

> *(j) Application of Federal Food, Drug, and Cosmetic Act*
> *The Federal Food, Drug, and Cosmetic Act [21 U.S.C. 301 et seq.] applies to a biological product subject to regulation under this section, except that a product for which a license has been approved under subsection (a) shall not be required to have an approved application under section 505 of such Act [21 U.S.C. 355].*

The applicable section of the Federal Food, Drug, and Cosmetic Act section 505 (21 U.S.C.355) has four paragraphs. The first paragraph states

- the authority for IND regulations,
- the requirement for preclinical studies to provide a scientific justification for a clinical study,
- the restriction on distribution of an investigational product to investigators under the supervision of the IND sponsor,
- the requirement for careful and complete records of clinical investigations,

- the requirement to submit a pediatric plan. The submission of a pediatric plan and initiation of either adult or pediatric studies are not necessarily concurrent.

The second paragraph contains
- statutory requirement for the 30 day review period for an IND submission
- the general data requirements for submitting an IND application.
- the requirement for primary data tabulations from animal or human studies. Generally summary data are insufficient for the FDA to make the necessary assessments; however, flexibility is inherent in the process and discussions directly with the relevant review Division in the FDA may provide further information.

The third paragraph outlines the statutory authority for clinical hold and the fourth paragraph is the statutory requirement for informed consent.

The original text that forms the basis for the IND regulations follows:

(i) Exemptions of drugs for research; discretionary and mandatory conditions; direct reports to Secretary

(1) The Secretary shall promulgate regulations for exempting from the operation of the foregoing subsections of this section drugs intended solely for investigational use by experts qualified by scientific training and
> *Such regulations may, within the discretion of the Secretary, among other conditions relating to the protection of the public health, provide for conditioning such exemption upon—*
>> *(A) the submission to the Secretary, before any clinical testing of a new drug is undertaken, of reports, by the manufacturer or the sponsor of the investigation of such drug, of preclinical tests (including tests on animals) of such drug adequate to justify the proposed clinical testing;*
>> *(B) the manufacturer or the sponsor of the investigation of a new drug proposed to be distributed to investigators for clinical testing obtaining a signed agreement from each of such investigators that patients to whom the drug is administered will be under his personal supervision, or under the supervision of investigators responsible to him, and that he will not supply such drug to any other investigator, or to clinics, for administration to human beings;*

The role of the FDA in cancer clinical trials 63

> *(C) the establishment and maintenance of such records, and the making of such reports to the Secretary, by the manufacturer or the sponsor of the investigation of such drug, of data (including but not limited to analytical reports by investigators) obtained as the result of such investigational use of such drug, as the Secretary finds will enable him to evaluate the safety and effectiveness of such drug in the event of the filing of an application pursuant to subsection (b) of this section; and*
>
> *(D) the submission to the Secretary by the manufacturer or the sponsor of the investigation of a new drug of a statement of intent regarding whether the manufacturer or sponsor has plans for assessing pediatric safety and efficacy.*

(2) Subject to paragraph (3), a clinical investigation of a new drug may begin 30 days after the Secretary has received from the manufacturer or sponsor of the investigation a submission containing such information about the drug and the clinical investigation, including—

> *(A) information on design of the investigation and adequate reports of basic information, certified by the applicant to be accurate reports, necessary to assess the safety of the drug for use in clinical investigation; and*
>
> *(B) adequate information on the chemistry and manufacturing of the drug, controls available for the drug, and primary data tabulations from animal or human studies.*

(3)
> *(A) At any time, the Secretary may prohibit the sponsor of an investigation from conducting the investigation (referred to in this paragraph as a "clinical hold") if the Secretary makes a determination described in subparagraph (B). The Secretary shall specify the basis for the clinical hold, including the specific information available to the Secretary which served as the basis for such clinical hold, and confirm such determination in writing.*
>
> *(B) For purposes of subparagraph (A), a determination described in this subparagraph with respect to a clinical hold is that—*
>
>> *(i) the drug involved represents an unreasonable risk to the safety of the persons who are the subjects of the clinical investigation, taking into account the qualifications of the clinical investigators,*

information about the drug, the design of the clinical investigation, the condition for which the drug is to be investigated, and the health status of the subjects involved; or

(ii) the clinical hold should be issued for such other reasons as the Secretary may by regulation establish (including reasons established by regulation before November 21, 1997).

(C) Any written request to the Secretary from the sponsor of an investigation that a clinical hold be removed shall receive a decision, in writing and specifying the reasons therefore, within 30 days after receipt of such request. Any such request shall include sufficient information to support the removal of such clinical hold.

(4) Regulations under paragraph (1) shall provide that such exemption shall be conditioned upon the manufacturer, or the sponsor of the investigation, requiring that experts using such drugs for investigational purposes certify to such manufacturer or sponsor that they will inform any human beings to whom such drugs, or any controls used in connection therewith, are being administered, or their representatives, that such drugs are being used for investigational purposes and will obtain the consent of such human beings or their representatives, except where it is not feasible or it is contrary to the best interests of such human beings.

8.2 IND Regulations

The IND regulations in 21 CFR Part 312 are divided into 5 Subparts- General Provisions (Subpart A), Investigational New Drug Application (Subpart B), Administrative Actions (Subpart C), Responsibilities of Sponsors and Investigators (Subpart D) all of which apply to all products and an additional section for products intended to treat life threatening and severely debilitating illnesses (Subpart E), which includes products intended to treat cancer.

In Subpart A is a section, 312.3 on General Definitions, of which a few excerpts will be cited to ensure clarity in the following sections. Underlined and bold text are intended for emphasis and are not part of the original regulations. As specified in the regulation, the term "drug" in the IND regulations applies to drugs and biologics.

Sec. 312.3 Definitions and interpretations.

(a) The definitions and interpretations of terms contained in section 201 of the Act apply to those terms when used in this part:

(b) The following definitions of terms also apply to this part:

__Act__ means the Federal Food, Drug, and Cosmetic Act (secs. 201-902, 52 Stat. 1040 et seq., as amended (21 U.S.C. 301-392)).

__Clinical investigation__ means any experiment in which a drug is administered or dispensed to, or used involving, one or more human subjects. For the purposes of this part, an experiment is any use of a drug except for the use of a marketed drug in the course of medical practice.

__IND__ means an investigational new drug application. For purposes of this part, ``IND'' is synonymous with ``Notice of Claimed Investigational Exemption for a New Drug.''

__Investigational new drug__ means a __new drug or biological drug__ that is used in a clinical investigation. The term also includes __a biological product that is used in vitro for diagnostic purposes__. The terms ``investigational drug'' and ``investigational new drug'' are deemed to be synonymous for purposes of this part.

__Investigator__ means an individual who actually conducts a clinical investigation (i.e., under whose immediate direction the drug is administered or dispensed to a subject). In the event an investigation is conducted by a team of individuals, the investigator is the responsible leader of the team. ``

__Subinvestigator__ includes any other individual member of that team.

The FDA publishes International Conference on Harmonization (ICH) documents as Guidance Documents in the Federal Register. ICH document E8, "General Considerations for Clinical Trials" (FR 62(242): 66113

December 17, 1997) notes that

> *For the sake of brevity, the term "drug" has been used in this document. It should be considered synonymous with "investigational (medicinal) product," "medicinal product," and "pharmaceutical," including vaccines and other biological products.*

8.3   When is an IND Needed?

The requirements as to when to file an IND and when an exemption from IND filing can be granted are outlined in Title 21 CFR 312. The specific sections are excerpted below. All investigational agents require an IND. The IND requirements that pertain to licensed marketed products depend upon the intent and circumstances. For example a new route of administration, new dose or different patient population that would potentially result in a different risk to benefit assessment than the already approved use and because the risk may be either unknown or increased, requires an IND. The term "indication" refers to the intended use of a product such as to prevent, treat or mitigate a disease or condition. The last subsection of the regulation notes that a sponsor may request FDA advice as to whether an IND is required.

Underlining and bolding, which are not in the original regulations, are added for emphasis of particular text.

> *Sec. 312.2 Applicability.*
>
> *(a) Applicability. Except as provided in this section, this part applies to all clinical investigations of products that are subject to section 505 of the Federal Food, Drug, and Cosmetic Act or to the licensing provisions of the Public Health Service Act (58 Stat. 632, as amended (42 U.S.C. 201 et seq.)).*
>
> *(b) Exemptions.*
>
> *(1) The clinical investigation of a drug product that <u>is lawfully marketed in the United States</u> is exempt from the requirements of this <u>part if **all** the following</u> apply:*
>
> *(i) The investigation is not intended to be reported to FDA as a well-controlled study in support of a new indication for use nor intended to be used to support any other*

> significant change in the labeling for the drug;
>
> (ii) If the drug that is undergoing investigation is lawfully marketed as a prescription drug product, the investigation is not intended to support a significant change in the advertising for the product;
>
> (iii) The investigation does not involve a route of administration or dosage level or use in a patient population or other factor that significantly increases the risks (or decreases the acceptability of the risks) associated with the use of the drug product;
>
> (iv) The investigation is conducted in compliance with the requirements for institutional review set forth in part 56 and with the requirements for informed consent set forth in part 50; and

Additional Note- Part 50 is the FDA regulation pertaining to informed consent and part 56 are the FDA regulations pertaining to IRBs

> (v) The investigation is conducted in compliance with the requirements of Sec. 312.7.

Additional Note- Section 21 CFR 312.7 pertains to promotion and charging for investigational products.

> (c) Bioavailability studies. The applicability of this part to in vivo bioavailability studies in humans is subject to the provisions of Sec. 320.31.

Additional Note- Section 21 CFR 320.31 notes that bioavailability investigations using new chemical entities, radioactive compounds, cytotoxic drugs and dosing regimens or schedules that are not part of any approved product labeling must be performed under an IND

> (d) Unlabeled indication. This <u>part does not apply</u> to the use in the practice of medicine for an <u>unlabeled indication of a new drug product approved under part 314 or of a licensed biological</u> product.

(e) Guidance. FDA may, on its own initiative, issue guidance on the applicability of this part to particular investigational uses of drugs. <u>On request, FDA will advise on the applicability</u> of this part to a planned clinical investigation.

The FDA issued a Guidance Document in January 2004 applying to both CDER and CBER that specifically addresses assessing the need for an IND for investigations using approved products in cancer patients. While the general conditions that apply to oncology products for filing an IND are no different than those that apply to other products, the needs of cancer patients and the risks that are generally acceptable in cancer therapy lead to a particular interpretation of the question of increased risk or decreased acceptability of risk.

Additional specific examples are cited in the Guidance Document, which may be found at http://www.fda.gov/cder/Guidance/6036fnl.pdf.

In summary, all unlicensed products require an IND and licensed products that are studied for unapproved uses or with new dosage forms, routes of administration, dosing regimens that are different than the approved regimen, or in new patient populations require filing an IND. In general, if the data using a licensed product could support a new use claim or if the risks are unknown or potentially greater than the approved use, an IND must be filed. Bioavailability studies on approved products that use particular product classes or dosing regimens that differ from the approved dosing regimen must also file an IND.

8.4 Pre-IND Consultation

Prospective IND sponsors have the option of receiving non-binding advice from the FDA on the structure and content of an IND submission for drugs/biologics intended to treat life threatening and severely debilitating illness (21 CFR 312.82). A prospective sponsor contacts the FDA review division with responsibility for the product to request a Pre-IND discussion. A formal meeting package prepared by the sponsor containing background information and specific questions is submitted to the FDA at least 30 days in advance of the meeting. Each FDA review discipline (product, pharmacology/toxicology, clinical and if necessary, biometrics) will review the meeting package and prepare specific answers to the questions as appropriate for that discipline. Supplemental comments in addition to answers to the questions may also be conveyed by the FDA to the sponsor.

To simplify the review process and responses, prospective sponsors are encouraged to separate questions into discipline specific topics.

Typical inquires are related to:

- Extent of product characterization
- Development of potency assays
- Product preparation procedures
- Product purity and methods for prevention and testing of contamination from infectious agents
- Appropriate non-clinical model systems to use
    o What and how many animal species
    o Number and extent of studies
        - Whether animal studies need to be Good Laboratory Practice (GLP) or if alternative procedures are possible
        - Length of studies
        - Extent of exposure
        - Extent and type of pathologic examinations
    o In general non-clinical studies should parallel intended clinical use with regard to exposure and number of doses
- Design of proposed clinical investigations
    o Justification of starting dose and dose escalation schema
    o Patient populations
    o Adequacy of safety monitoring
    o Length and type of follow up

Generally an internal FDA meeting (pre-meeting) occurs to discuss draft answers to the questions and reach consensus prior to the sponsor meeting. The sponsor meeting with the FDA may occur either in person or by telephone.

8.5　IND Filing

Each IND requires a sponsor. A sponsor must assume responsibility for the investigations and may be an individual or an organization. If the sponsor is an organization, there must be a designated point of contact within the organization. If an individual both initiates and conducts an investigation (21 CFR 312.3), the individual has the dual role of being a Sponsor-Investigator. This requires that the individual be attune to responsibilities designated to both sponsors and investigators (21 CFR Subpart D). The FDA does not disclose any information regarding an IND including the existence of an

IND, which is prohibited by Chapter III Section 301 of the FD&CA, unless there is a significant public health issue.

All IND inquiries and filing are made with the appropriate FDA review division. For combination products, a sponsor may consult the FDA Office of Combination Products, regarding which Center has review jurisdiction for the specific product. A combination product is defined in 21CFR Section 2.3 and consists of:

1) A product comprised of two or more regulated components, i.e., drug/device, biologic/device, drug/biologic, or drug/device/biologic, that are physically, chemically, or otherwise combined or mixed and produced as a single entity;

(2) Two or more separate products packaged together in a single package or as a unit and comprised of drug and device products, device and biological products, or biological and drug products;

(3) A drug, device, or biological product packaged separately that according to its investigational plan or proposed labeling is intended for use only with an approved individually specified drug, device, or biological product where both are required to achieve the intended use, indication, or effect and where upon approval of the proposed product the labeling of the approved product would need to be changed, e.g., to reflect a change in intended use, dosage form, strength, route of administration, or significant change in dose; or

(4) Any investigational drug, device, or biological product packaged separately that according to its proposed labeling is for use only with another individually specified investigational drug, device, or biological product where both are required to achieve the intended use, indication, or effect.

Additional information including details on determination of which FDA Center or Centers will be involved in the review of a combination product and what role each will have in combination product regulation can be found at http://www.fda.gov/oc/combination/

General instructions on filing an IND may be found at http://www.fda.gov/cber/ind/ind.htm and at http://www.fda.gov/cder/regulatory/applications/ind_page_1.htm.

The role of the FDA in cancer clinical trials 71

In FDA, CBER IND original submissions and amendments may be submitted electronically instead of by paper. For general information and guidance pertaining to the electronic submission of regulatory documents to CBER, refer to the CBER website at http://www.fda.gov/cber/esub/esub.htm.

8.6 Contents of an IND Application

The contents of an IND are outlined in 21CFR 312.23 and include the following nine components:

1. Cover sheet of a Form 1571 filled out by the sponsor. Each Associate investigator must have an additional Form designated as 1572. Both forms are available at http://forms.psc.gov/forms/FDA/fda.html
2. Table of contents
3. Introductory statement and summary of general investigational plan
4. Investigator's Brochure if the planned investigation will occur at multiple sites and the sponsor is not a sponsor-investigator. Most academic investigator initiated studies that file for an IND are considered sponsor-investigator studies and will not require an Investigator's Brochure unless the product is supplied by a third party. The regulations refer to the requirements for Investigator Brochure in two sections- 21CFR312.23 (a) (5) and in addition 21CFR312.55. The information is complementary and both sections apply.
5. Clinical protocols. Specific listings and requirements are noted in the regulations for various protocol types.
6. Product information including chemistry, manufacturing and control information.
7. Pharmacology and toxicology information
8. Summary of prior human experience with the product, if applicable.
9. Special topic information such as dependence or abuse potential, radioactive information, and plans for pediatric studies.

An FDA Guidance for Phase I studies for drugs and well characterized biotechnology products was published in 1995 (http://www.fda.gov/cder/Guidance/clin2.pdf). A clarification issued in 2000(http://www.fda.gov/cber/gdlns/qaind1.htm) addresses when updated toxicology reports are due. The Guidance emphasizes the graded nature of the product information that is expected during the course of clinical development. In general, characterization and specifications for a product are expected to become more precise as the development program advances. For early phase studies, product characterization expectations are less stringent. (http://www.fda.gov/cber/gdlns/indcgmp.htm) The Guidance also comments on expectations pertaining to pharmacologic and toxicologic data, noting that preliminary reports may be sufficient to initiate the review process and that final quality assured reports may be submitted subsequently. The intent is not to delay the submission of an IND application and hence the initiation of a clinical program pending preparation of the final quality assured reports with the expectation that the conclusions from the preliminary reports and the final reports will be the same.

Cellular based products have particular challenges including, but not limited to, lot size, timing of administration, stability, reproducibility, sterility, and consistency. For example, the definition of a lot may be a single dose, or multiple doses to treat a single patient. Anticipation of lot size and specifications, including potential stability concerns, must be addressed early in product development. A related issue is maintaining consistency and reproducibility between different lots.

The timing of patient administration may be determined by the stability of the product and the potential for preservation. A product that has limited stability may require administration shortly after preparation. This, in turn, would require approaches for lot release that require testing results to be available in a timely manner.

Cellular products may have limited storage or holding potential and knowing the critical parameters is essential to maintain quality of the product. Stability should be thoroughly investigated early in product development. Independent of the manufacturing approach, aseptic processing must be maintained throughout manufacture.

Cell-device combinations may result in additional considerations. These include the impact of the device upon the biologic such as genotypic or phenotypic stability of cells and tissues and modification of survival and metabolism. The biologic product may impact the device through degradation of components, clogging of filters or mechanisms, or transmission of adventitious agents.

Additional comments and recommendations may be found in the following Guidance Documents:

- Guidance for Industry: Guidance for Human Somatic Cell Therapy and Gene Therapy, 1998.(http://www.fda.gov/cber/gdlns/somgene.pdf)

- Points To Consider in the Characterization of Cell Lines to Produce Biologicals, CBER, FDA, 1993. (http://www.fda.gov/cber/gdlns/ptccell.pdf)
- ICH Harmonized Tripartite Guideline: Viral Safety Evaluation of Biotechnology Products Derived from Cell Lines of Human or Animal Origin,-1998 (http://www.fda.gov/cber/gdlns/virsafe.pdf)
- Draft Guidance for Reviewers: Instructions and Template for Chemistry, Manufacturing, and Control (CMC) Reviewers of Human Somatic Cell Therapy Investigational New Drug Applications (INDs), 2003 (http://www.fda.gov/cber/gdlns/cmcsomcell.htm)

Gene therapy has additional considerations for regulatory review including interactions with the National Institutes of Health (NIH), Office of Biotechnology Activities (OBA). In a letter sent by CBER to IND sponsors and principal investigators for gene therapy studies in November 1999 (http://www.fda.gov/cber/ltr/gt110599.htm) the following procedures were outlined. The original letter, cited below, refers to the NIH Office of Recombinant DNA (ORDA); however subsequently the Office name changed to the Office of Biotechnology Activities (OBA) (http://www4.od.nih.gov/oba/rac/patterson2-00.pdf). The process remains the same.

- The documentation required in Appendix M-I of the current *NIH Guidelines* should be submitted to NIH/OBA prior to the submission of an IND to FDA. This will help to ensure that novel issues will be identified and discussed publicly in a timely manner.
- FDA will notify NIH/OBA of the receipt of a gene therapy IND to assist NIH/OBA in monitoring investigator compliance with the *NIH Guidelines*.
- In accordance with the FDA regulations found at US Code of Federal Regulations, Title 21, part 312.32 "IND Safety Reports" and *NIH Guidelines, Appendix M-VII-C "Adverse Event Reporting,"* investigators/sponsors are expected to report all serious adverse events to both the FDA and NIH.
- FDA will notify NIH/OBA of the receipt of an adverse event report on a gene therapy IND to enhance investigator compliance with the *NIH Guidelines*.
- Within 15 working days after receipt by NIH/OBA of a complete submission, the Recombinant DNA Advisory Committee (RAC) will determine whether a protocol is novel and, therefore, requires public RAC review. NIH/OBA will notify FDA within one working day of the RAC's decision regarding the necessity for full public

review of a gene therapy protocol. The FDA will request that the sponsor delay initiation of, or suspend an ongoing protocol until the RAC has determined whether the protocol requires public review. Failure to comply can result in removal of NIH funding to the investigators institute. Also any investigator that works at an institute that receives NIH funding for recombinant DNA research must submit their clinical protocol to OBA for review prior to initiation of their trial.
- If the RAC decides that full public review is warranted, the FDA will request, at the completion of its IND review (within 30 days of receipt of the IND or when the IND is allowed to proceed by FDA), that sponsors delay initiation of the protocol until after completion of the RAC review process.

In addition to addressing the procedures for public review by the Recombinant DNA Advisory Committee, gene therapy investigators must address issues such as qualification of components used for product manufacture, quality assurance throughout the manufacture process, the production of replication competent viruses through contamination, the potential for permanent alteration to somatic or germline DNA, abuse potential, and long-term toxicity.

In March 2000, FDA CBER issued a letter to all investigators and sponsors for gene therapy products outlining a series of quality assurance and monitoring requirements. The letter is posted on the CBER internet site (http://www.fda.gov/cber/ltr/gt030600.htm) and FDA refers all Sponsors of gene therapy products to this letter and its requirements.

A Draft Guidance was issued in 2005 on Observing Participants for Delayed Adverse Events in Gene Therapy Trials (http://www.fda.gov/cber/gdlns/gtclin.htm) that outlines delayed adverse event considerations that apply to various populations, including cancer patients.

Additional comments and recommendations can be found in the following Guidance Documents:

- Guidance for Industry: Guidance for Human Somatic Cell Therapy and Gene Therapy – 1998
(http://www.fda.gov/cber/gdlns/somgene.pdf)
- Guidance for Industry: Supplemental Guidance on Testing for Replication Competent Retrovirus in Retroviral Vector Based Gene Therapy Products and During Follow-up of Patients in Clinical Trials Using Retroviral Vectors - 2000
(http://www.fda.gov/cber/gdlns/retrogt1000.htm)
- Draft Guidance for FDA Review Staff and Sponsors: Content and Review of Chemistry, Manufacturing, and Control (CMC)

Information for Human Gene Therapy Investigational New Drug Applications (INDs) 2004 – (http://www.fda.gov/cber/gdlns/gtindcmc.htm)

8.7 The IND Review Process

Upon receipt of an IND application, the FDA will issue an Acknowledgement Letter that informs the sponsor of the IND number and outlines general procedures. Unless the sponsor is contacted and informed of deficiencies, an IND is considered in effect 30 days after the IND application has been received by the FDA.

The FDA has teams of technical experts that are assigned to each IND submission. In general, the primary review disciplines are product, pharmacology/toxicology, clinical and biometrics. Administrative coordination is provided by a Regulatory Project Manager, who functions as the point of contact between the FDA and the IND sponsor. The general principles of IND review are outlined in the regulations and are cited here with additional underlining to emphasize selected text.

Sec. 312.22 General principles of the IND submission.

> *(a) FDA's primary objectives in reviewing an IND are, in all phases of the investigation, to assure the safety and rights of subjects, and, in Phase 2 and 3, to help assure that the quality of the scientific evaluation of drugs is adequate to permit an evaluation of the drug's effectiveness and safety. Therefore, although FDA's review of Phase 1 submissions will focus on assessing the safety of Phase 1 investigations, FDA's review of Phases 2 and 3 submissions will also include an assessment of the scientific quality of the clinical investigations and the likelihood that the investigations will yield data capable of meeting statutory standards for marketing approval.*

Not all clinical studies conform to the nomenclature of phases 1, 2 or 3 to indicate the stage of development. For example, ICH Document E8 "General Considerations of Clinical Trials" presents an alternative nomenclature based on study objectives and classifies studies as Human Pharmacology, Therapeutic Exploratory, Therapeutic Confirmatory and Human Use (http://www.fda.gov/cder/guidance/1857fnl.pdf).

In general, FDA reviews early phase studies to determine if the risks are acceptable for the type of product and patient population and that the rights of patients are protected.(21 CFR 312.42) Later phase clinical studies are reviewed with additional considerations of design in addition to safety and patient protection.

According to regulation, the FDA review team will attempt to work with the sponsor during the 30 day review process to clarify questions and, if needed, seek modifications, in order to allow the investigation to proceed after 30 days. If no deficiencies are identified or discussion of the deficiencies is not possible, the IND is either considered active following the 30 day review period, and may begin enrolling patients following IRB approval or is placed on clinical hold.

Title 21 CFR Subpart C Section 312.42 (c) states:

> c) *Discussion of deficiency. Whenever FDA concludes that a deficiency exists in a clinical investigation that may be grounds for the imposition of clinical hold FDA will, unless patients are exposed to immediate and serious risk, attempt to discuss and satisfactorily resolve the matter with the sponsor before issuing the clinical hold order.*

8.8 Clinical Hold

If deficiencies cannot be resolved during the 30 day review period, a clinical hold will be issued. A clinical hold is defined as the delay or suspension of clinical work requested under an IND (21 CFR 312.42).

The relevant grounds for clinical hold in 21 CFR 312.42, with underlining specific words for emphasis, follow:

> *Sec. 312.42 Clinical holds and requests for modification.*
> *(a)__General__. A clinical hold is an order issued by FDA to the sponsor to delay a __proposed__ clinical investigation or to suspend an __ongoing__ investigation. The clinical hold order may apply to one or more of the investigations covered by an IND. When a proposed study is placed on clinical hold, subjects may not be given the investigational drug. When an ongoing study is placed on clinical hold, no new subjects may be recruited to the study and placed on the investigational drug; patients already in the study should be taken off therapy involving the investigational drug unless specifically permitted by FDA in the interest of patient safety.*
> *(b)__Grounds for imposition of clinical hold__—*
> *(1)Clinical hold of a __Phase 1 study__ under an IND.*

> *FDA may place a proposed or ongoing Phase 1 investigation on clinical hold if it finds that:*
>
> > *Human subjects are or would be exposed to an <u>unreasonable and significant risk</u> of illness or injury;*
> >
> > *The clinical <u>investigators</u> named in the IND are <u>not qualified</u> by reason of their scientific training and experience to conduct the investigation described in the IND;*
> >
> > *The <u>investigator brochure is misleading, erroneous, or materially incomplete</u>; or*
> >
> > *The IND <u>does not contain sufficient information</u> required under Sec. 312.23 to assess the risks to subjects of the proposed studies.*

Additional Note: The requirements in Section 312.23 are cited in an earlier section of this chapter.

An additional reason for placing a study on clinical hold, not cited here, is if there is gender exclusion and the disease occurs in both men and women. 312.42(b)(1)(v)

Later phase studies may be placed on clinical hold for any of the above reasons and, in addition, if a design deficiency would not allow the study to meet its stated objectives. 312.42(b)(2)

Additional hold criteria apply to studies that are <u>not</u> designed to be adequate and well controlled that may interfere with ongoing adequate and well controlled studies, particularly if there are limitations on product supply or numbers of patients or if adequate and well controlled studies have already shown lack of effectiveness or if alternative therapies are considered to have a better benefit to risk profile.

CBER informs IND sponsors by telephone or other means of rapid communication of the clinical hold and a letter is sent to the sponsor within 30 days of the telephone call. In the letter, the sponsor is instructed why the IND is on hold and what additional information or changes are required to remove the hold. Additional non-hold comments which are not binding but intended to improve the protocol may also included in the letter. If the IND is allowed to proceed and not placed on hold, the FDA may still send a letter containing only non-hold comments/recommendations.

The sponsor may reply to a hold letter at any time by submitting an IND amendment which must be marked as a Complete Response to Clinical Hold. The FDA review team will review the response to hold and must make a determination and issue a written reply by 30 days after receipt of the

Complete Response to Clinical Hold. The outcomes of a Complete Response to Clinical Hold letter are that either

- the hold issues were adequately addressed and the hold is removed, in which case the sponsor is informed by telephone and a letter stating that the clinical hold is removed is issued, or;
- the issues were not adequately addressed or the revised submission contains new deficiencies, in which case the sponsor is informed by telephone and a Continued Hold letter is issued with the reasons for continuing hold and what the sponsor must do to remove the hold.

The procedures are based on the regulation cited in 21 CFR 312.42. Underlining is for emphasis and is not included in the original text.

> *(e)Resumption of clinical investigations*. *An investigation may only resume after FDA* (usually the Division Director, or the Director's designee, with responsibility for review of the IND) *has notified the sponsor that the investigation may proceed*. *Resumption of the affected investigation(s) will be authorized when the sponsor corrects the deficiency(ies) previously cited or otherwise satisfies the agency that the investigation(s) can proceed. FDA may notify a sponsor of its determination regarding the clinical hold by telephone or other means of rapid communication.*
>
> *If a sponsor of an IND that has been placed on clinical hold requests in writing that the clinical hold be removed and submits a complete response to the issue(s) identified in the clinical hold order, FDA shall respond in writing to the sponsor within 30-calendar days of receipt of the request and the complete response. FDA's response will either remove or maintain the clinical hold, and will state the reasons for such determination. Notwithstanding the 30-calendar day response time, a sponsor may not proceed with a clinical trial on which a clinical hold has been imposed until the sponsor has been notified by FDA that the hold has been lifted.*
>
> *If the sponsor disagrees with the reasons cited for the clinical hold, the sponsor may request reconsideration of the decision in accordance with Sec. 312.48.*

Section 312.42 contains additional text that notes that if clinical hold deficiencies are not addressed within a year, the IND may be placed on inactive status.

The role of the FDA in cancer clinical trials 79

> *(g) Conversion of IND on clinical hold to inactive status. If all investigations covered by an IND remain on clinical hold for 1 year or more, the IND may be placed on inactive status by FDA under Sec. 312.45.*

Further information on responding to clinical hold can be found in an FDA Guidance Document published in 2000 "Submitting and Reviewing Complete Responses to Clinical Holds" (http://www.fda.gov/cber/gdlns/clinhld1000.htm).

The FDA may place an investigation on clinical hold at any time. If only part of the clinical work under an IND is delayed or suspended, for example one of several protocols or one arm of a multi-arm study, the action is termed a Partial Hold. The procedures for removing a partial hold are similar to removing a complete hold. A representative scenario for when the FDA may place an ongoing study on clinical hold would be the occurrence of adverse events that would trigger a re-evaluation of the risks and monitoring procedures.

8.9 Shipping Investigational Products

The regulations pertaining to use of an investigational agent note that the product may be shipped 30 days after the FDA receives the IND application but may not be administered until the IND is in effect. Underlined text is for emphasis and not included in the original regulations.

> *Sec. 312.40 General requirements for use of an investigational new drug in a clinical investigation.*
>
> *a) An investigational new drug may be used in a clinical investigation if the following conditions are met:*
>
> *(1) The sponsor of the investigation submits an IND for the drug to FDA; the IND is in effect under paragraph (b) of this section; and the sponsor complies with all applicable requirements in this part and parts 50 and 56 with respect to the conduct of the clinical investigations;*
> *and*
> *(2) Each participating investigator conducts his or her investigation in compliance with the requirements of this part and parts 50 and 56.*

Additional Note: parts 50 and 56 refer to Title 21 of the Code of Federal Regulations Parts 50 (Protection of Human Subjects) and 56 (Institutional Review Boards).

b) An IND goes into effect:

(1) Thirty days after FDA receives the IND, unless FDA notifies the sponsor that the investigations described in the IND are subject to a clinical hold under Sec. 312.42;
or
(2) On earlier notification by FDA that the clinical investigations in the IND may begin.

(c) A sponsor may ship an investigational new drug to investigators named in the IND:

(1) Thirty days after FDA receives the IND;
or
(2) On earlier FDA authorization to ship the drug.

(d) An investigator may not administer an investigational new drug to human subjects until the IND goes into effect under paragraph (b) of this section.

8.10 IND Amendments

Subsequent to the initial filing of an IND, further submissions to the IND are termed amendments and are numbered by the FDA in order of receipt.

Some of the applicable regulations with formatting and underlining specific words for emphasis, are noted. For a new protocol or changes in an existing protocol, a sponsor needs to notify the FDA by submission of the protocol or revised protocol prior to proceeding, except for safety changes, which can be implemented prior to FDA notification. Following notification, a sponsor does not need to wait for FDA comment to proceed but IRB approval is always required. The FDA may place an ongoing study on clinical hold at any time if any of the criteria for clinical hold are met.

Sec. 312.30 Protocol amendments.

Once an IND is in effect, a sponsor shall amend it as needed to ensure that the clinical investigations are conducted according to protocols included in the application. This section sets forth the provisions under which new protocols may be submitted and changes in previously submitted protocols may be made.

Whenever a sponsor intends to conduct a <u>clinical investigation with an exception from informed consent for emergency research</u> as set forth in Sec. 50.24 of this chapter, the sponsor shall submit <u>a separate IND</u> for such investigation.

(a) New protocol. Whenever a sponsor intends to conduct a study that is not covered by a protocol already contained in the IND, the sponsor shall submit to FDA a protocol amendment containing the protocol for the study. Such study may begin provided two conditions are met:
(1) The <u>sponsor has submitted the protocol to FDA</u> for its review; and
(2) the <u>protocol has been approved by the Institutional Review Board</u> (IRB) with responsibility for review and approval of the study in accordance with the requirements

(b) Changes in a protocol.
(1) A sponsor shall submit a <u>protocol amendment describing any change in a Phase 1 protocol that significantly affects the safety of subjects</u> or any change in a <u>Phase 2 or 3 protocol that significantly affects the safety of subjects, the scope of the investigation, or the scientific quality of the study</u>. Examples of changes requiring an amendment under this paragraph include:
(i) Any increase in drug dosage or duration of exposure of individual subjects to the drug beyond that in the current protocol, or any significant increase in the number of subjects under study.
(ii) Any significant change in the design of a protocol (such as the addition or dropping of a control group).
(iii) The addition of a new test or procedure that is intended to improve monitoring for, or reduce the risk of, a side effect or adverse event; or the dropping of a test intended to monitor safety.

(2)

(i) A protocol change under paragraph (b)(1) of this section may be made provided two conditions are met:

(a) The sponsor has submitted the change to FDA for its review; and

(b) The change has been approved by the IRB with responsibility for review and approval of the study. The sponsor may comply with these two conditions in either order.

(ii) Notwithstanding paragraph (b)(2)(i) of this section, a protocol change intended to eliminate an apparent immediate hazard to subjects may be implemented immediately provided FDA is subsequently notified by protocol amendment and the reviewing IRB is notified in accordance with Sec. 56.104(c).

(d) Content and format. A protocol amendment is required to be prominently identified as such (i.e., ``Protocol Amendment: New Protocol'', ``Protocol Amendment: Change in Protocol'', or ``Protocol Amendment: New Investigator''), and to contain the following:

(1)

(i) In the case of a new protocol, a copy of the new protocol and a brief description of the most clinically significant differences between it and previous protocols.

(ii) In the case of a change in protocol, a brief description of the change and reference (date and number) to the submission that contained the protocol.

(iii) In the case of a new investigator, the investigator's name, the qualifications to conduct the investigation, reference to the previously submitted protocol, and all additional information about the investigator's

study as is required under Sec. 312.23(a)(6)(iii)(b).
(e) When submitted. A sponsor shall submit a protocol amendment for a new protocol or a change in protocol before its implementation. Protocol amendments to add a new investigator or to provide additional information about investigators may be grouped and submitted at 30-day intervals. When several submissions of new protocols or protocol changes are anticipated during a short period, the sponsor is encouraged, to the extent feasible, to include these all in a single submission.

8.11 IND Investigator Responsibilities

In addition to compliance with the relevant laws and regulations regarding human subject protection and filing protocols and amendments, an IND holder is expected to submit to the FDA expedited reports of serious and unexpected adverse events and an annual report containing summaries of all clinical investigations under an IND.

An adverse event is defined in ICH E2a published in 1994 and the concurrent FDA Guidance Document published in 1995 (http://www.fda.gov/cder/guidance/iche2a.pdf) as "Any untoward medical occurrence in a patient or clinical investigation subject administered a pharmaceutical product and which does not necessarily have to have a causal relationship with this treatment."

Other relevant definitions can be found in the FDA Regulations 21CFRPart 312 Section 312.32. Underlined text and formatting is for emphasis and clarity and not part of the original regulation.

Sec. 312.32 IND safety reports.

(a) Definitions. The following definitions of terms apply to this section:-
 Associated with the use of the drug. *There is a reasonable possibility that the experience may have been caused by the drug.*
 Disability. *A substantial disruption of a person's ability to conduct normal life functions.*
 Life-threatening adverse drug experience. *Any adverse drug experience that places the patient or subject, in the view of the investigator, at immediate risk of death from the reaction as it*

occurred, i.e., it does not include a reaction that, had it occurred in a more severe form, might have caused death.

Serious adverse drug experience*: Any adverse drug experience occurring at any dose that results in any of the following outcomes:*

<u>*Death,*</u>

A <u>life-threatening</u> adverse drug experience,

<u>*inpatient hospitalization*</u> *or prolongation of existing hospitalization,*

a <u>persistent or significant disability</u>/incapacity, or

a <u>congenital anomaly</u>/birth defect.

<u>*Important medical events*</u> *that may not result in death, be life-threatening, or require hospitalization may be considered a serious adverse drug experience when, based upon appropriate medical judgment, they <u>may jeopardize the patient</u> or subject and may <u>require medical or surgical intervention to prevent one of the outcomes</u> listed in this definition.*

Examples of such medical events include allergic bronchospasm requiring intensive treatment in an emergency room or at home, blood dyscrasias or convulsions that do not result in inpatient hospitalization, or the development of drug dependency or drug abuse.

Unexpected adverse drug experience*: <u>Any adverse drug experience, the specificity or severity of which is not consistent with the current investigator brochure</u>; or, if an investigator brochure is not required <u>or</u> available, <u>the specificity or severity of which is not consistent with the risk information described in the general investigational plan</u> or elsewhere in the current application, as amended. For example, under this definition, hepatic necrosis would be unexpected (by virtue of greater severity) if the investigator brochure only referred to elevated hepatic enzymes or hepatitis. Similarly, cerebral thromboembolism and cerebral vasculitis would be unexpected (by virtue of greater specificity) if the investigator brochure only listed cerebral vascular accidents. ``Unexpected,'' as used in this definition, refers to an adverse drug experience that has not been previously observed (e.g., included in the investigator brochure) rather than from the perspective of such experience not being anticipated from the pharmacological properties of the pharmaceutical product.*

A sponsor must notify the FDA and all participating investigators in writing of adverse events that are both serious and unexpected within 15 calendar days of receipt of the information. If the event is an unexpected death or life threatening event, notification is expected by facsimile or telephone within 7 calendar days to be followed by a written report within 8 calendar days following the initial rapid communication. The total number of days for filing a written report for a death or life threatening adverse event is 15 days, the same as for all serious and unexpected adverse events.

Findings from non-clinical studies that suggest significant risk for humans such as animal studies demonstrating mutagenicity, teratogenicity or carcinogenicity must also be reported to the FDA and participating investigators within 15 calendar days.

An event that initially was not considered both serious and unexpected but subsequently determined to meet the criteria must follow the same procedure of notification and a written report within 15 calendar days after the reclassification.

Collectively such IND safety reports are termed expedited safety reports. ICH expectations are summarized in the E2a Guideline and the relevant FDA Guidance Document regarding the content and format of expedited safety reports (http://www.fda.gov/medwatch/report/iche2a.pdf).

Expedited safety reporting requirements are summarized in the following table:

Table 3. Requirements for expedited safety reports

Adverse Event	Filing	Time Frame
Serious and unexpected	Written Report to FDA and notification of participating investigators	15 calendar days from receipt of information
Unexpected death or life threatening event	Initial telephone or facsimile report to FDA and notification of participating investigators	7 calendar days from receipt of information
Unexpected death or life threatening event	Written Report to FDA and notification of participating investigators	15 calendar days from receipt of information
Non-clinical data that suggests serious risk to humans	Written Report to FDA and notification of participating investigators	15 calendar days from receipt of information
Adverse event subsequently determined to meet criteria of serious and unexpected	Written Report to FDA and notification of participating investigators	15 calendar days from receipt of information

Each written safety report must identify all prior safety reports filed with the IND concerning a similar adverse experience and an analysis of the new event in the context of the previous reports. No language in the regulations imposes a requirement of causality or relatedness to the investigational product for expedited reporting. The expectation and requirement is that <u>all</u> serious and unexpected adverse events will be reported with a written report within 15 calendar days. Follow up safety reports based on the initial expedited report are expected when the information becomes available.

The important terms in filing an expedited report are serious <u>and</u> unexpected. If a serious event is expected, then it does not meet the criteria. As an example, patients with leukemia not in remission can experience many serious adverse events. If these adverse events are known and expected and noted in the study protocol, then when they occur, they would not trigger an expedited report. However, if the frequency, severity or duration exceeded what is expected, then the events would require expedited reporting.

Adverse events that do not meet the criteria for expedited reporting may be filed as either an information amendment to the IND or incorporated into the IND annual report. For oncology studies, as for any other disease, events that are considered to be expected based on their nature, severity, duration and frequency as part of the natural history of the disease, are not considered to meet the criteria for filing an expedited safety report. Noting in the study protocol serious adverse events that are expected from the underlying disease and any other therapeutic regimens, as well as the toxicities of the investigational product generally assists in clarifying which adverse events are unexpected and serious.

If a clinical study under an IND uses a product that is already marketed, adverse events occurring under the relevant IND need to be filed as adverse event reports to that IND. Adverse events for the marketed product that occur in other settings outside the IND that are serious and unexpected or not part of the approved product labeling would be filed through the appropriate reporting mechanisms and in addition would be submitted to the IND as an information amendment, with changes in the Informed Consent form and study protocol if warranted.

The FDA, or the sponsor with FDA agreement, may alter the safety reporting procedures under an IND to alternate schedules and procedures to ensure patient safety.

The absence of a requirement for reporting an adverse event and relatedness to the IND product is underscored by a disclaimer noted in the last section of 21CFR312.32.

(e) Disclaimer. A safety report or other information submitted by a sponsor under this part (and any release by FDA of that report or information) does not necessarily reflect a conclusion by the sponsor or FDA that the report or information constitutes an admission that the drug caused or contributed to an adverse experience. A sponsor need not admit, and may deny, that the report or information submitted by the sponsor constitutes an admission that the drug caused or contributed to an adverse experience.

9. ANNUAL REPORTS

An IND sponsor must file within 60 days of the anniversary date that an IND went into effect an annual report to the FDA summarizing progress to date. The contents of an IND annual report to the FDA are outlined in 21CFR Subpart B Section 312.33 and include the following 7 components:

- Individual study information- a brief summary of each study completed and those in progress including demographic information
- Summary information on all studies, both clinical and non-clinical, including integrated summaries of adverse events, deaths, safety reports, drop outs, bioavailability studies and manufacturing changes.
- Description of the general investigational plan for the coming year that includes
    o The rationale for the drug or the research study;
    o the indication(s) to be studied;
    o the general approach to be followed in evaluating the drug;
    o the kinds of clinical trials to be conducted
    o the estimated number of patients to be given the product in those studies; and
    o any risks of particular severity or seriousness anticipated on the basis of the toxicological data in animals or prior studies in humans with the product or related products.
- Current investigator's brochure, if revised, with a description of any revisions
- Description of significant Phase 1 protocol modifications that were not previously submitted as protocol amendments
- Summary of significant foreign marketing developments
- Any outstanding FDA related business matters

10. PATIENT ACCESS TO INVESTIGATIONAL PRODUCTS

A common method for patients to access investigational products is to enroll in a clinical study.

Sponsors with open protocols are required to list their studies based on the Food and Drug Administration Modernization Act (Public Law 105-115 Section 112 Subsection (d)) within 21 days after the protocol goes into effect on a Federal web site known as Clinicaltrials.gov. Section 113 of the Food and Drug Modernization Act requires you to submit information to the data bank about a clinical trial conducted under an investigational new drug (IND) application if it is for a drug to treat a serious or life-threatening disease or condition and it is a trial to test effectiveness (42 U.S.C. 282(j)(3)(A)). Specific information regarding the resource and listing studies can be found at http://www.clinicaltrials.gov.

Potential difficulties to enrolling on a clinical protocol include factors such as not meeting eligibility criteria and geographic distance from a study site. Alternatives to enrolling on a clinical protocol are participating in a protocol as a special exception, a single patient protocol under an existing IND or a single patient IND. Each of these approaches is intended to overcome enrollment impediments using different administrative mechanisms. All require IRB approval. No matter which mechanism is selected, use of the investigational product is dependent upon the willingness of the manufacturer or distributor to supply it. Include some type of statement that FDA encourages treatment under multiple patient protocols. The features of each are listed in the following table.

Table 4. Regulatory mechanisms to access investigational products

Administrative Mechanism	General Procedure
Existing clinical protocol	Patient enrolls at approved protocol site
Exception to existing protocol based on altered eligibility criteria	Product sponsor, principal investigator, IRB and FDA agreement
Single patient protocol under existing IND	• Product sponsor, principal investigator, treating physician, IRB and FDA agreement • Sponsor must file new protocol as IND amendment with treating physician as principal investigator
Single patient IND	• Product sponsor, treating physician, IRB and FDA agreement • Treating physician must file new IND with FDA and become principal investigator

An additional mechanism to provide an indeterminate number of patients access to an investigational product is termed a Treatment Protocol or a Treatment IND, which is explained in detail below. The former is a protocol under an existing IND while the latter is a new IND opened for the purpose of expanded access. In either case, a protocol is written that does not have a specific target number of patients, but allows all patients that meet the eligibility criteria to enroll. The number of study sites may be predetermined and limited or may also be flexible.

The Food, Drug and Cosmetic Act was amended in 1997 in Chapter 9, Subchapter V Part E Section 561 through the Food and Drug Administration Modernization Act Section 402 (Public Law 105-115) to address expanded access to investigational therapies and diagnostics.

The major provisions of the statutory change are:

- The Secretary of Health and Human Services (or designate) can authorize emergency shipment of an investigational product under conditions determined by the Secretary for the diagnosis, monitoring, or treatment of a serious disease or condition
- Any person, acting through a physician licensed in accordance with State law, may request from a manufacturer or distributor, and any manufacturer or distributor may provide to a requesting licensed physician an investigational drug or investigational device for the diagnosis, monitoring, or treatment of a serious disease or condition if five (5) conditions are met:
    o the licensed physician determines that the person has no comparable or satisfactory alternative therapy available to diagnose, monitor, or treat the disease or condition involved, and
    o the probable risk to the person from the investigational drug or investigational device is not greater than the probable risk from the disease or condition;
    o the Secretary of HHS (or designate) determines that there is sufficient evidence of safety and effectiveness to support the use of the investigational drug or investigational device; and
    o the Secretary of HHS (or designate) determines that provision of the investigational drug or investigational device will not interfere with the initiation, conduct, or completion of clinical investigations to support marketing approval; and
    o the sponsor, or clinical investigator submits to the FDA a clinical protocol consistent with existing laws and

regulations describing the use of the investigational drug or investigational device in a single patient or a small group of patients.

As with all protocols, IRB approval is also required prior to enrollment.
- A Treatment IND can be initiated by a physician or sponsor for expanded access to a product if all of the following nine (9) conditions are met (http://www.fda.gov/CDER/guidance/105-115.htm#SEC.%20402):
  o The use of the product is intended for use in the diagnosis, monitoring or treatment for a serious or immediately life threatening disease or condition
  o No comparable or satisfactory alternative is available
  o The product is under investigation in a controlled clinical trial for the intended use or all clinical trials necessary to support licensing have been completed
  o The sponsor of the product is actively pursuing marketing approval of the product for the intended use with due diligence
  o The expanded access program will not interfere with enrollment in other ongoing clinical investigations
  o Sufficient evidence of safety and effectiveness supports the intended use
  o The totality of available scientific evidence provides a reasonable basis to conclude that the product _may_ be effective for the intended use
  o The totality of available scientific evidence provides a reasonable basis to conclude that the product would not expose patients to unreasonable risk or injury
  o The expanded access protocol complies with the relevant laws and regulations

The conditions cited in the law for either individual patient access or a treatment IND are consistent with a product in a late stage of development and that marketing approval is contemplated in the near future. An expanded access protocol or treatment IND is intended to be open for a limited time.
- The Secretary of HHS (or designate) can inform professional societies and medical associations about the expanded access program for a product with some restrictions
- If any of the requirements for expanded access are no longer in effect, the Secretary of HHS (or designate) can terminate expanded access for the product

The role of the FDA in cancer clinical trials 91

Within the FDA Commissioner's Office is the Office for Special Health Issues (OSHI). OSHI assists patients and others with questions regarding access to investigational products and participation in FDA process and procedures. Further information regarding their programs can be found at http://www.fda.gov/oashi/home.html.

11. EXPORT AND IMPORT OF INVESTIGATIONAL PRODUCTS

The regulation of exporting investigational products is determined by United States Federal laws and regulations and laws and regulations of the country or jurisdiction that is receiving the product.

U.S. requirements for exporting an investigational product, as noted in the Code of Federal Regulations Title 21 Section 312.110, are:
- the investigational product has an active IND
- each person receiving the product is an investigator named in the IND
- prior authorization from the FDA for use in a clinical investigation is obtained.

The applicable laws and regulations regarding importation of investigational products vary by region. Compliance with all local laws and regulations is expected.

The Food Drug and Cosmetic Act in section 331 prohibit the interstate shipment or importation of unapproved products, whether for personal or investigational use. The IND regulations describe, in 21CFR Section 312.110, conditions under which an investigational product may be imported under an IND.
- The IND for the product is currently in effect (active)
- The recipient is either the IND sponsor, a qualified investigator named in the IND, or the assigned domestic agent of a foreign sponsor as named in an IND
- The IND describes the actions to be taken with the imported product

11.1 Charging for Investigational Products

The IND regulations, in 21 CFR 312.7, address the issue of charging for investigational products. Although commercialization and marketing are prohibited, a sponsor may charge for an investigational product, with the charges limited to cost recovery for manufacture, research, development and handling of the product. Charging for ancillary services and the cost of care routinely provided for treatment of the underlying disease or condition are not regulated by the FDA.

Two cases for charging are noted in the regulation. The first is that for any clinical trial under an IND, a sponsor requires prior authorization to charge by submitting to the FDA a full written explanation of why charging is necessary to undertake or continue the study and why provision of the product is not considered part of the normal cost of doing business. The FDA will make a determination and inform the sponsor in writing if the request to charge has been granted.

The second case is for a Treatment Protocol or Treatment IND. A sponsor may charge for product if the following four (4) conditions are met:

- Ongoing clinical investigations have adequate enrollment
- Charging does not constitute commercial marketing (all marketing prior to approval is prohibited)
- The product is not commercially advertised or marketed
- The sponsor is actively pursuing marketing approval with due diligence

The same regulation (21 CFR312.7) notes that once results of clinical investigations have sufficient data to support a marketing application, an ongoing investigation should not be unduly prolonged nor should a product be commercially distributed or test marketed. Commercial distribution and marketing are distinguished from exchange of scientific information and dissemination of scientific findings. Commercial marketing is intended to represent a claim of safety and effectiveness while scientific findings provide data, but do not make a claim.

12. SPECIAL TOPICS

12.1 Orphan Drugs

In 1983 Congress passed the Orphan Drug Act, which was signed into law by President Ronald Reagan. The Act defines a designation, termed Orphan Designation, that applies to the combination of a product and an intended indication if the indication has a prevalence of less than 200 000 people in the United States or if there is no reasonable expectation that the costs of development could be recovered from sales in the United States within 5 years of marketing approval. The fact that the designation applies to the combination of the product and intended indication means that a product could have multiple Orphan designations or could have Orphan designation and also be developed for regular marketing approval for another use. The requirement of a combination of product and intended indication for Orphan designation also means that one indication can have several products associated with it, each with a separate Orphan designation.

The determination of Orphan designation is made by the Office of Orphan Product Development located in the FDA Commissioner's Office. Once a product with an intended indication receives Orphan Designation, it can qualify for a longer period of marketing exclusivity (7 years versus the standard 5 years for regular marketing approval) and can qualify for financial assistance through a competitive grant program administered by the FDA. Additional incentives include tax credits, exemption from FDA User Fees associated with filing a product licensing application, and exemption from complying with the pediatric mandate (discussed below). Many malignancies could meet the criteria for Orphan Designation. Further information regarding the application process to receive Orphan Designation and the additional incentives can be found at http://www.fda.gov/orphan/index.htm.

12.2 Pediatric Programs

Since the 1970's there has been public discussion of the lack of adequate testing and labeling for products that are used in children. The reasons for specific labeling for product use for children are because the physiology, surface to mass ratio and development of children is a changing continuum from premature infants to adolescents and results in different processing, pharmacokinetics, and product activation in different age groups. The adverse events profile and dosing for a product need to be determined for each relevant pediatric population.

Several Federal initiatives have been attempted over the last two decades culminating in the codification of an incentive program and a mandate. The incentive program is a component of the Best Pharmaceuticals for Children Act (BPCA), which is Public Law No. 107-109 and available at: http://www.fda.gov/cder/pediatric/PL107-109.pdf. The BPCA was signed by President George W. Bush in 2002.

The major provisions of the Act are outlined in the following table.

Table 5. Major Provisions of the Best Pharmaceuticals for Children Act

Continuation of the pediatric incentive program until October 2007
Establishment of procedure to study medications for pediatric use that lack exclusivity or are off patent
Establishment of procedures to ensure proper pediatric labeling
Adverse event reporting and tracking for pediatric use
Requirement for a pediatric plan for availability of investigational drugs for INDs
Reports to Congress on by Institute of Medicine on pediatric study practices, the General Accounting Office on enrollment of minority children and pediatric exclusivity and the FDA on patient access to new cancer therapeutics
Establishment of FDA Office of Pediatrics
Establishment of a dispute resolution mechanism for pediatric labeling
Establishment of new advisory committee for pediatric pharmacology and endorsement of two existing pediatric subcommittees
Establishment of partnership with the National Institutes of Health for pediatric research
No waiver of user fees for pediatric submissions for marketing applications
Pediatric submissions for marketing applications receive 6-month priority review

The incentive for developing products for pediatric use is only available to drug products and is not available for biologicals, devices, or certain antibiotics. The incentive consists of a 6 month extension to marketing exclusivity to be added to whatever existing exclusivity a product has. It applies to all dosage forms and formulations of the product. The mechanism to gain the incentive is that the FDA will send a Written Request to a sponsor outlining what type of pediatric data are considered a public health need for the product. The pediatric data do not need to be in the same indication as the adult indication. The Written Request will outline the types of data requested and time frame for submitting the data to the FDA. The time frame is determined by the estimated time for answering the scientific questions and is independent of and not related to the expiry date for any existing exclusivity. A sponsor may submit to the FDA a proposal for a pediatric Written Request to initiate the process, although not all proposals are converted into Written Requests and not all Written Requests are preceded by proposals.

If the studies are performed as requested and submitted prior to or by the due date, then the study reports are reviewed internally by the FDA and submitted to a Review Board that makes a determination based on whether the Written Request was fairly responded to. If the determination is affirmative, the 6 month extension is applied to existing exclusivity. Further information on this program may be found at the FDA Guidance Document on qualifying for pediatric exclusivity which is available at http://www.fda.gov/cder/guidance/2891fnl.htm.

The pediatric mandate is contained in the Pediatric Research Equity Act, Public Law 108-155, which was signed into law by President George W. Bush in December 2003. The law states that if a product, which includes biologics as well as drugs, represents either a meaningful therapeutic benefit or will be used by a substantial number of children in a disease or condition that exists in both adults and children, then the FDA can mandate pediatric studies. The penalty is that the product would be considered misbranded. Meaningful therapeutic benefit is defined as a significant improvement in the diagnosis, treatment or prevention of a disease compared with products that are adequately labeled for the relevant pediatric population or if the drug or biological is in a class of products for which additional therapeutic options are needed. Substantial use is defined as greater than 50 000 children based on the threshold for Orphan Designation of 200 000 people and the estimate that 25% of the United States population are children.

While the pediatric studies must be completed, they do not need to be completed concurrent with the adult studies, so as not to delay the marketing approval of a product. The pediatric studies may be deferred until a date that the FDA designates or, depending upon the indication and the population, may be waived for some or all age groups.

Depending upon the nature of the product, it may be possible to comply with the pediatric mandate and also receive the incentive. Further information about the Pediatric Research Equity Act may be found in the FDA Guidance Document on complying with the Act at http://www.fda.gov/cder/guidance/6215dft.pdf.

The mandate and the incentive program are compared in the following table.

Table 6. Comparison of FDA Pediatric Initiatives

Pediatric Mandate (Pediatric Research Equity Act)	Pediatric Incentive Program (Best Pharmaceuticals for Children Act)
Applies to all drugs and biologics except Orphan Designation	Biologics and some drugs excluded but includes Orphan Designation
Only applies to the drug product and indication under review	Applies to all products with same active moiety
Only applies if an approved or pending indication occurs in adults and children	Eligible indications for study must occur in pediatric populations
Only applies if there is a therapeutic advance or widespread use	Only applies when there is underlying patent or exclusivity protection
May be used more than once for a product if a public health need is identified	Limited use in a product lifetime
Mandatory- compliance expected	Voluntary – no compliance required
No expiration stated in legislation	Program expires in 2007

13. MEETING WITH THE FDA

One of the most effective mechanisms to exchange information and receive regulatory guidance during the evolution of a drug development plan is to meet with the FDA. There is no charge for meeting with the FDA, but there are expectations and requirements. The FDA can accommodate meetings in person, by teleconference, or by prior arrangement, by videoconference. Meetings, like all communications with the FDA, are confidential.

Meeting requests may be initiated by the sponsor by submitting a meeting request to the FDA. The usual timing for meeting requests are at developmental landmarks. Prior to submitting an IND, the sponsor may request a pre-IND meeting/telcon. For an active IND common meetings include meeting to discuss confirmatory efficacy study design at the end of Phase 2, content and format of a marketing application at the conclusion of clinical development, and chemistry and manufacturing issues when product development indicates. Product development issues should be resolved prior to beginning any confirmatory efficacy study.

Administratively, meetings are categorized as one of three (3) types as outlined in the Prescription Drug User Fee Act II which was part of the Food and Drug Administration Modernization Act of 1997 (Public Law 105-115) (http://www.fda.gov/CBER/genadmin/pdufago111297.htm). A type A meeting is considered urgent and critical with the goal of moving a stalled development program forward. A type A meeting is expected to be scheduled within 30 days of receipt of the meeting request. A type B meeting is considered a developmental landmark type of meeting such as preIND, End of Phase 2, or premarketing application. Type B meetings are expected to be scheduled within 60 days of receipt of the meeting request. Typically a sponsor can expect one type B meeting per landmark. All other types of meetings are classified as type C and are expected to be scheduled within 75 days of receipt of the meeting request. An FDA guidance document can be found at http://www.fda.gov/cber/gdlns/mtpdufa.htm. The types of meetings are summarized in the following table

Table 7. Types of Meetings

Meeting Type	Purpose	Scheduling Time
A	Urgent request to address stalled development program	Within 30 days
B	Address major clinical development landmarks	Within 60 days
C	All other issues not considered type A or B	Within 75 days

A meeting request should contain:

- A brief statement of the purpose and type of meeting
- A requested range of meeting dates based on the type of meeting
- A listing of the specific objectives and anticipated outcomes
- A proposed agenda, including estimated times needed for each agenda item;
- A listing of planned attendees including all consultants and any requested FDA participants by name or discipline type
- The approximate time that supporting documentation for the meeting will be sent to the Center
  - Supporting documentation is expected to be received at the FDA 30 days in advance of the meeting except for type A meetings, when the supporting documentation is expected 14 days in advance

The supporting documentation, or meeting package, is required to be submitted by the sponsor a specified period of time in advance of the meeting to allow adequate time for FDA review and to allow discussion at an internal FDA premeeting to reach consensus on the advice to be offered to the sponsor.

The sponsor meeting documentation should contain

- a brief statement of the meeting purpose including
  o general nature of the questions being asked
  o context of the meeting in the overall development plan
- summary of the product characteristics
- summary of regulatory history
- a summary of completed or planned studies or data that are the focus of the meeting
- proposed agenda with time estimates
- detailed questions grouped according to review discipline (product, preclinical, clinical)

Due to resource and time constraints, a sponsor should not plan extensive presentations. In addition, any data, questions, or topics to be discussed should be included in the meeting package. Any new data or questions introduced during the course of the meeting cannot be answered because the FDA will not have the opportunity to review and discuss the new information.

The more detailed the questions, the more specific the advice the FDA can offer. Broad questions may not yield sufficient specific information in a reply. Speculative questions such as will marketing approval be granted are considered review issues that can only be determined after all studies are complete and the data thoroughly evaluated.

Further advice and details may be found in the FDA Guidance Document Formal Meetings With Sponsors and Applicants for PDUFA Products, 2000 (http://www.fda.gov/Cber/gdlns/mtpdufa.pdf).

An additional type of meeting, termed an Advisory Committee meeting is one convened by the FDA to solicit advice on an issue or product. FDA Advisors are nominated and selected on criteria described in the Federal Advisory Committee Act of 1972 (Public Law 92-463, 5 USC Appendix). The Federal government can formally only receive advice from chartered advisory committees that hold public meetings. The dates and topics of the meetings are announced in the Federal Register.

The advice provided by a chartered advisory committee is considered a recommendation and is not binding. If the topic the FDA is seeking advice on pertains to a marketing application for a particular product, then the sponsor of the product is invited to the meeting to make a presentation. The contents of the presentation must be submitted to the FDA in advance and are posted, along with FDA review materials, on the FDA website 24 hours before the public meeting occurs.

14. SPECIAL PROTOCOL ASSESSMENTS

A program based in the 1997 FDA Modernization Act (Public Law 105-115 Section 119) established a mechanism for reaching agreement between the FDA and a sponsor on the design of a protocol intended to support marketing approval. Three classes of protocols have been designated as qualifying for special protocol assessment:

- Carcinogenicity protocols
- Stability protocols
- Clinical protocols intended to form the primary basis of an efficacy claim

The outcome of a Special Protocol Assessment is a binding agreement between the FDA and the sponsor that the design of the protocol is acceptable. Submission of a Special Protocol Assessment should be marked as such and must contain specific questions for the FDA to address. The regulatory due date for the FDA to concur or not concur with the study design and send written responses to the questions is 45 days after receipt. The FDA may also provide additional comments. A Special Protocol Assessment is intended to be an interactive process. If, on the basis of an interaction, the sponsor submits a revised protocol, the previous submission is no longer considered active and the new protocol submission would reset the regulatory clock to 45 days after receipt. The FDA has the option of seeking consultation from Special Government Employees who serve on Advisory Committees. In such a case, FDA will notify the sponsor that an advisory committee or a selected member will review the protocol, and will advise the sponsor of the expected date of that consultation and the reason for seeking outside review.

To anticipate the possibility of protocol revisions, a sponsor should submit a protocol for Special Protocol Assessment at least 90 days in advance of when the protocol is anticipated to begin. The FDA will not review a protocol for Special Protocol Assessment once patient screening or enrollment begins. A protocol may still be reviewed by the FDA; however, it does not qualify for Special Protocol Assessment.

For a clinical protocol, the sponsor should include information to assess the role of the trial in the overall clinical development plan. Included in the protocol should be information supporting the trial design, the power calculations, choice of study endpoints, and other critical design features such as choice of control, duration, assessment methods, complete statistical analytic plan, and description and charter for any independent data monitoring or endpoint committees.

In addition, for a clinical protocol, a description of any anticipated regulatory outcome such as a specific claim or potential product labeling that the sponsor intends the study to support should be included.

For a stability protocol the sponsor should include information such as product characterization, relevant manufacturing data, specifications, container closure, and the retest period or shelf life anticipated at the time of filing a marketing application.

For further details, refer to the FDA Guidance Document on Special Protocol Assessments at http://www.fda.gov/cber/gdlns/protocol.htm.

15. FAST TRACK

The Food and Drug Administration Modernization Act of 1997 (Public Law 105-115 Section 112) described a program intended to structure interactions between a sponsor and the FDA for INDs that meet certain criteria. The designation is granted for the combination of a product and a potential claim that would address a serious aspect of a serious or life threatening disease or condition that represents an unmet medical need.

A request for Fast Track designation may be submitted at the time of the original submission of your IND or at any time thereafter prior to receiving marketing approval. When designated as Fast Track an application be considered for the accelerated and priority review programs (although fast track designation is not needed for these programs), in addition to having the ability to submit a BLA in portions (Submission of Portions of an Application = SoPA). SoPA may only be available if designated as Fast Track.

Fast Track designation is requested by the IND sponsor and the FDA must respond to the request within 60 days after receipt. Fast Track designation based on the law results in efforts to expedite development and review of a marketing application. This translates into holding landmark meetings, allowing clinical development using surrogate markers, and allowing a marketing application to be submitted in reviewable sections based on a prospective mutually agreeable schedule. The Fast Track mechanism formalized the approach for a subset of drugs.

An application for Fast Track designation should contain information that addresses:

- How the aspect of the condition to be treated is serious and life threatening
- The potential the product has, given its stage of clinical development, for treating the serious aspect of the serious and life threatening disease or condition
- Description of a specific clinical development program designed to determine whether the product will affect a serious aspect of the condition. The details and specifics of the description should be commensurate with the stage of development and should include the major outcome variables to be assessed.
- Description of any accepted or approved therapies for the same aspect of the serious or life threatening disease or condition. If so, the proposed development program should support how an unmet medical need will be addressed.

Further information can be found in the FDA Guidance Document Fast Track Drug Development Programs: Designation, Development and Application Review 2006 (http://www.fda.gov/cber/gdlns/fsttrk.pdf).

16. PREPARATION AND REVIEW OF MARKETING APPLICATIONS

Products that are designated as being subject to Section 351 of the Public Health Service Act are reviewed for marketing under the provisions of the Public Health Service Act, the Food Drug and Cosmetic Act and Sections 314 and 601 of Title 21 of the Code of Federal Regulations. As a point of contrast, drug products do not address the purity and potency requirement noted in the Public Health Service Act; otherwise the laws and regulations are the same.

The criteria for approving a license application for a biologic are stated in the Public Health Service Act Title 42 - Chapter 6a Subchapter II - Part F - Sec. 262. Subsection (2)(B) Underlining and formatting is for emphasis and not in the original text.

> – *The Secretary shall approve a biologics license application on the basis of a demonstration that the biological product that is the subject of the application is* **_safe, pure, and potent;_**

The requirement for effectiveness, as well as safety and the submission of full study reports is contained in the Food Drug and Cosmetic Act as

Amended Title 21 - Chapter 9 - Subchapter V - Part A - Section 355 Subsection 1(A) which states

*full **reports of investigations** which have been made **to show** whether or not such drug is safe for use and **whether such drug is effective in use**;.*

The applicable regulation for Biologics is in the Code of Federal Regulations Title 21 Part 601 Section 601.25

— *__Proof of effectiveness shall consist of controlled clinical investigations__ as defined in Sec. 314.126 of this chapter, **unless this requirement is waived on the basis of a showing that it is not reasonably applicable to the biological product or essential to the validity of the investigation, and that an alternative method of investigation is adequate to substantiate effectiveness.***

Code of Federal Regulations Title 21 Parts 314 and 601 are devoted to licensing applications. Part 601 cross references Part 314. The subparts are devoted to particular topics as listed in the following table.

Table 8. Organization of Regulations for Marketing Authorization

Subparts of Part 314 of Title 21 Chapter I Subchapter D of the Code of Federal Regulations		Subparts of Part 601 of Title 21 Chapter I Subchapter F of the Code of Federal Regulations
Subpart	Topic in 314 (Summarized)	Topics in 601 (Summarized)
A	General Provisions	General Provisions
B	Applications	Reserved
C	Abbreviated Applications	Biologics Licensing
D	FDA Action on Applications and Abbreviated Applications	Diagnostic Radiopharmaceuticals
E	Hearing Procedures	Accelerated Approval
F	Reserved	Confidentiality of Information
G	Miscellaneous Provisions	Postmarketing Studies
H	Accelerated Approval	Approval When Human Efficacy Studies are not Ethical or Feasible
I	Approval When Human Efficacy Studies are not Ethical or Feasible	

Section 314.50 describes the content and format of a licensing application. Section 314.126 in Subpart D elaborates on adequate and well controlled studies, and among the characteristics described, are that

- *The purpose of conducting clinical investigations of a drug is to distinguish the effect of a drug from other influences, such as spontaneous change in the course of the disease, placebo effect, or biased observation....*
- *Reports of **adequate and well-controlled investigations** provide the primary basis for determining whether there is ``substantial evidence" to support the claims of effectiveness for new drugs...*
- *The **methods of assessment** of subjects' response are **well-defined and reliable.** The protocol for the study and the report of results should explain the variables measured, the methods of observation, and criteria used to assess response.*

A successful clinical development program will set as a goal the characteristics of adequate and well controlled studies described in these regulations. Additional guidance on establishing effectiveness can be found in the FDA Guidance Document on Providing Clinical Evidence of Effectiveness for Human Drugs and Biological Products (http://www.fda.gov/cber/gdlns/clineff.pdf) and specific guidance on statistical principles can be found in the ICH E9 document "Statistical Principles for Clinical Trials" (http://www.fda.gov/cber/gdlns/ichclinical.pdf).

The general expectation is that at least two studies will demonstrate safety and effectiveness to provide a measure of replicability in the findings; however, the FDA guidance on clinical evidence of effectiveness notes that a single multicenter study that provides highly reliable and statistically strong evidence of an important clinical benefit, such as prolongation of survival, and in which confirmation of the result in a second trial would be practically or ethically impossible could provide sufficient evidence. To support marketing approval, the data submitted should be sufficient in quality and quantity to establish the safety and effectiveness of the product with a high level of confidence, as required by law and scientific expectations.

Regulatory decisions are made on the basis of a risk to benefit determination. Because acceptable risk and benefit are different for anticancer therapies than for other therapeutic products, FDA guidance directed to new cancer treatment uses for marketed drugs and biological products was published in 1999 (http://www.fda.gov/cber/gdlns/canctreat.pdf) and subsequent draft guidance for clinical trial endpoints for the general licensure of cancer drugs and biologics was published in 2005 (http://www.fda.gov/cber/gdlns/clintrialend.pdf).

A well constructed product development plan will address each of the sections of the product label or approved package insert. These sections are described in Title 21 Code of Federal Regulations Part 201 and are summarized in the following table based on 21 CFR 201.56 and 201.57:

Table 9. Sections of a Product Label (Summarized)

Highlights of Prescribing Information
Indications and Usage
Dosage and Administration
Dosage Forms and Strengths
Contraindications
Warnings and Precautions
Adverse Reactions
Use in Specific Populations
Abuse and Dependence
Overdosage
Description
Clinical Pharmacology
Non-clinical toxicology
Clinical Studies
References
How Supplied/Storage and Handling
Patient Counseling and Information

The safety data in the product label is graded from most severe (contraindications) to least severe (general adverse reactions). If a product has a particularly notable warning, the text is placed at the top of the label and surrounded by a dark border. Such a warning is referred to as a Black Box Warning.

The assessment of effectiveness has been guided by recommendations from Advisory Committees and has been interpreted as showing clinical benefit. Clinical benefit is generally interpreted as living longer (survival advantage) or living better (such as symptom relief or delay of worsening of the disease or condition) without compromising overall survival (21 CFR 601.41).

An application for a marketing claim can be approved if the submitted data support the claim and if the benefit to risk is favorable and the product meets the statutory standards for safety and effectiveness, manufacturing and controls, and labeling (21CFR 314.105). An application that is not approved may be approvable if the product substantially meets the requirements for approval and the FDA believes that the product can be approved if specific additional information is submitted or specific conditions such as a change in the product labeling are agreed to by the applicant (21CFR 314.110).

A marketing application may not be approved if any of the 18 reasons listed in 21CFR 314.125, as summarized in the following table, apply.

Table 10. Summary of Reasons for not approving an application for marketing

Inadequate manufacturing, processing, packing or holding methods to maintain Identity, strength, quality purity, stability and bioavailability
Inadequacy of tests for safety
Safety testing is indeterminate or shows the product is unsafe
Insufficient safety information
Lack of substantial evidence consisting of adequate and well controlled investigations that the product will have the claimed effect
False or misleading labeling
Untrue statement of material fact in the application
Proposed labeling is not in compliance with labeling requirements in 21 CFR 201
Lack of bioavailability or bioequivalence data required in 21CFR320
An uncorrected deficiency in filing the application
Manufacture or processing in an unregistered establishment that is not exempt based on applicable regulations
Denial of an adequate opportunity to inspect facilities, controls and records of an authorized inspector
Lack of good manufacturing process for methods, facilities and controls
An omission of a report of any investigation using the drug that is not explained in the submission
A nonclinical laboratory study to support safety that is not conducted under good laboratory practice (GLP) without an adequate explanation for non-compliance with GLP
A clinical investigation involving human subjects that is not in compliance with the institutional review board or informed consent regulations
Refusal to permit inspection of facilities or records by an applicant or contract research organization of bioavailability or bioequivalence studies
Failure to include relevant patent information

Once a marketing application is approved, the use claim provides 5 years of marketing exclusivity and additional claims, submitted as efficacy supplements, receive 3 years marketing exclusivity (21CFR 314.108).

16. ACCELERATED APPROVAL

The accelerated approval program was initiated in the 1990s as a mechanism to allow promising products intended to treat serious or life threatening diseases that provide meaningful therapeutic benefit to patients over existing treatments (21CFR 601.40) . Meaningful therapeutic benefit means treating patients whose disease has not responded to available therapy or patients who do not tolerate or the response is an improvement over available therapy. The phrase "available therapy" should be interpreted as therapy that is specified in the approved labeling of regulated products, with only rare exceptions, as described in the 2004 FDA Guidance Document on Available Therapy (http://www.fda.gov/cber/gdlns/availther.htm). To demonstrate the meaningful therapeutic benefit, the studies using the product may use a surrogate likely to predict clinical benefit in place of a direct demonstration of clinical benefit. The determination of the utility of the likely surrogate is made on a case by case basis, often in consultation with an Advisory Committee. The absence of a direct demonstration of clinical benefit results in restrictions on advertising and a mandatory commitment following marketing approval to perform additional studies to show clinical benefit. The program is termed accelerated because the licensing is based on a stage of clinical development prior to direct demonstration of clinical benefit.

Another and different criterion for approval under accelerated approval would be if a product can be safely used only if distribution and use is restricted. Examples would be to facilities or physicians with special resources and training of the use is conditioned on the performance of specified medical procedures.

17. PRIORITY REVIEW

The time a marketing application is under FDA review is by law targeted to be 10 months (Prescription Drug User Fee Act II which was part of the Food and Drug Administration Modernization Act of 1997 (Public Law 105-115). If a product is determined to be a significant improvement compared to marked products in the treatment, diagnosis or prevention of a life threatening disease, it can be eligible for Priority Review, which reduces the FDA review time to 6 months (http://www.fda.gov/cder/mapp/6020-3.pdf). Priority applications are designated at the time of your pre-BLA meeting or as soon as possible after receipt of your BLA.

The terms Fast Track, Accelerated Approval and Priority Review are contrasted in the following table.

Table 11. Comparison of Regulatory Terms

Term	Applicability	Criteria
Fast Track	IND program designed to facilitate communication between the FDA and the sponsor and provide flexibility in submitting a licensing application	Product addresses a serious aspect of a serious or life threatening illness that represents an unmet medical need
Accelerated Approval	Overall product development program that allows filing a licensing application based on studies using a surrogate likely to predict clinical benefit prior to direct demonstration of clinical benefit. May also apply to restricted distribution	Product provides a meaningful therapeutic benefit over existing treatments for a serious or life threatening illness
Priority Review	Reducing review time for a licensing application from 10 months to 6 months	Product provides a significant improvement compared to marked products in the treatment, diagnosis or prevention of a life threatening disease

Note that Fast Track addresses unmet medical needs while Accelerated Approval and Priority Review address meaningful therapeutic benefit over existing treatments.

18. SUPPLEMENTAL MARKETING CLAIMS

The guidance on new cancer treatment uses for marketed products builds on the principles of the clinical evidence of effectiveness guidance, and describes several scenarios of the type and quantity of the clinical evidence that may be adequate to support approval for additional use claims. All are based on the determination that the product is safe and effective in at least one cancer indication.

A single adequate and well controlled multicenter study with appropriate endpoints demonstrating safety and effectiveness may be sufficient to support additional labeling:

- If the approved indication is for an advanced refractory stage of a malignancy, then for an earlier stage of the same malignancy
- If another form of cancer that is known to have a generally similar pattern of responsiveness to therapy as the approved indication
- For a product that ameliorates adverse effects of other cancer treatments without compromising the effectiveness of the other cancer treatments in a palliative setting (not life prolonging or potentially curative). If the other cancer treatment were life prolonging or potentially curative additional studies to verify preservation of treatment effectiveness would usually be needed.

A single adequate and well controlled study with appropriate endpoints to demonstrate safety and effectiveness may be sufficient for:

- A new dosing regimen or change in schedule
- Extending labeling in an indication to combination therapy when a product is already approved for monotherapy and the other products to be used in the combination have demonstrated safety and effectiveness in the same indication
- Extending labeling to monotherapy in the same indication when a product is approved for an indication in combination therapy
- Extending labeling to a different combination in the same indication

A single study demonstrating safety, dosing and response rate may be sufficient when extending labeling to a biologically similar type of cancer in children as in the approved adult indication when the proposed pediatric use is in a setting where known curative treatments are unavailable.

Supplemental claims that address an entirely new use are expected to meet the same requirements for demonstrating safety and effectiveness as original submissions.

Depending upon the extent of prior data, extending labeling to additional indications may need limited or no additional safety, pharmacokinetic, product-interaction, or usage data based on age, gender, race or co-existing diseases.

For further details refer to "Guidance for Industry: FDA Approval of New Cancer Treatment Uses for Marketed Drug and Biological Products (http://www.fda.gov/cber/gdlns/canctreat.pdf)."

19. CONCLUSION

The responsibilities of the FDA are extensive and the levels of potential interaction for an investigator or sponsor can be multiple. Topics such as auditing procedures, inspections, post marketing surveillance, safety analysis, preclinical data expectations, pharmacokinetics recommendations, Institutional Review Boards, Good Laboratory Practice, Good Manufacturing Practice, Good Clinical Practice and policy development have not been broached in this brief review. The focus has been on the origin of the fundamental principles of biologic regulation and their applicability for the oncology clinical investigator.

The FDA has unique resources in terms of expertise and institutional experience, and has well defined mechanisms for interaction. Product development is viewed as a shared responsibility and the FDA can be an important and supportive partner in the process.

The author gratefully acknowledges the careful reading and comments on this manuscript by Ashok Batra, MD, Peter Bross, MD, Deborah Lavoie, JD, Stephanie Simek, PhD, Celia Witten, PhD, MD and Robert Yetter, PhD.

Chapter 5

THE ROLE OF COOPERATIVE GROUPS IN CANCER CLINICAL TRIALS

Ann M. Mauer, MD, Elizabeth S. Rich, MD, PhD and Richard L. Schilsky, MD
Cancer and Leukemia Group B, Central Office of the Chairman, Chicago, Illinois, USA

1. INTRODUCTION

The Cooperative Group Program of the National Cancer Institute (NCI) was founded in 1955 when several pioneering cancer researchers approached the United States Congress for increased financial support for the study of chemotherapy for cancer. In response to this request, $5 million was appropriated to the NCI to establish the Chemotherapy National Service Center.[1] By the late 1950s, the program included seventeen NCI-funded groups that were engaged in the study of new agents from the NCI's drug development program. In the past six decades, the NCI Cooperative Group Program has evolved and presently includes 10 organizations (Table 1). Several cooperative groups focus on specific cancer populations, cancer sites, or treatment modalities, while the larger cooperative groups are fully multidisciplinary. Over the years, the research mission of the Cooperative Groups has broadened to include the prevention of cancer and the optimization of survival and quality of life for persons with cancer. Since the formation of the Cooperative Group Program, over 500,000 individuals have participated in more than 4,000 cooperative group trials.[2] These trials have led to remarkable advances in the treatment of all forms of pediatric and adult cancer.

Each cooperative group consists of a large network of physicians, statisticians, nurses, clinical research associates, pharmacists, and other affiliated investigators, including patient advocates, who collaborate to conduct cancer clinical trials in multi-institutional settings. More than

16,000 investigators from over 2,000 unique institutions - including comprehensive cancer centers, academic medical centers, community hospitals and physician practices - participate in this system of organized research. Over 25,000 new patients are enrolled onto cooperative group treatment studies annually, representing the majority of all patients enrolled in publicly and privately sponsored cancer trials in the United States.[3] Approximately $150 million in annual funding is provided to the cooperative groups by the NCI.[4]

2. THE COOPERATIVE GROUP PROCESS

The design, management, and conduct of cooperative group trials is a collaborative effort among multiple parties, including primarily the cooperative group investigators and staff and the NCI, but also the pharmaceutical industry and federal regulatory agencies. The Cancer Therapy Evaluation Program (CTEP) is the program within the Division of Cancer Treatment and Diagnosis (DCTD) of the NCI that oversees the research activities of the cooperative groups. Through a peer review process, the NCI provides public funds to the cooperative groups to develop new studies within their particular areas of interest and expertise and within the national priorities for cancer treatment and prevention research. The cooperative group structure and funding are not generally linked to specific clinical trials. This mechanism allows flexibility in resource allocation and promotes the rapid testing of promising new cancer therapies in large patient populations.

CTEP also facilitates collaborations between the research community and the pharmaceutical/biotechnology industry to develop new cancer treatments. CTEP currently sponsors more than 160 Investigational New Drug applications (INDs) and is involved in more than 50 collaborative agreements with pharmaceutical companies. One of the primary objectives underlying the formation of the groups continues to be the conduct of large, multicenter trials for the investigational agents sponsored by CTEP. The conduct of these trials through the cooperative group mechanism allows rapid accrual of patients while reducing the possible bias of studies carried out at a single or a few institutions.

All cooperative groups have a similar structure that includes an operations office overseen by the group chair and a statistical center directed by the group statistician. The groups are comprised of institutions that have applied for membership and have met the membership criteria of the respective group. Membership standards, based on policies determined by each group, include verification of credentials, assessment of site preparedness, accrual potential and the ability to comply with group standards and Federal requirements. The participants are designated as main members, affiliates of a main member institution, or members of a participating Community Clinical Oncology Program (CCOP). Main Member institutions are largely academic or major medical centers that make significant contributions to Group activities. Main member institutions provide substantial accrual to Group protocols, contribute institutional scientific expertise and resources to Group activities, and hold responsibility for mentoring and monitoring affiliate institutions. Affiliate institutions represent sites of clinical expertise that main member institutions have determined contribute significantly to Group activities. Such institutions are often community-based or are institutions with lower accrual rates. Affiliates administratively function and interact with the cooperative group through the main member institution. CCOPs function as an outreach initiative to expand access of clinical trials to community physicians and their patients. CCOPs are comprised of any of the following: hospitals, clinics, health maintenance organizations (HMO), groups of practicing physicians or a consortium that agrees to work with a principal investigator through a single administrative unit. Each cooperative group institution is represented by a principal investigator who oversees the institution's activities within the Group. The principal investigators of the main member institutions comprise a committee that provides governance of the group, including formulation of group policy and oversight of membership.

To maintain membership, each institution must meet a minimum level of patient accrual to clinical trials. Institutional performance is appraised annually by a committee of principal investigators and administrative personnel. Each main institution and its affiliate institutions undergo an audit overseen by CTEP at regular intervals to review the primary records for compliance with federal regulations and the individual group's protocol requirements.

Investigators participating in cooperative group research may come from a wide variety of academic and practice settings. Emphasis is placed on definitive, randomized phase III studies and the developmental efforts preliminary to them. In addition, the cooperative groups are uniquely suited to conduct phase I and phase II trials efficiently and also to evaluate treatments for patients with unusual tumor types or for special populations, such as the elderly, minority patients, or patients with organ dysfunction.

The development of cooperative group clinical trials is a collaborative effort among many parties, with multiple levels of review and oversight (see Figure 1). The process of study development typically begins when a scientific committee comprised of investigators with expertise in a particular area generates an idea and develops a study concept. This concept undergoes internal peer review, and for phase III trials, review by CTEP. Once the concept is approved, the study protocol is developed by the study chair with the input of other cooperative group investigators, the scientific committee leadership, statisticians, protocol coordinators, pharmacists, clinical research associates, and data managers. Protocols are then submitted for approval to CTEP and, if applicable, the Food and Drug Administration (FDA). Phase III trials are also reviewed by the Central Institutional Review Board (CIRB) prior to final approval by CTEP. For institutions that do not utilize the CIRB, further approval is required by the local institutional review board (IRB) to ensure compliance with local standards.

The enrollment of patients on cooperative group trials is governed by rigid standards. All eligibility criteria must be fulfilled, and patients must be informed of the potential risks and benefits of the study and alternative options for treatment. An IRB-approved, informed consent document must be signed by the patient and the investigator prior to registration. The multicenter nature of cooperative group clinical trials presents a variety of challenging methodological problems regarding assurance of quality and consistency in study conduct. The need for formal mechanisms of medical review and quality assurance is obvious. The cooperative groups have developed a number of approaches to address these issues.

The groups frequently work together under the auspices of "Intergroup Committees" to pool resources in order to answer an important research question more efficiently and effectively. This process also allows the completion of trials in rare diseases or disease subsets when one group may not have sufficient patient accruals to complete the trial. The Intergroup process was initiated with the breast committees and presently there is an Intergroup committee for each of the major diseases. The collaborations may also extend beyond the NCI-sponsored cooperative groups to include clinical trial groups outside North America. Other advantages of the Intergroup system are the facilitation of communication between the groups to minimize redundancy in group studies; the identification of areas of unmet need; and the identification of areas where a collaborative effort would be necessary to answer a particular question. Based on recommendations of the Clinical Trials Working Group convened by the National Cancer Advisory Board (integratedtrials.nci.nih.gov), the intergroup committees will be converted to multi-disciplinary Scientific Steering Committees in the coming years that will be responsible for the review, development and prioritization of all concepts for phase III trials in a given disease area.

The NCI's Community Clinical Oncology Program (CCOP) and Cancer Trials Support Unit (CTSU)[5] have enhanced access by physicians and patients to clinical trials within the community. CCOPs are community-based organizations that participate in treatment protocols and cancer prevention and control research studies developed by cooperative groups or cancer centers. They submit data in the same format and according to the same standards as any other member or affiliate investigator. CCOPs are funded by the NCI Division of Cancer Prevention (DCP) through a competitive peer-reviewed grant program.

The CTSU is an administrative unit sponsored by the NCI for the support of a national network of physicians to participate in NCI-sponsored Phase III cancer treatment trials developed by the adult cancer cooperative groups. The objectives of the CTSU are to increase physician and patient access to NCI-sponsored clinical trials; to streamline and standardize data collection and reporting; and to reduce regulatory and administrative burdens on investigators participating in NCI-sponsored cooperative group clinical trials. Nearly all cooperative group Phase III treatment trials in breast, gastrointestinal, genitourinary, and lung cancers, as well as adult leukemia and sarcoma are available to CTSU investigators. Participation in the CTSU is available to main members and affiliates of the cooperative groups. Additionally, non-Group aligned sites and investigators may participate as a CTSU Independent Clinical Research Site (CICRS). Non-Group associated physicians must meet standards similar to those for Cooperative Group members before they may enroll patients on CTSU trials.

3. ACCOMPLISHMENTS AND CURRENT ACTIVITIES

The Cooperative Groups have been instrumental in the development of new standards of cancer patient management and in the development of sophisticated clinical investigation techniques. In addition to providing data important for improving treatment of specific tumors and obtaining regulatory approval of new drugs, Cooperative Group trials have made many important contributions to the practice of oncology and the principles and methods of clinical investigation. The identification of histologic subtypes of tumors and the recognition of prognostic variables have permitted refinements in diagnosis and treatment of both solid tumors and hematologic malignancies. By exploring novel strategies for the integration of different therapeutic modalities, the Groups have identified indications for the use of adjuvant and neoadjuvant chemotherapy and concurrent chemoradiotherapy for solid tumors. Refinements in the utilization of chemotherapy have been made possible by the evaluation of new agents and the study of dose intensity.

Through cooperative group phase III trials, new cancer treatments have been rigorously compared to best available treatments in hypothesis-driven clinical trials. The Cooperative Groups have also played an important role in the development of novel therapeutic agents in phase I and phase II trials. A listing of cooperative group accomplishments between 1986 and 2001 is available at the CTEP website (http://ctep.cancer.gov/resources/coop2.html). Major advances credited to the cooperative groups, emphasizing those of the past decade that have altered clinical practice and led to the identification of promising basic science findings and translation into clinical research, include treatment of childhood cancer, adjuvant therapy for adult solid tumors, and combined modality therapy.

3.1 Cancer Treatment

Childhood Cancer

In 2001, the Children's Oncology Group was formed by the merger of the four major pediatric clinical trials groups based in North America: the Children's Cancer Group, the Pediatric Oncology Group, the National Wilms' Tumor Study Group, and the Intergroup Rhabdomysosarcoma Study Group. The collective achievements of these groups over the past four decades have lead to effective treatments for childhood cancers that have significantly improved the cure rates for childhood malignancies, including leukemia, rhabdomyosarcoma and Wilms' tumor.[6,7] The 5-year survival of children and adolescents with solid tumors increased from 27% to 80% between 1960 and 2000.[6,8] The slope of the curve demonstrates that the change in survival over this period is remarkably constant, reflecting the nature of progress made through clinical trials. Pediatric cooperative group clinical trials have also been instrumental in defining the late effects of treatment in children, investigating the causes of childhood cancer through epidemiologic studies, and stimulating the close collaboration of basic and clinical investigators.

Adult Solid Tumors

In addition to providing data important for refining the treatment of specific tumors, Cooperative Group trials have made many important contributions to the practice of oncology. The identification of histologic subtypes and the recognition of prognostic variables have permitted refinements in diagnosis and treatment of both solid tumors and hematological malignancies. Many standard elements of cancer clinical trials were first introduced in cooperative group studies including defined response criteria, standard toxicity definitions, explicit eligibility criteria and routine assessment of performance status. By exploring novel strategies for the integration of different therapeutic modalities, Cooperative Group trials have identified indications for the use of adjuvant and neoadjuvant chemotherapy and concurrent chemoradiotherapy for solid tumors. Improvements in systemic therapy have been made possible by the evaluation of new agents, the study of dose intensity and dose density, and the use of the "window of opportunity" and other novel study designs[9] to identify active agents for tumors for which there is no effective treatment.

Adjuvant Therapy for Solid Tumors

The significant experience, expertise, and broad base of scientific resources of the Cooperative Groups are illustrated by studies of adjuvant and neoadjuvant therapy for solid tumors. Adjuvant therapy trials require large numbers of patients, significant data management effort and statistical support and the collaboration of multiple oncology specialists. Thus the cooperative group mechanism, with Intergroup collaboration, is uniquely suited for the conduct of such trials. Cooperative group trials have demonstrated that adjuvant therapy improves survival in patients with early stage breast, lung[10,11], colon[12-14], and gastric cancer[15] as well as melanoma[16].

Cooperative group trials have contributed significantly to the contemporary surgical management of breast cancer. Landmark trials conducted by the National Surgical Adjuvant Breast and Bowel Project (NSABP) demonstrated equivalent survival between patients undergoing mastectomy and lumpectomy followed by radiation therapy.[17] Additional trials have validated the sentinel lymph node procedure.[18,19] Research activities from several cooperative groups have contributed significantly to the development of adjuvant chemotherapy and hormone therapy for breast cancer. Recent trials have investigated the integration of taxanes into doxorubicin based chemotherapy regimens,[20,21] and examined the value of chemotherapy dose intensity and density.[22,23] Two recent cooperative group trials demonstrated that the addition of trastuzumab to paclitaxel after a regimen of doxorubicin and cyclophosphamide reduced the rates of recurrence by half in women with HER-2 positive breast cancer.[24]

Combined Modality Therapy

Major advances in combined modality therapy are attributable to the multidisciplinary organization and expertise of the Cooperative Groups. Early Cooperative Group trials established the superiority of combined chemotherapy and radiotherapy compared with radiotherapy alone in treatment of locally advanced non-small cell lung cancer (NSCLC).[25] Subsequent Cooperative Group trials of combined modality treatment in

NSCLC investigated the relative benefits of induction chemotherapy and surgical resection to determine optimal treatment strategy for locally advanced disease.[26,27 28]

Several cooperative group trials have demonstrated the benefit of combined radiotherapy and chemotherapy in locally advanced cervical cancer, which lead to the adoption of combined modality therapy as standard for women with localized cervical cancer.[23,29-31]. Cooperative group studies have also established the benefit of combined modality approaches for the treatment of cancers of the esophagus[32], head and neck[33-35], and rectum[36].

FDA approval of drugs and diagnostics

Cooperative group trials have played an important role in supporting FDA approval of drugs and diagnostics (Table 2). For example, in May 2004, the FDA approved azacitidine, the first drug approved for use in patients with myelodysplastic syndromes (MDS). Approval was based in part on response rates supported by improved survival, reduced risk of transformation to acute leukemia, and improved quality of life as demonstrated in CALGB 9221, a randomized trial of 5-azacitidine versus best supportive care in patients with all subtypes of MDS.[37] In October 2005, FDA approved marketing of nelarabine for patients with refractory T cell leukemia and lymphoma based on data from trials conducted by CALGB in collaboration with SWOG and COG.

3.2 Cancer Prevention

Cooperative group trials have significantly advanced the field of cancer prevention, with several studies demonstrating a significant reduction in cancer risk. Based on results of the Breast Cancer Prevention Trial, tamoxifen became the first FDA-approved agent for reducing cancer risk.[38] Another randomized trial established that the daily use of aspirin is associated with a significant reduction in the incidence of colorectal adenomas in patients with previous colorectal cancer.[39] Results of the Prostate Cancer Prevention Trial (PCPT) demonstrated that the use of finasteride resulted in a significant reduction in prostate cancer risk, although the trial also revealed an increase in the risk of high-grade prostate cancer for patients treated with finasteride.[40] The successor trial to the PCPT, The Selenium and Vitamin E Cancer Prevention Trial (SELECT), was planned by investigators from the five major U.S. NCI Cooperative Groups. SELECT is a phase III randomized, placebo-controlled study of selenium and/or vitamin E supplementation in 32,400 men for prostate cancer prevention.[41] Major themes of cancer prevention have recently been reviewed in detail by Lippman and Levin.[42]

3.3 Correlative Science

A major goal of Cooperative Group studies has been to better understand the biological factors that determine prognosis or predict response to therapy of various tumor types. The Cooperative Groups have organized the infrastructure necessary to conduct correlative science studies in a coordinated system that includes the centralized collection of leukemia and solid tumor specimens, appropriate storage, tracking, and use of specimens.[43] These specimens, with matched clinical data, are among the most valuable assets of the Cooperative groups. With the increasing availability of therapies directed against specific intracellular targets, research efforts have focused on whether tumor expression, amplification or mutation of these targets is predictive of a tumor's response to the targeted therapy. Results of a prospectively designed validation study of a multigene-expression assay in a large, multicenter clinical trial (NSABP B-17) have shown that the multigene assay predicts recurrence and survival in women with node-negative breast cancer who have received tamoxifen treatment.[44] A cooperative group study demonstrated that fluorescence *in situ* hybridization (FISH) to assess HER2/neu positivity in breast cancer patients is a reliable method to predict clinical outcome following adjuvant doxorubicin-based therapy for stage II breast cancer patients and led to FDA approval of a new diagnostic standard.[45]

The cooperative groups have been actively involved in the study of novel anti-cancer agents with distinctive molecular targets, mechanisms of action, or properties including vaccines, monoclonal antibodies, anti-angiogenesis agents, tyrosine kinase inhibitors, and other agents that target signal transduction pathway proteins. In addition to identifying new agents for further evaluation, correlative science studies have also identified biologic characteristics of tumors that may be exploited in clinical trials. Samples collected over years of cooperative group leukemia trials have yielded fundamentally important cytogenetic information that has impacted on the treatment of leukemia. A risk-adapted approach is being studied for patients with Philadelphia chromosome-positive acute lymphoblastic leukemia and in age- and cytogenetic-adapted modifications to treatment of patients with acute myeloid leukemia.[46] In addition to risk stratifying patients according to cytogenetics, the cooperative groups have been leaders in designing trials using tissue and molecular microarrays and imaging to determine individual patient and tumor profiles with the ultimate aim of individualizing therapy.

3.4 Symptom Control/ Quality of Life/ Survivorship

Cooperative group trials have also addressed complex questions regarding symptom control and quality of life in patients receiving therapy or palliative care. Quality of life scores have been used to determine if control of symptoms – pain, fatigue, nausea, anorexia and cachexia, chemotherapy-related anemia, depression, hot flashes – translates to an improvement in quality of life. For example, contrary to anecdotal reports and some small studies, results of a North Central Cancer Treatment Group Study suggested that megestrol acetate is superior to dronabinol for the treatment of cancer-associated anorexia and/or weight loss.[47] Companion studies to treatment trials, such as those evaluating 5-azacitidine, have also prospectively analyzed the impact of therapy on quality of life.[48]

As recently reviewed, a growing body of literature, including seminal research from Cooperative Group trials,[49,50] has examined the physical, mental, and emotional sequelae of cancer treatment on long-term survivors. Late physical effects include premature ovarian failure in women and its consequences, including sexual dysfunction, osteoporosis, hot flashes, and the risk of infertility. Other outcomes include growth retardation in pediatric patients, late cardiac effects, steroid-related diabetes mellitus, the effects on cognition following whole brain radiation, therapy-related second malignancies, economic consequences of survivorship[51], and general physical and social functioning. Many of these effects would not have been detected without the cooperative group infrastructure to enable long term follow-up of patients treated with defined regimens in clinical trials.

3.5 Economic Outcomes Research

The Cooperative Groups are in a unique position to integrate health outcomes and economic measures into their research activities. During the 1990's the NCI actively supported efforts to integrate economic analyses into cancer clinical trials. Conferences were convened with experts from the cooperative groups, cancer centers, and experts in the field of health economics to discuss the implementation of economic evaluation in cancer clinical trials. A workbook was published in 1998 to serve as a practical reference for economic analyses of cancer clinical trials.[52]

The first set of economic analyses of cooperative group clinical trials were published between 1997 and 2002 and have been reviewed in detail.[53] These studies were based primarily on retrospective economic analyses, with the exception of one study by the Southwest Oncology Group. Several of the studies compared the use of colony-stimulating factors to placebo, illustrating the application of economic assessments of the cost of cancer care when significant resources are being used, in this case for supportive care agents[54,55].

Cost–effectiveness analyses provide information on the value of an intervention or therapy in relation to its costs when compared to a competing alternative treatment. Studies such as these are particularly important with the recent introduction of exceptionally expensive new agents that produce only modest improvements in survival for patients with advanced cancer. The impact of the widespread use of such drugs on the healthcare system can only be determined with carefully conducted economic analyses along side definitive clinical trials. The Cooperative Groups are well suited to undertake such studies which are often of low priority for pharmaceutical industry sponsors.

4. STRENGTHS

The major scientific strength of the Cooperative Groups remains their portfolio of randomized phase III trials that have the potential to change medical practice. Cooperative group clinical trials remain critical for the systematic evaluation of the effectiveness of new anti-cancer agents with the goal of creating new knowledge to advance the field of cancer therapy to benefit patients. These trials are conducted in a rigorous manner that reflects the Groups' expertise in statistics and data management, with strong input as well from patient advocacy groups. The collective scientific and clinical expertise of Cooperative Group members has resulted in successful collaborations in multimodality trials with important adjunct studies, including correlative science, quality of life, and economic outcomes. The inherent diversity of the Groups results in objectivity and different perspectives that reflect the interests and opinions of a broad range of investigators and health care professionals from private, academic, and community institutions, as well as a large and diverse patient base. This diversity has also made possible the study of special populations, including patients with rare tumor types, of different ages, and belonging to diverse racial/ethnic groups. Promoting international cooperation and collaboration has also been an aim of the Cooperative Groups.

Matched clinical and pathologic data from Cooperative Group trials is a valuable resource that allows for retrospective analysis of clinical and non-clinical factors that impact cancer prognosis and survivorship. Clinical trial databases have proved useful for the study of the relationship between race/ethnicity or age and prognosis. Several retrospective analyses examining the outcomes of different racial/ethnic groups and cancer outcomes have been undertaken.[56-58] Analysis of outcome based on age is part of ongoing trials in adult acute leukemia.

The cooperative group infrastructure has also facilitated the study of cancer in particular populations. The NCI has developed an infrastructure to promote the accrual of minorities to clinical trials. The NCI Minority Accrual Initiative that was conceived in 1990 has lead to an increase in the accrual of racial/ethnic minority patients onto Group clinical trials with a goal of investigating the basis for observed differences in cancer outcome among different racial and ethnic groups. Activities supported through this program include reimbursement of performance sites for increased accrual of minority patients over previously established baselines; translation of patient education materials into languages other than English; training for investigators to enhance skills for recruiting minority patients; and the recruitment of translators and patient advocates to help with accrual and follow-up of minority patients.

The Cooperative Groups actively support educational activities for their members and research staff and the mentoring of young investigators. The Cooperative Group infrastructure is particularly important in the training of investigators to conduct clinical research as no other venue brings together senior clinical investigators, experienced biostatisticians, data management experts, clinicians from all oncology specialties as well as laboratory and population scientists to focus on solving contemporary problems in cancer diagnosis, treatment and prevention.

5. CHALLENGES

The major challenge facing the Cooperative Groups involves improving efficiency and productivity of the cancer clinical trials system - given limited resources - while preserving and enhancing its strengths and the quality of its work.

There is an urgent need to enhance the timeliness of clinical trial accrual to accelerate drug and device development and expand access to new therapies. The existing regulatory structures for the oversight of clinical research are complex and often of uncertain value. Ideally the federal government should unify and streamline its regulations. The challenge lies in how best to: 1) Increase efficiency by improving the scientific and bioinformatics infrastructure for clinical studies. 2) Reduce the auditing, monitoring, and regulatory burden on clinical trials sites by coordinating requirements of the NCI, FDA and OHRP in order to identify specific changes that can eliminate redundancy and reduce costs. 3) Streamline protocol development and standardize clinical trial procedures and clinical research tools. 4) Enhance access to the scientific infrastructure to facilitate the conduct of high priority correlative studies to translate new discoveries into clinical practice.

Overall, enrollment in cancer cooperative group trials is slow and race-, gender-, and age-based disparities in cancer trial participation still exist.[59,60] Further studies are needed to better understand the social economic, logistical, and other factors that contribute to low accrual rates of racial and ethnic minorities, women, and elderly on clinical trials.

6. FUTURE DIRECTIONS AND GOALS

The long-established, comprehensive national infrastructure of the cooperative groups has led to many outstanding achievements in cancer treatment and prevention. Increasing economic pressures have forced the strategic reassessment of priorities while continuing to support high quality clinical and correlative science research that have been the hallmark of cooperative group trials. Recently, the National Cancer Institute convened the Clinical Trials Working Group (CTWG) to make recommendations on how to improve the national cancer clinical trials program. The CTWG report has been accepted by the National Cancer Advisory Board and is publicly available at www.cancer.gov. Among the recommendations is the formation of disease strategy groups to prioritize phase II trials and to review phase III concepts. Major improvements in efficiency are called for in the CTWG report to reduce duplication of effort and cost. Greater collaboration with industry and possible mergers may be necessary to consolidate resources.

Annual budgets for initiatives to understand cancer biology, examine health outcomes and perform economic analyses are called for in the CTWG report and will help to ensure sustained activity in these areas in a time of limited resources. A clinical trials database and specimen inventory management system would ideally provide investigators with access to comprehensive and current information about ongoing and completed trials and specimens available for study.

To remain viable and competitive, the cooperative groups need to resolve several issues regarding protocol management. The time it takes to begin a trial, standardization of protocols for purposes of streamlining implementation, payment for research-related clinical tests, and institutional overhead are all issues that are prolonging the approval, initiation, and conduct of trials. One strategy to increase participation in clinical trials with more diverse participation would be to improve efficiency in protocol activation and post-activation management through systematic management at various stages of protocol development. Management methods and communication tools would be applied in order to maximize efficiency and resources to speed protocol activation and accrual.[61]

The cooperative group system must respond to the exponential increase in new therapeutics and new technology in a changing fiscal and health care environment. The clinical research community must find productive ways to respond to economic pressures by reducing the costs of research through efficiencies and by redefining study parameters, endpoints, and outcomes. In sum, the forces of expanding opportunities and contracting resources call for a new approach to setting priorities for, developing, and conducting clinical trials.

Table 1. NCI-Sponsored Cancer Cooperative Groups

American College of Radiology Imaging Network (ACRIN) (www.acrin.org)
American College of Surgeons Oncology Group (ACOSOG) (www.acosog.org)
Cancer and Leukemia Group B (CALGB) (www.calgb.org)
Children's Oncology Group (COG) (www.childrensoncologygroup.org)
Eastern Cooperative Oncology Group (ECOG) (www.ecog.org)
Gynecologic Oncology Group (GOG) (www.gog.org)
North Central Cancer Treatment Group (NCCTG) (ncctg.mayo.edu)
National Surgical Adjuvant Breast and Bowel Project (NSABP) (www.nsabp.pitt.edu)
Radiation Therapy Oncology Group (RTOG) (www.rtog.org)
Southwest Oncology Group (SWOG) (www.swog.org)

Table 2. FDA Approvals of Drugs and Diagnostics Based on Cooperative Group Data

Cisplatin for non-small cell lung cancer
Paclitaxel ovarian and non-small cell lung cancer
Paclitaxel as adjuvant therapy for breast cancer
Tamoxifen for breast cancer prevention
Interferon as adjuvant therapy for high risk melanoma
5-azacytidine for myelodysplastic syndrome
Oxaliplatin for metastatic colorectal cancer
Docetaxel for metastatic hormone refractory prostate cancer
FISH probe for HER2/neu (PathVysion™) determination
Multigene assay (Oncotype DX™) as a predictor of recurrence/survival in breast cancer

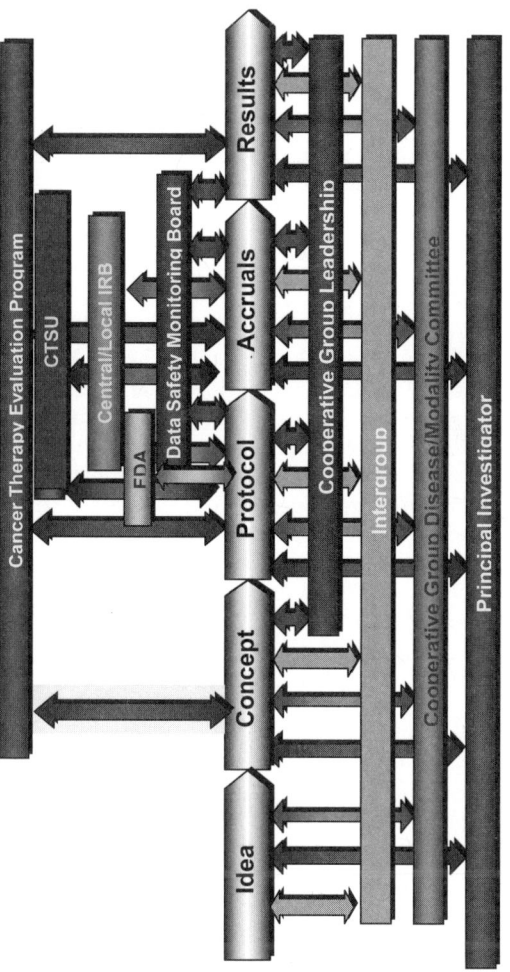

Figure 1. Cooperative Group Clinical Trial Development. The development of cooperative group clinical trials is a collaborative effort among multiple parties, including the cooperative group, the Intergroup, and government research and regulatory agencies.

REFERENCES

1. Keating P, Cambrosio A: From screening to clinical research: the cure of leukemia and the early development of the cooperative oncology groups, 1955-1966. Bull Hist Med 76:299-334, 2002
2. Kelahan AM, Catalano R: The history, structure, and achievements of the cancer cooperative groups. Managed Care & Cancer:28-33, 2001
3. NCI's Clinical Trials Cooperative Group Program
4. National Cancer Institute FY 2004 NCI Fact Book
5. Cancer Trials Support Unit
6. Lukens JN: Progress resulting from clinical trials. Solid tumors in childhood cancer. Cancer 74:2710-8, 1994
7. Ruymann FB, Grovas AC: Progress in the diagnosis and treatment of rhabdomyosarcoma and related soft tissue sarcomas. Cancer Invest 18:223-41, 2000
8. Ries LAG, Eisner MP, C.L. K: SEER Cancer Statistics Review, 1975-2000., (ed http://www.seer.cancer.gov/csr/1975_2002), National Cancer Institute
9. Stadler WM, Rosner G, Small E, et al: Successful implementation of the randomized discontinuation trial design: an application to the study of the putative antiangiogenic agent carboxyaminoimidazole in renal cell carcinoma--CALGB 69901. J Clin Oncol 23:3726-32, 2005
10. Strauss GM, Herndon J, Maddaus MA, et al: Randomized clinical trial of adjuvant chemotherapy with paclitaxel and carboplatin following resection in Stage IB non-small cell lung cancer (NSCLC): Report of Cancer and Leukemia Group B (CALGB) Protocol 9633. Journal of Clinical Oncology, 2004 ASCO Annual Meeting Proceedings (Post Meeting Edition) 22, 2004
11. Winton T, Livingston R, Johnson D, et al: Vinorelbine plus cisplatin vs. observation in resected non-small-cell lung cancer. N Engl J Med 352:2589-97, 2005
12. Haller DG, Catalano PJ, Macdonald JS, et al: Phase III study of fluorouracil, leucovorin, and levamisole in high-risk stage II and III colon cancer: final report of Intergroup 0089. J Clin Oncol 23:8671-8, 2005
13. Mamounas E, Wieand S, Wolmark N, et al: Comparative efficacy of adjuvant chemotherapy in patients with Dukes' B versus Dukes' C colon cancer: results from four National Surgical Adjuvant Breast and Bowel Project adjuvant studies (C-01, C-02, C-03, and C-04). J Clin Oncol 17:1349-55, 1999
14. Moertel CG, Fleming TR, Macdonald JS, et al: Intergroup study of fluorouracil plus levamisole as adjuvant therapy for stage II/Dukes' B2 colon cancer. J Clin Oncol 13:2936-43, 1995
15. Macdonald JS, Smalley SR, Benedetti J, et al: Chemoradiotherapy after surgery compared with surgery alone for adenocarcinoma of the stomach or gastroesophageal junction. N Engl J Med 345:725-30, 2001
16. Kirkwood JM, Manola J, Ibrahim J, et al: A pooled analysis of eastern cooperative oncology group and intergroup trials of adjuvant high-dose interferon for melanoma. Clin Cancer Res 10:1670-7, 2004
17. Fisher B, Anderson S, Bryant J, et al: Twenty-year follow-up of a randomized trial comparing total mastectomy, lumpectomy, and lumpectomy plus irradiation for the treatment of invasive breast cancer. N Engl J Med 347:1233-41, 2002

18. Mamounas EP, Brown A, Anderson S, et al: Sentinel node biopsy after neoadjuvant chemotherapy in breast cancer: results from National Surgical Adjuvant Breast and Bowel Project Protocol B-27. J Clin Oncol 23:2694-702, 2005
19. White RL, Jr., Wilke LG: Update on the NSABP and ACOSOG breast cancer sentinel node trials. Am Surg 70:420-4, 2004
20. Henderson IC, Berry DA, Demetri GD, et al: Improved outcomes from adding sequential Paclitaxel but not from escalating Doxorubicin dose in an adjuvant chemotherapy regimen for patients with node-positive primary breast cancer. J Clin Oncol 21:976-83, 2003
21. Mamounas EP: NSABP Protocol B-27. Preoperative doxorubicin plus cyclophosphamide followed by preoperative or postoperative docetaxel. Oncology (Williston Park) 11:37-40, 1997
22. Citron ML, Berry DA, Cirrincione C, et al: Randomized trial of dose-dense versus conventionally scheduled and sequential versus concurrent combination chemotherapy as postoperative adjuvant treatment of node-positive primary breast cancer: first report of Intergroup Trial C9741/Cancer and Leukemia Group B Trial 9741. J Clin Oncol 21:1431-9, 2003
23. Peters WA, 3rd, Liu PY, Barrett RJ, 2nd, et al: Concurrent chemotherapy and pelvic radiation therapy compared with pelvic radiation therapy alone as adjuvant therapy after radical surgery in high-risk early-stage cancer of the cervix. J Clin Oncol 18:1606-13, 2000
24. Romond EH, Perez EA, Bryant J, et al: Trastuzumab plus adjuvant chemotherapy for operable HER2-positive breast cancer. N Engl J Med 353:1673-84, 2005
25. Sause WT, Scott C, Taylor S, et al: Radiation Therapy Oncology Group (RTOG) 88-08 and Eastern Cooperative Oncology Group (ECOG) 4588: preliminary results of a phase III trial in regionally advanced, unresectable non-small-cell lung cancer. J Natl Cancer Inst 87:198-205, 1995
26. Albain KS, Rusch VW, Crowley JJ, et al: Concurrent cisplatin/etoposide plus chest radiotherapy followed by surgery for stages IIIA (N2) and IIIB non-small-cell lung cancer: mature results of Southwest Oncology Group phase II study 8805. J Clin Oncol 13:1880-92, 1995
27. Albain KS, Crowley JJ, Turrisi AT, 3rd, et al: Concurrent cisplatin, etoposide, and chest radiotherapy in pathologic stage IIIB non-small-cell lung cancer: a Southwest Oncology Group phase II study, SWOG 9019. J Clin Oncol 20:3454-60, 2002
28. Vokes EE, Herndon JE, 2nd, Crawford J, et al: Randomized phase II study of cisplatin with gemcitabine or paclitaxel or vinorelbine as induction chemotherapy followed by concomitant chemoradiotherapy for stage IIIB non-small-cell lung cancer: cancer and leukemia group B study 9431. J Clin Oncol 20:4191-8, 2002
29. Morris M, Eifel PJ, Lu J, et al: Pelvic radiation with concurrent chemotherapy compared with pelvic and para-aortic radiation for high-risk cervical cancer. N Engl J Med 340:1137-43, 1999
30. Keys HM, Bundy BN, Stehman FB, et al: Cisplatin, radiation, and adjuvant hysterectomy compared with radiation and adjuvant hysterectomy for bulky stage IB cervical carcinoma. N Engl J Med 340:1154-61, 1999
31. Rose PG, Bundy BN, Watkins EB, et al: Concurrent cisplatin-based radiotherapy and chemotherapy for locally advanced cervical cancer. N Engl J Med 340:1144-53, 1999
32. al-Sarraf M, Martz K, Herskovic A, et al: Progress report of combined chemoradiotherapy versus radiotherapy alone in patients with esophageal cancer: an intergroup study. J Clin Oncol 15:277-84, 1997

33. Al-Sarraf M, LeBlanc M, Giri PG, et al: Chemoradiotherapy versus radiotherapy in patients with advanced nasopharyngeal cancer: phase III randomized Intergroup study 0099. J Clin Oncol 16:1310-7, 1998
34. Forastiere AA, Goepfert H, Maor M, et al: Concurrent chemotherapy and radiotherapy for organ preservation in advanced laryngeal cancer. N Engl J Med 349:2091-8, 2003
35. Adelstein DJ, Li Y, Adams GL, et al: An intergroup phase III comparison of standard radiation therapy and two schedules of concurrent chemoradiotherapy in patients with unresectable squamous cell head and neck cancer. J Clin Oncol 21:92-8, 2003
36. O'Connell MJ, Martenson JA, Wieand HS, et al: Improving adjuvant therapy for rectal cancer by combining protracted-infusion fluorouracil with radiation therapy after curative surgery. N Engl J Med 331:502-7, 1994
37. Silverman LR, Demakos EP, Peterson BL, et al: Randomized controlled trial of azacitidine in patients with the myelodysplastic syndrome: a study of the cancer and leukemia group B. J Clin Oncol 20:2429-40, 2002
38. Fisher B, Costantino JP, Wickerham DL, et al: Tamoxifen for prevention of breast cancer: report of the National Surgical Adjuvant Breast and Bowel Project P-1 Study. J Natl Cancer Inst 90:1371-88, 1998
39. Sandler RS, Halabi S, Baron JA, et al: A randomized trial of aspirin to prevent colorectal adenomas in patients with previous colorectal cancer. N Engl J Med 348:883-90, 2003
40. Thompson IM, Goodman PJ, Tangen CM, et al: The influence of finasteride on the development of prostate cancer. N Engl J Med 349:215-24, 2003
41. Lippman SM, Lee JJ, Karp DD, et al: Randomized phase III intergroup trial of isotretinoin to prevent second primary tumors in stage I non-small-cell lung cancer. J Natl Cancer Inst 93:605-18, 2001
42. Lippman SM, Levin B: Cancer prevention: strong science and real medicine. J Clin Oncol 23:249-53, 2005
43. Schilsky RL, Dressler LM, Bucci D, et al: Cooperative group tissue banks as research resources: the cancer and leukemia group B tissue repositories. Clin Cancer Res 8:943-8, 2002
44. Paik S, Shak S, Tang G, et al: A multigene assay to predict recurrence of tamoxifen-treated, node-negative breast cancer. N Engl J Med 351:2817-26, 2004
45. Dressler LG, Berry DA, Broadwater G, et al: Comparison of HER2 status by fluorescence in situ hybridization and immunohistochemistry to predict benefit from dose escalation of adjuvant doxorubicin-based therapy in node-positive breast cancer patients. J Clin Oncol 23:4287-97, 2005
46. Kolitz JE, George SL, Dodge RK, et al: Dose escalation studies of cytarabine, daunorubicin, and etoposide with and without multidrug resistance modulation with PSC-833 in untreated adults with acute myeloid leukemia younger than 60 years: final induction results of Cancer and Leukemia Group B Study 9621. J Clin Oncol 22:4290-301, 2004
47. Jatoi A, Windschitl HE, Loprinzi CL, et al: Dronabinol versus megestrol acetate versus combination therapy for cancer-associated anorexia: a North Central Cancer Treatment Group study. J Clin Oncol 20:567-73, 2002
48. Kornblith AB, Herndon JE, 2nd, Silverman LR, et al: Impact of azacytidine on the quality of life of patients with myelodysplastic syndrome treated in a randomized phase III trial: a Cancer and Leukemia Group B study. J Clin Oncol 20:2441-52, 2002
49. Ganz PA: A Teachable Moment for Oncologists: Cancer Survivors, 10 Million Strong and Growing! J Clin Oncol, 2005
50. Demark-Wahnefried W, Aziz NM, Rowland JH, et al: Riding the Crest of the Teachable Moment: Promoting Long-Term Health After the Diagnosis of Cancer. J Clin Oncol, 2005

51. Hensley ML, Dowell J, Herndon JE, 2nd, et al: Economic outcomes of breast cancer survivorship: CALGB study 79804. Breast Cancer Res Treat 91:153-61, 2005
52. Integrating economic analysis into cancer clinical trials: the National Cancer Institute-American Society of Clinical Oncology Economics Workbook. J Natl Cancer Inst Monogr:1-28, 1998
53. Bennett CL, Golub R, Waters TM, et al: Economic analyses of phase III cooperative cancer group clinical trials: are they feasible? Cancer Invest 15:227-36, 1997
54. Bennett CL, Stinson TJ, Tallman MS, et al: Economic analysis of a randomized placebo-controlled phase III study of granulocyte macrophage colony stimulating factor in adult patients (> 55 to 70 years of age) with acute myelogenous leukemia. Eastern Cooperative Oncology Group (E1490). Ann Oncol 10:177-82, 1999
55. Bennett CL, Hynes D, Godwin J, et al: Economic analysis of granulocyte colony stimulating factor as adjunct therapy for older patients with acute myelogenous leukemia (AML): estimates from a Southwest Oncology Group clinical trial. Cancer Invest 19:603-10, 2001
56. Dignam JJ: Efficacy of systemic adjuvant therapy for breast cancer in African-American and Caucasian women. J Natl Cancer Inst Monogr:36-43, 2001
57. Dignam JJ, Ye Y, Colangelo L, et al: Prognosis after rectal cancer in blacks and whites participating in adjuvant therapy randomized trials. J Clin Oncol 21:413-20, 2003
58. McCollum AD, Catalano PJ, Haller DG, et al: Outcomes and toxicity in african-american and caucasian patients in a randomized adjuvant chemotherapy trial for colon cancer. J Natl Cancer Inst 94:1160-7, 2002
59. Murthy VH, Krumholz HM, Gross CP: Participation in cancer clinical trials: race-, sex-, and age-based disparities. Jama 291:2720-6, 2004
60. Hutchins LF, Unger JM, Crowley JJ, et al: Underrepresentation of patients 65 years of age or older in cancer-treatment trials. N Engl J Med 341:2061-7, 1999
61. Demmy TL, Yasko JM, Collyar DE, et al: Managing accrual in cooperative group clinical trials. J Clin Oncol 22:2997-3002, 2004

Chapter 6

THE ADVOCATE ROLE IN CLINICAL STUDY DEVELOPMENT AND PARTNERING WITH PATIENT ADVOCATES IN YOUR LOCAL INSTITUTION

Barbara Parker

Breast Cancer SPORE and American College of Surgeons Oncology Group
Duke University Medical Center, Durham, NC, USA

1. INTRODUCTION

Patient advocates have been associated with clinical study development for more than a decade. Their participation brings special challenges while it adds value to the clinical research enterprise. Advocates may vary in number, function and level of involvement, but they are all patient focused individuals who are willing to make a personal commitment to work with clinical researchers within a cooperative group.

2. HISTORY

Grace Monaco was the first patient advocate to work with a pediatric cancer group in 80s. Martha Romans was the first GOG advocate in the early 90s, followed by Mary Lou Smith and Mike Katz with ECOG, and Deborah Collyar with CALGB in the mid 90s. Pat Halpin-Murphy began working with NSABP and Wayland Eppard with NCCTG in the late 90s. ACOSOG (Barbara Parker) and ACRIN (Barbara LeStage) are the most recent cooperative groups to create patient advocate committees. Currently eight of the nine* Cooperative Group patient advocate committee chairs are members of the Patient Advisory Board (PAB) in the Coalition of National Cancer Cooperative Groups (CNCGG).

*ACOSOG – American College of Surgeons Oncology Group
ACRIN – American College of Radiology Imaging Network
CALGB - Cancer and Leukemia Group B
COG – Children's Oncology Group
GOG – Gynecology Oncology Group
ECOG – Eastern Cooperative Oncology Group
NCCTG – North Central Cancer Treatment Group
NSABP – National Surgical Adjuvant Breast and Bowel Project
RTOG – Radiation Therapy Oncology Group
SWOG – Southwest Oncology Group

3. BACKGROUND

The patient advocate collaboration with clinical researchers is unique in several ways and brings unique challenges for both advocate and clinician. A patient advocate usually enters this collaboration untrained in the language and concepts of clinical research. Historically the patient relationship with clinicians has been 'unequal,' the patient deferential to the clinician. Finally, s/he might be dealing with advanced or metastatic disease – and sometimes dies. These factors influence how advocates and clinical researchers interact. While the fact of advanced disease and death is the raison d'etre for clinical cancer research and reminds us of the need for clinical research, it can lead to instability in advocate participation. Vis-à-vis customary patient – clinician boundaries, an effective advocate is willing to move beyond boundaries into collegial relationships. This effort can be helped or hindered by a clinician's response. Fortunately, the need for training about clinical research has been addressed by the CNCCG.

4. TRAINING

To address the paucity of knowledge about clinical research among neophyte advocates, the Coalition has supported the development of a patient advocate training program that includes self study modules on cooperative groups, clinical trials, drug development, surgery and radiation therapies, protecting research participants and the use of tissue in research. Designed to be used individually or as a syllabus for group study, these comprehensive, user friendly modules have attracted great interest beyond the cooperative group setting as an introduction to various issues in clinical research. Together, these education modules help patient advocates become familiar with the language and concepts of clinical research and form a framework within which they can more comfortably raise patient issues in clinical research discussions.

4.1 Number

The number of advocates in each cooperative group varies. ECOG and RTOG support about seven or eight advocates while CALGB and ACOSOG have about twice that many, and the other Groups are in between. Most advocates are survivors, including two childhood cancer survivors in COG, but some are family members (e.g., in COG, most of the advocates are parents of children with cancer).

4.2 Function-Basic

Although advocate roles and titles differ slightly from one cooperative group to another depending on the structure and specific needs of the group, their function is comparable from group to group. In all the cooperative groups patient advocates sit on and participate in disease committee activities, including discussion and comment on ideas and concepts presented to a committee, protocol development, conference calls, reviewing informed consent documents and committee decision making regarding prioritization of studies. Advocates are also part of administrative and modality committee activities, playing an active role in education, ethics, quality of life, cancer control/prevention and diversity committees among others. The degree of participation among advocates varies according to the experience and assertiveness of the advocate, the culture of the committee and the committee chair's comfort level with advocate participation.

4.3 Function-Sophisticated

The scope of advocate involvement beyond disease and administrative committees depends on the cooperative group. In some groups, patient advocates participate in scientific direction committees and data safety monitoring committees in addition to disease committees. In others, the patient advocate committee chair is a member of the Executive Committee and participates in prioritization of protocols and group policy decisions. In CALGB and ECOG, groups with a longer advocate history, advocates have made plenary presentations. In many groups, the scope of activity includes group wide as well as disease specific issues. The patient representatives in ECOG organized a teleconference focus group among myeloma patient group leaders and PIs to address protocol design issues and a breast focus group is planned. ACOSOG advocates plan to form a group wide unit to focus on accrual. COG advocates are studying how group approved informed consent forms are modified in IRB reviews. They have persuaded COG to include in informed consents the fact that a copy of the protocol is available by request. CALGB advocates regularly speak during CRA training ensuring that awareness of patient perspectives is part of their preparation. ECOG patient representatives regularly update clinicians on current patient issues (e.g., osteonecrosis of the jaws as an occasional consequence of bisphosphonate use). NSABP has a formal advisory interaction between advocates and clinicians to discuss current oncology issues (e.g., implications for and opinions of patients about Vioxx). Because NCCTG is organized as a hub (Mayo) and spoke (community medical sites) system rather than an association of institutions, academic centers and health systems, the advocacy program is organized similarly, with a hub of research advocates and a larger group of member site advocates. The research advocate activities in NCCTG include the basic functions described above, and also include active interactions, training and mentoring of member site advocates. The research advocates hold annual training seminars, quarterly meetings and telephone mentoring for member site advocates and provide them with site visits and a listserv for communication. Their 2004 ASCO poster devoted to this advocacy template aroused considerable interest among clinicians.

Activities of trained advocates include, but are not limited to, meeting with newly diagnosed patients, presentation of general clinical trials information to community groups and speaking to cancer support groups. (For more information on how patient advocates at a local site can be involved in clinical trial advocacy, see "Partnering with Patient Advocates at your Local Institution.")

5. GRANTS

The Coalition small grant program has enabled some advocate groups to initiate research projects. CALGB advocates surveyed patient advocates about why they did or did not participate in clinical trials. ACOSOG advocates will pair a seasoned advocate with the clinical research staff at several clinical trial sites to interface between potential patient participants and the research staff. NSABP advocates developed an educational brochure for patients highlighting the importance of quality of life research. ACRIN advocates will develop patient educational materials that are expected to increase understanding, satisfaction, accrual, and retention in a specific ACRIN study. Materials may include explanatory letter, study brochure, study flowchart of patient requirements, "Tips for your Procedure," and follow-up and thank you letters.

6. ACCRUAL

An initial rationale for including advocates in the cooperative group system was help with increasing accrual to trials. Groups hoped that advocates would publicize open trials within the patient community. ACRIN advocates are doing exactly that: placing significant emphasis on communicating to and through patient groups to inform patients about imaging clinical trials. Many patient advocate committees have links with patient support and advocacy groups through Internet communication, newsletters and public speaking. NSABP advocates developed a poster for clinical offices as a reminder to discuss clinical trials. In some cases advocates have provided a liaison to patient groups in the unlikely event of study problems that impact accrual. Some advocate activities with other goals may impact accrual. For instance, the ACRIN project mentioned in the paragraph above is likely to have a positive effect on accrual.

7. INFORMED CONSENT

Another logical role for advocates is to make sure informed consent explanations are at an appropriate literacy level, reflect cultural sensitivities and are written in 'plain language' as much as possible. Advocates also review the protocol to ensure that the template consent form cooperative groups use includes all aspects of the protocol, with special note of issues important to patients. These may include what costs the patient will be responsible for, how many visits will be necessary, what treatments or tests are required, what side effects are possible, likely, etc.

8. STUDY DEVELOPMENT-PLUS

Groups have found value in advocate involvement beyond these two readily understood roles. When advocates are 'at the table' early in the study development process – during presentation of ideas, discussion of concepts, development of protocols (all stages of study development before informed consent review and thoughts about accrual) – they have an opportunity to 'weigh in' about issues such as likely patient reaction to the proposed design, patient burdens, quality of life component, clinical significance (for *patients,* not scientists), barriers to enrollment, etc. Other aspects of advocate participation, done in parallel to the study development process, have proven valuable. ECOG advocates partnered with Y-ME providing patient education materials for trials that they felt were asking questions important to patients. This initiative included a nursing committee survey about the materials and follow up calls to the trial sites monthly to encourage and track accrual as well as an evaluation component. ACOSOG advocates developed a talking points document for CRAs working on a study in which accrual was difficult. CALGB advocates have made helpful suggestions for studies where accrual was slow. Advocate input has improved education materials for patients. Advocate-developed decision aids for a difficult ACRIN study resulted in higher than expected accrual and retention. After studies are open advocates can continue to add value. They have worked to analyze accrual trends (making suggestions for improvement when needed and investigating reasons when accrual is faster than expected), tracking protocol distribution, monitoring IRB review, etc.

9. INDEPENDENT PROJECTS

Advocate initiated, patient focused research projects have become part of the cooperative group picture as patient advocates have become more integrated. Among these are a pilot project in CALGB sending recently enrolled participants a letter thanking them for enrolling in a clinical trial, ECOG advocates' development of early trial closure notification guide lines (adopted by the Coalition which recommends these to its Cooperative Group membership), a pilot project on patient notification of trial findings – a high priority issue for most patients and a low priority one for most researchers) in CALGB and ECOG, a template for advocate involvement in protocol development in RTOG and a brochure developed in ECOG describing the advocate-researcher relationship.

Inviting to the table of research decisions some of the people for whom this work is done is important and has proven increasingly valuable.

10. PARTNERING WITH PATIENT ADVOCATES AT YOUR LOCAL INSTITUTION

When thinking about launching a clinical trial in your community, consider creating partnerships with local Patient Advocates. Such partnerships can be advantageous for all concerned. As partners in clinical research, patient advocates can be a conduit for the flow of information between the medical community and the patient community. Consider this:

in a 2001 Harris Interactive Survey, 87% of patients said that they would very much or somewhat trust information about a trial which came from patient groups – double the level of trust they would have in PHARMA or the government. Patient Advocates also can bring to the medical community information from the patient community about barriers, concerns and questions the patient community has about enrolling in a trial. Advocates can brainstorm with the medical community on effective ways to overcome barriers or respond to concerns. The Patient Advocate role is not to be a recruiter, but to be a clinical trials educator/and or navigator for patients. This might include helping a patient determine that a particular trial is not suitable for his/her needs. For instance, if a man had a clear dislike for travel and a trial for which he qualified was an hour's drive away, it might not meet his needs. Another example: A woman's choice of a mastectomy over lumpectomy might be based on her decision that maintaining her schedule, which is not consistent with daily radiation, is more important than maintaining her breast.

The Patient Advocate committee has several suggestions on ways Investigators can partner with local Patient Advocates. Most communities have some organized patient groups. But if yours doesn't, look for some among your patients. (One member of our group began her advocacy activities after being invited to contribute a patient perspective at the meeting of oncologists and third party payors.) The qualities that make an effective advocate are evidence of initiative, emotional distance from and ability to see beyond his/her own experience (usually a couple years after diagnosis), willingness to learn, and an ability to communicate and interact with people. Advocates bring a host of talents, skills, experiences and passion to the clinical trials community.

10.1 Invite advocates for discussion

The single most effective way to publicize a study is to create a partnership with patient advocates that will facilitate any of the other suggestions below. Partnering with Patient Advocates will pay dividends over time. They typically have extensive contacts with patient groups, they are highly motivated to 'make a difference' for other patients, and frequently have good ideas for improving procedures that are important to patients. Getting to know the local advocates 'up front' will enable you to gauge who is a good communicator or who is a leader and so forth and build on those strengths. Setting up a process to bring an appropriate advocate group together with an Investigator and/or the study team does not have to be time consuming: meeting over dinner or for a weekend breakfast periodically will do the trick.

10.2 Partner with local patient networks

Sharing information about a clinical trial in your community with local patient networks is a good way to get the news out to your target population. This can be: a member of your study team speaking to groups that have regular meetings, providing flyers or brochures for them to distribute, (*requires advance IRB approval) writing an article for their newsletter, informing 'hotline' volunteers (if they have one) about the study, or posting information about the study on the group's website (if they have one) with a link to the NCI website or the CNCCG website where all cooperative group trials are listed. These are all things a local Patient Advocate can do outside the medical setting. Besides 'getting the word out' about a particular study – your primary objective, these suggestions achieve what might be termed a secondary objective - planting the seed about clinical trials in general and about you and your institution specifically as a resource for clinical trials.

10.3 Create an information flyer or brochure*

You may want to develop a flyer or brochure about a particular study that fits your local community. For instance, a story telling format would be an effective approach to Native Americans and a brochure in this format might increase chances of successful recruitment. Any materials developed at the local institution would require IRB approval before it can be disseminated, although materials developed independently by an advocate group does not. The education committee of ACOSOG also can – and does – develop educational material for specific trials – brochures, videos, etc. If this mechanism of sharing information interests you and there is not already material available, check with the Education committee to see if they have something 'in the works' or can adapt something else for the study of interest to you. Your local Patient Advocate may be interested in working on this, or in reviewing and critiquing a draft before it is final.

10.4 Develop a "patient to patient" letter*

This suggestion, similar to a flyer or brochure, is much more personal. First developed by breast cancer Patient Advocates at UCSF as a general information piece about clinical trials, this deceptively simple mechanism of sharing information has proved extremely successful. Such a document is available through the ACOSOG Education Committee. It capitalizes on the high level of trust that patients have of information endorsed by other patients (demonstrated by the Harris Interactive Survey). The ACOSOG

Education committee is exploring the idea of adapting the UCSF template for some trials with trial specific as well as general clinical trial information.

11. Q & A FOR CRA USE WITH PATIENTS*

Many CRAs will tell you it would be helpful to have something that would help them answer questions patients have about a study that are not addressed in the informed consent process or document and become apparent after the study is open. A local Advocate could be influential in the development of a reference piece for CRAs - not an extended informed consent.

12. ADVOCATE TO EXPLAIN STUDY PROCESS (NOT MEDICAL INFORMATION)

As 'navigators,' Patient Advocates are sometimes seen as more approachable by patients, and are perceived as having more time to spend with the patient. Patients know the advocates have 'walked in their shoes' which is probably responsible for the high degree of trust they have in clinical trial information that comes from fellow patient groups. As collaborators with the clinical research team, navigators might provide information about the informed consent process, explain concepts like randomization, follow-up and risk of recurrence. They could also identify for the patient sources of information about treatment options, local support, etc. They might offer to assist the patient with logistics of participation in a study (transportation, scheduling, etc.). Finally they could assist patients in identifying areas of concern and share their personal experiences with patients and their families.

13. SEEK OUT LOCAL MEDIA

Local media health reporters (newspaper, radio, TV) might be interested in reporting on -and thus publicizing - a clinical trial with a local advocate 'angle.' Sometimes advocates already have a connection with the media health reporters who call them for opinions or quotes about health stories. Taking advantage of this, or facilitating the creation of such a relationship, can pay big dividends by expanding the credibility of a study in a particular community. Advocates could make themselves available to the local press working in conjunction with the physician. Sometimes the advocate may be interviewed for a human interest story; other times the advocate could be a liaison to the PI, providing contact information for physician interviews or physician quotes on the status of clinical trials in the area.

13.1 Medical and community outreach

A Patient Advocate might be willing to attend local medical meetings (e.g., nurses, oncologists, surgeons) to 'exhibit' or make available information to health professionals about particular clinical trials. A patient advocate can make sure that information about the study is available in cancer patient education resource rooms or areas. A Patient Advocate might speak to 'target' community groups about clinical trials in general, e.g., retirement communities, or other groups with a heavy concentration of older people (more likely to contract cancer than younger people).

13.2 Identify barriers to accrual in community

Sometimes when clinical trials are activated and opened with little input from Patient Advocates during their development, barriers become apparent after the fact. For instance at a (non-ACOSOG) trial in Chicago, one of the criteria was that future care be transferred to the trial site which was located in the midst of a heavily trafficked, congested area of the city. Patient Advocates could have anticipated the reticence of suburbanites to visit this area on a regular basis and could have helped the CRA address these concerns in screening conversations. Validated parking receipts, an offer of transportation schedules, or mid-day appointments all would have been helpful to accrual.

13.3 Identify local community norms

In communities with a significant 'special population' (African American, Hispanic, Native American), patient advocates can be particularly helpful in helping to identify community norms and function as an intermediary with the community. For instance, in many Native American traditions, important information is communicated not through a newspaper or other media, but through word of mouth and through story telling by a trusted community 'elder.' An important source for credible information in some African American communities is the local church. (This is fairly well recognized now and many churches have come to feel burdened with the expectations placed on them to be 'all things to all [their] people.') In first Hispanic and Asian communities, family priorities take precedence over individual needs, so it is important to communicate the value of a clinical trial to the family.

13.4 Identify internet information sources for patients

At a recent medical meeting it was noted that 11% of patients being treated in a clinical trial found their trial through the Internet. A web savvy patient advocate could assume responsibility for making sure the trial is posted on all the Internet web sites commonly used by patients (including local hospital or medical center websites) and notifying the PI or other designated person if the information about their site was incorrect (e.g., wrong contact name or information) or missing (e.g., study is open in local site, but is not listed on a web site).

ACKNOWLEDGMENTS

Thanks to the Patient Advisory Board (both Chairs from each Cooperative Group) for their work representing patients in clinical research. (ACOSOG: Barbara Parker and Jim Williams; ACRIN: Barbara Le Stage and Peggy Devine; CALGB: Deborah Collyar and Sandra Batte; COG: John Mussman and Missy Layfield; ECOG: Mary Lou Smith and Mike Katz; GOG: Martha Romans and Susan Scherr; NCCTG: Wayland Eppard and Cynthia Chauhan; NSABP: Pat Halpin-Murphy, RTOG: Hank Porterfield and Pam McAllister).

Chapter 7

THE NATIONAL BREAST CANCER COALITION: SETTING THE STANDARD FOR ADVOCATE COLLABORATION IN CLINICAL TRIALS

Fran Visco

National Breast Cancer Coalition, Washington, DC, USA

1. INTRODUCTION

The National Breast Cancer Coalition Fund (NBCCF) has had a profound influence on breast cancer clinical trials. By educating advocates and ensuring their involvement in all aspects of the clinical trial process, NBCCF is recognized in the scientific, industry, medical and advocacy communities as a leader in progressing breast cancer clinical trials. Founded in 1991, NBCCF has grown to a network of hundreds of organizations and tens of thousands of individuals across the country. The Coalition has one mission: to eradicate breast cancer through *action* and *advocacy*. To achieve this mission, NBCCF focuses on three main goals:

- **Research:** Increasing appropriations for high-quality, peer-reviewed research, and ensuring that the funding is well spent. NBCCF works with the scientific community to focus research efforts on well-designed clinical studies that have a meaningful impact on breast cancer prevention and care.
- **Access:** Increasing access for all women to high quality treatment and care, and to breast cancer clinical trials.
- **Influence:** Increasing the influence of women living with breast cancer and other breast cancer activists in the decision making that affects all issues surrounding the disease.

This chapter explores the ways in which NBCCF pursues these goals through its Clinical Trials Initiative.

2. THE COLLABORATIVE ROLE OF ADVOCATES IN CLINICAL TRIALS: A VITAL PERSPECTIVE

From the beginning, NBCCF recognized that advocates offer something few scientists can bring to the table: the unique and personal perspective of being diagnosed with breast cancer, the experience of treatment and its aftermath and a point of view outside of the scientific and health care system. NBCCF's grassroots network represents the diversity of breast cancer in every way, including geography, race, socio-economics, age, sexual orientation and perspective, among others. Equally as important, NBCCF's network incorporates the perspective of those with the disease. NBCCF educates and trains this network and then brings that educated power to the research and health care communities. In fact, the Coalition trains advocates who have been affected by breast cancer—in most cases those who have had the disease—in order to represent a genuine patient-centered approach in clinical trial design, oversight and implementation.

Due to NBCCF's work, advocates now contribute to aspects of clinical trials that were once the sole province of scientific and health care professionals. They sit on trial steering committees, attend investigator meetings, participate in Data Safety Monitoring Boards and Institutional Review Boards, assist with protocol and informed consent design, and coordinate the outreach to and accrual of participants. They analyze trials and report to the public and policy makers from an informed patient perspective. They address the public policy issues that surround scientific and health care decisions, from barriers to access to care to the design and reporting of trials.

Many advocates have had breast cancer or have been affected by the disease in some way, which enables them to raise questions or evaluate data with the perspective of "having been there." This is invaluable to creating an authentic patient-centered approach.

2.1 A Groundbreaking Initiative

Recognizing the complexity of the clinical trial system and process, NBCCF approaches its clinical trials work with an integrated strategy, combining education and training, legislation and public policy change, and collaborations on specific clinical trials. All components of the strategy are required to advance the search for meaningful solutions to breast cancer.

2.2 Why Clinical Trials?

The grassroots advocates who make up NBCCF recognize that clinical trials provide the most effective venue to determine how to prevent, treat, and cure breast cancer. We often hear the statistic that less than three percent of adult cancer patients in the United States currently participate in clinical trials. Many trials either take too long, or are not long enough. Some never accrue a sufficient number of patients to adequately inform – or even begin – the trial. NBCCF asked the question: What percentage of patient participation should we achieve? What are the clinical trials we should be interested in? How many trials warrant patient participation? Which should get financial support? NBCCF refused to support the notion that any and all breast cancer clinical trials should move forward. NBCCF developed its Clinical Trials Initiative to help change the system and address these and other issues within the clinical trial process.

2.3 NBCCF's Clinical Trials Initiative

NBCCF's Clinical Trials Initiative incorporates the belief that advocate involvement is imperative to changing clinical trials. Therefore, the Initiative's strategies are based on the rich potential of connecting the power and perspective of trained advocacy with the expertise of science and health care.

To put the Initiative into action, the Coalition developed programs to equip advocates with the information needed to participate fully in all aspects of the clinical trial process. Advocates now provide important insights into the research and design of trials, and also work to heighten awareness about the trials within the breast cancer community.

The Clinical Trials Initiative is defined by three approaches:

1. Education: Educating advocates about the science, processes and policies behind clinical trials;
2. Public Policy: Designing and supporting legislative and public policy approaches to support appropriate clinical trials; and
3. Scientific Collaboration: Collaborating with researchers and industry to design, oversee and implement meaningful clinical trials.

3. EDUCATION

NBCCF's integrated strategy includes educational programs that inform advocates about all aspects of clinical trials. These programs help advocates understand all phases of the clinical trial process and enable them to prioritize and decide which clinical trials warrant their participation and/or support. Educational materials also teach advocates how trials are designed and how to critically analyze trial data. NBCCF's clinical trial education programs address a comprehensive range of topics and are accessible to all advocates – from beginner to advanced.

A. Project LEAD®

Advocates need specific skills and knowledge to participate constructively in the wide range of forums that often influence decisions on breast cancer research. To provide advocates with these tools, the Coalition developed Project LEAD® – an acronym for Leadership, Education, Advocacy and Development – which is an extensive four-day program now recognized for innovation and excellence by the medical, science, research and advocacy communities.

The Coalition recruits motivated applicants for the LEAD training, as the coursework is demanding. NBCCF also seeks out students to participate in LEAD who will provide a diverse perspective to the clinical trial process. Applicants must demonstrate experience in activism and interest in medical research to be selected. NBCCF also accepts a large number of applications from advocates abroad. As of the spring of 2005, more than one thousand advocates – including 50 international students – have participated in the program.

The LEAD program is offered multiple times a year around the United States, and has been offered internationally. The program's curriculum is drawn from open communication among scientists, researchers, policymakers, and consumers nationwide. Faculty members include renowned scientists from academic and research institutions such as Brown University, Harvard University, University of California at Los Angeles and the National Institutes of Health, and provide expertise in such topics as:

- Basic science, such as the biology of cancer, basic genetics, the roles of DNA, RNA and proteins and development of cancer at the molecular level;
- Basic epidemiology such as biostatistics, descriptive studies, analytic studies, clinical trials, causality and screening; and
- Leadership and advocacy development skills.

Project LEAD® also includes a special session devoted specifically to clinical trials and their purpose, design and limitations, and includes information on systematic review and meta-analysis.

Advocates leave Project LEAD® armed with the expertise and insights needed to make a meaningful contribution to the clinical trials research process. They are well prepared to influence the work of trial investigators at pharmaceutical and biotechnology companies, as well as at the National Cancer Institute (NCI) and other research institutions around the country.

B. Project LEAD®: Clinical Trials

To provide intensive training for advocates in all the important aspects of clinical trial design, implementation and oversight, NBCCF designed its Clinical Trials Project LEAD® course. Developed as an advanced training program for Project LEAD® graduates, this course covers the scientific, ethical and practical aspects of the clinical trials process. Graduates of this course are expected to participate in NBCCF's Clinical Trials Initiative and representative NBCCF in partnerships with clinical researchers. Clinical Trials Project LEAD® graduates participate in peer review programs, present at scientific meetings and function as members of scientific committees.

The Clinical Trials Project LEAD® curriculum includes courses such as:

-Role of Clinical Trials in Breast Cancer and the Research Protocol
-Key components of Clinical Trials: Phases 1-4
-Overview of the Drug Development, Approval, and Regulatory Processes
-Measurement of Quality of Life Issues
-Endpoints, Interim Results and other Methodological Issues
-Clinical Trials Issues in the Metastatic and Adjuvant Settings
-Ethical Issues in Clinical Trials

C. Annual Advocacy Training Conference

In addition to the LEAD educational seminars, NBCCF also hosts an annual advocacy training conference. The event draws more than 700 breast cancer advocates, caregivers, researchers and industry representatives to participate in plenary sessions and workshops on the latest information in breast cancer research, legislation and quality care issues.

Conference faculty members are experts in the fields of medicine, science and advocacy. A sample of research-related sessions illustrates the range of topics explored:

- Breast Cancer Care: Who Decides and How Safe Are We?
- New Trends in Breast Cancer Research
- Clinical Trials and Advocate Involvement
- Advanced Topics in Epidemiology
- Race, Ethnicity and the Science of Breast Cancer
- Science and the Controversy of Biomarkers
- Breast Cancer Treatment: New and Emerging Therapies
- Clinical Trials and Informed Consent
- Clinical Trials and Public Policy
- Evidence-based Medicine and its Implications

D. Fact Sheets, Position Papers and Analyses

To continually educate advocates, and the general public, about the latest in ongoing and upcoming clinical trials and to help them analyze trials, NBCCF publishes Fact Sheets, Position Papers and Analyses on its web site (www.stopbreastcancer.org).

Some examples of these materials include:

Fact Sheets:

- *Outcomes in Breast Cancer Clinical Trials*

    o This fact sheet provides some basic background information about the endpoints or outcomes that are selected for measurement in breast cancer clinical trials. It explains sample size and selection of outcome measures and describes the concept of interim results.

- *Early Stopping of Clinical Trials*

    o This fact sheet explains the benefits and detriments of stopping of breast cancer clinical trials early. It describes the problem of "cross over" and the lost opportunity to gather information about long-term side effects and the fact that small but statistically significant increases in the time to recurrence may or may not be associated with longer or healthier life.

Position Papers

- *Access to Investigational Interventions Outside of Clinical Trials*

    o This position paper explains NBCCF's belief that access to investigational interventions undermines the clinical trials system and the principle of evidence-based medicine and that such access should only be allowed in very limited circumstances.

- *Mammography Screening*

    o This paper lays out the scientific, thorough reasoning behind NBCCF's position that there is insufficient evidence to recommend for or against screening mammography in any age group of women.

Analyses

- *Clinical Trial Comparing Breast Cancer Screening Options*

    o NBCCF's analysis examines the first breast cancer screening trial that compared mammography plus physical examination to physical examination alone in 50-59 year-old women.

- *Aspirin Use and Breast Cancer Risk*

    o NBCCF analyzed a study that examined the association between aspirin use and breast cancer risk. This was the first study to explore whether the protective effect of nonsteroidal anti-inflammatory drugs (NSAIDs) varied by estrogen or progesterone receptor status.

4. PUBLIC POLICY

Another way in which advocates influence clinical trials is by impacting legislation that plays a role in breast cancer research. In order to conduct these lobbying efforts, NBCCF – which is classified as a 501(c)(3) educational non-profit – relies on its sister organization, the National Breast Cancer Coalition (NBCC) – which is classified as a 501(c)(4) – its lobbying arm.

The work of advocates under the umbrella of NBCC focuses on legislative priorities that will increase funding for breast cancer research, including clinical trials, provide access to high quality health care and clinical trials, and expand the influence of advocacy in all aspects of the breast cancer decision-making process. The accomplishments of these efforts to date are impressive: NBCC advocates have created an increase in annual federal funding for breast cancer research by more than 800 percent, from less than $200 million before 1991 to more than $14 billion in 2005, including a cumulative appropriation of $1.75 billion for the Department of Defense Peer Reviewed Breast Cancer Research Program.

One of NBCC's most sweeping legislative achievements is the development of the Department of Defense Breast Cancer Research Program (DOD BCRP). The project was created as a result of NBCC's 1993 "$300 Million More" campaign. NBCC launched this campaign after holding a series of research hearings at which fifteen of the nation's most prominent scientists working in the field of breast cancer testified. As a result of the hearings, the Coalition told Congress that an additional $300 million would be needed in 1993 for breast cancer research, for a total of $430 million. This total appropriation comprised the first significant increase in federal breast cancer research funding.

The DOD BCRP forged the way for new and innovative directions in breast cancer research. The program is renowned for its efficient use of resources – more than 90% of the funds go directly to research grants – and a unique part of the program has been the participation of advocates at every level. Since 1992, more than 600 breast cancer survivors have served on the BCRP review panels that determine which research proposals receive funding based on scientific merit.

The DOD BCRP has supported several mechanisms to advance meaningful breast cancer clinical trials including, for example, support for Clinical Translational Research, Centers of Excellence and Clinical Bridge Awards. The Clinical Translational Research Awards are designed to sponsor innovative research that will result in substantial improvements over current approaches to breast cancer chemoprevention and therapy by accelerating the progression of recent, highly promising findings in preclinical breast cancer research from the laboratory to the clinic. The Centers of Excellence Awards are intended to support the establishment of multi-institutional collaborations among highly accomplished scientists from diverse backgrounds to focus on a major scientific problem in breast cancer. And the Clinical Bridge Awards support critical pre-clinical or post-clinical trial research with high potential for imminent clinical application.

Recognizing that support for researchers designing and implementing clinical trials is not the only answer, NBCC developed strategies to help patients interested in trials.

If the public, including patients, doctors and researchers, do not have access to information about trials, then treatment decisions and research are impeded, health care costs are affected and lives are lost. NBCC recognized the need to focus on ensuring that individuals have access to critical information on ongoing clinical trials and to the results from those trials. In 2005, NBCC set the Fair Access to Clinical Trials Act (FACT) as one of its legislative priorities. FACT would create two publicly available sets of information provided in the national data bank of trials: a registry of clinical trials and a results database. The registry would include information on all trials for drugs, biologics or devices to treat serious and/or life-threatening diseases. The results database would require that all trials (except Phase I) testing the safety or effectiveness of any drug, biologic or device, report specific information including a summary of results regardless of whether the results were published in a journal.

Financial burdens for patients and access to information can also create barriers to clinical trials; NBCC pursued various public policy approaches to alleviate these problems. On a federal level, in 1999, one of NBCC's priorities was the Medicare Cancer Clinical Trials Coverage Act that would provide Medicare coverage of routine patient care costs associated with clinical trials. While that bill did not become law, NBCC was instrumental in the Clinton Administration's resolution of this issue through an executive memorandum in June 2000. In large part due to NBCC's advocacy, routine care costs such as tests, procedures and doctors visits that are normally covered will also be covered for Medicare recipients participating in clinical trials. On a state basis, NBCC published model state legislation and helped its grassroots network work within their home states to get meaningful laws enacted that would require insurance companies to cover these patient costs incurred in clinical trials.

5. SCIENTIFIC COLLABORATION

The third component of NBCCF's clinical trials initiative involves collaborating with researchers and industry on specific trials - but not all trials. In fact NBCCF's Board of Directors, made up of 25 organizations from across the country that reflect the diversity that is breast cancer, developed criteria for NBCCF participation.

Once a trial meets NBCCF criteria, advocates work alongside scientific and medical professionals in every step of the trial process.

5.1 High Standards for Clinical Trials

When NBCCF chooses to participate in a clinical trial, they bring the power and the trust of a nationwide grassroots advocacy network. Therefore, before engaging in a collaboration, NBCCF evaluates every clinical trial according to rigorous principles. To enter into a partnership with NBCCF, the study must:

- Be designed to answer an important, novel question relevant to breast cancer;
- Be a well-designed clinical trial that is scientifically rigorous, employing appropriate and meaningful outcomes;
- Be conducted in an ethical manner, with data to support efficacy and safety standards sufficient for reasonable people to believe the trial should proceed;
- Provide participants with sufficient information to provide meaningful informed consent; and
- Receive approval from the Institutional Review Board.

The trial must also employ mechanisms to provide adequate protection for participants' privacy and confidentiality. And, there must be a system in place—such as a Safety Monitoring Committee—for evaluating the protocol and patient safety as the trial proceeds.

In addition, the research agreements between the trial sponsor and any academic or independent investigators must adhere to all of the guidelines for sponsorship, authorship and accountability outlined by the 2004 International Committee of Medical Journal Editors' "Uniform Requirements for Manuscripts Submitted to Biomedical Journals."[1] The academic or independent research institutions participating in the study must be involved in the design, recruitment and data interpretation for the trial.

A mechanism must also be in place to adequately address NBCCF's concerns about the payment of costs for the trial participants' patient care. The trial must adequately address NBCCF's concerns about the inclusion of diverse populations and inappropriate exclusion of specific populations, as well, and must meet NBCCF's expectations regarding partnerships.

NBCCF also expects the trial sponsor to provide the Coalition with the following:

- Opportunities for meaningful input into study design and implementation;
- Opportunities for meaningful review of and input regarding safety data;
- Information about every breast cancer clinical trial it is conducting; and,
- Updates, to the extent feasible, on the trial's progress, status and results—even if the trial is cancelled or ends early.

In addition, NBCCF expects the primary results of the study to be published in full form in a respected peer-reviewed journal. The findings are to be disseminated regardless of final FDA approval, the strength or direction of the results, or findings of significant adverse events.

Because of these high standards, the Coalition's participation has become an indication of a clinical trial's excellence within advocacy communities.

The clinical trial that paved the way for the role of breast cancer advocates in this process took place between NBCCF and the biotechnology firm, Genentech. In 1996, Genentech was poised to bring Herceptin® to trial. The drug was developed to improve the survival and disease progression rates in women with metastatic breast cancer who overexpress HER2. The company had already invested in the early stages of a trial design, but they were unable to recruit breast cancer patients to participate. Based on NBCCF's strong reputation for coordinating outreach at the grassroots level, officials from Genentech contacted the Coalition. NBCCF responded by initiating a groundbreaking collaboration between advocates and industry.

Before recruiting patients to participate, NBCCF wanted to ensure the quality and potential of the trial. NBCCF representatives sat on the trial's Data and Safety Monitoring Committee and its Steering Committee. They sent advocates to all major principal investigator meetings and NBCCF's advocates reviewed and helped revise the trial protocol. Once they were satisfied with each step of the trial, the Coalition mobilized their grassroots network to recruit cancer patients to participate. NBCCF's role led to the

U.S. Food and Drug Administration's (FDA) rapid approval of the first monoclonal antibody treatment for metastatic breast cancer.

This experience established a standard of excellence for other medical industries seeking to collaborate with advocacy organizations. In today's research circles, the high criteria and stringent requirements that NBCCF requires of clinical trials have made their participation highly sought-after.

5.2 Ongoing Trials

NBCCF has partnered on a number of clinical trials since initiating the collaborative model in 1996. In each case, they ensure that the most strategic and necessary questions are asked, and that trials include enough participants – with an equitable representation of the diverse patient population – to explore these questions effectively. And, to maintain a strident level of objectivity, NBCCF does not accept compensation from industry for any of its work on clinical trials. These trials include the following:

- A partnership with BCIRG (The Breast Cancer International Research Group, a not-for-profit academic, global, cooperative group of oncology researchers) on a phase III clinical trial. The trial was fully enrolled as of spring 2004, and as of 2005 was in the data collection phase. NBCCF was involved in many aspects of the design and implementation of this adjuvant trial. Representatives of NBCCF served on the Steering Committee, attended and participated in the investigator meetings and served on the Data and Safety Monitoring Committee. Outreach on the part of NBCCF allowed the trial to achieve its enrollment goal of 3,150 women more quickly than expected.

- NBCCF is partnering with a biopharmaceutical company on its investigational drug being tested in breast cancer patients with brain metastases to improve the effectiveness of radiotherapy and to increase survival. The drug showed promise for patients with breast cancer during a Phase II trial of several types of cancer. As of spring 2005, the company was conducting a confirmatory Phase III breast cancer trial. Protocol and consent materials have been reviewed and amended, and outreach efforts are in the initial phase in 15 cities. NBCCF representatives sit on the Data Safety Monitoring Board and participate at investigator's meetings. In addition, the Coalition has engaged its network to help with trial outreach.

- A continuing collaboration with one company has led to a Phase III clinical trial of an anti-angiogenic therapy. This therapy is being studied in a variety of tumor types including breast, colorectal and lung cancers. The clinical trial offers standard treatment while also helping the cancer community evaluate the safety and efficacy of a potential new treatment. The trial enrolled approximately 400 patients across the United States. It was an open-label, active-controlled trial that evaluated the safety, efficacy and pharmacokinetics of one drug in combination with another in patients with previously treated metastatic breast cancer. NBCCF was involved in all aspects of the trial, from targeting specific sites for accrual to serving on review boards and the Data Safety Monitoring Committee.

- NBCCF partnered with a company on a pivotal Phase III trial of a vaccine for women with metastatic breast cancer. The potential of the drug was promising, but the clinical trial revealed obstacles that indicated the drug was not ready for general use. This case demonstrates that, while clinical trials are intended to test unproven treatments, positive treatment results are never a certainty. Despite the outcome, however, there was valuable knowledge gained about the drug through the trial process.

6. CONCLUSION

The National Breast Cancer Coalition Fund revolutionized the model of educated advocates and clinical trials. Through the Clinical Trials Initiative and ongoing efforts, the Coalition educates, empowers and enables advocates to make a meaningful contribution to the clinical trials research process, and sets the standard for excellence in those trials through their stringent evaluation process.

Despite the impressive accomplishments of the Coalition, neither the best treatments nor the cure for breast cancer is known. Breast cancer remains the most commonly diagnosed cancer among women in the United States and worldwide (excluding skin cancer). In 2005, it is estimated that 269,730 new cases of breast cancer will be diagnosed among women in the United States. Breast cancer is also the second leading cause of cancer death for women in the U.S (after lung cancer); approximately 40,410 women in the U.S. will die from the disease in 2005.

These numbers will only decrease when prevention and a cure for the disease are found. Until then, the National Breast Cancer Coalition Fund will continue to bring the power of advocacy to influence science and industry in the pursuit of ending breast cancer.

REFERENCE

1. International Committee of Medical Journal Editors (ICMJE), *Uniform requirements for manuscripts submitted to biomedical journals: writing and editing for biomedical publication.* ICMJE, 2005. www.ICMJE.org

Chapter 8

THE ROLE OF THE PRINCIPAL INVESTIGATOR IN CANCER CLINICAL TRIALS

Stanley P. L. Leong, MD, FACS
University of California San Francisco, San Francisco, California, USA

1. INTRODUCTION

The principal investigator (PI) is the most important person in the creation and conduct of a clinical trial. Clinical scientists strive to develop better treatments for their patients by generating hypotheses and proving them through well-designed clinical trial protocols. Therefore, being a PI should be a cherished and noble goal. However, challenges for a PI are multifaceted. The purpose of this chapter is to discuss these challenges, as well as strategies to overcome them in order to make the day-to-day conduct of clinical trials more user-friendly.

2. OBLIGATIONS FOR THE PI

In general, clinicians are well trained to practice their medical specialties. When they join the staff of an accredited hospital, they are given the bylaws of the hospital so that they understand what is expected of them. However, when a clinician steps into the world of clinical research as the PI of a research study, he or she assumes responsibilities that are new and at times foreign.

The first and foremost step that a PI must take is to observe an urgent clinical problem and develop a hypothesis to explain the observation. He or she must then write a protocol which is a plan to test the hypothesis by well-defined methods to reach a conclusion (Figure 1). The protocol is a contract between the PI and the Institutional Review Board (IRB), which the PI will adhere to in carrying out the clinical trial. In doing so, the PI enters the world of clinical research, which is different from that of clinical practice (Figure 2). The challenge is to minimize the differences between these two worlds. These worlds have different rules and regulations, both of which must be understood in great detail. Therefore, a PI often requires further training to conduct clinical research or else risk a major blunder during the course of running a clinical trial.

The art of striking a balance between being a clinician and being a PI in a clinical trial is sometimes not easy. The current environment for conducting clinical research dictates that the PI considers every patient in a clinical trial as a "subject". By definition, that means the PI cannot maneuver around any treatment options that are part of the protocol, even if the PI thinks it would be in the best interest of the patient. The fact that clinical trials treat "subjects" rather than patients renders the physician-patient relationship devoid of individuality and compassion. Therefore, it is important for the PI to function in a different and detached mode to be sure that he or she conducts the trial in compliance with all applicable regulatory requirements, state laws, and institutional policies and guidelines. Conducting the study in an ethical manner that protects the rights and welfare of human subjects who are involved in the study requires a different mindset (Table 1) than acting as a clinician who makes on the spot decisions based on the best interests of a patient at the moment. However, despite the effort to separate clinical practice and clinical research, complete separation is not possible (Figure 2). When the PI interacts with the Food and Drug Administration (FDA) regarding a new investigation or new drug (Chapter 4), the PI is now also a "sponsor" whose responsibilities are listed in Table 2.

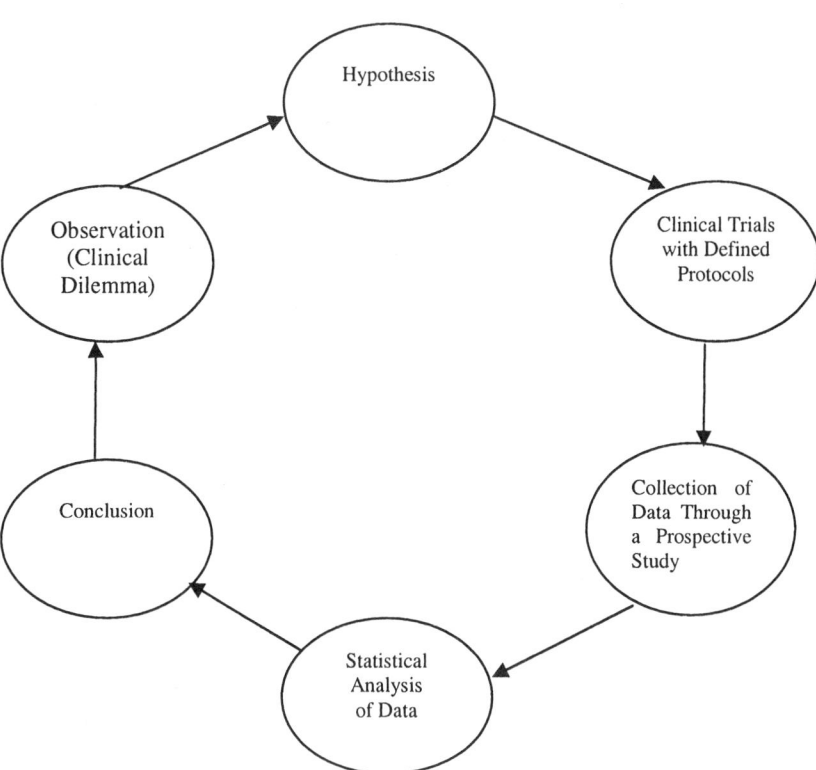

Figure 1. Clinical research is just like basic research, whereby a hypothesis is generated based on an observation or a clinical dilemma. Clinical trials are conducted to prove or disprove the hypothesis. Reliable methods should be used to conduct the trial and collect data. Results should be analyzed independently and impartially to reach a scientific conclusion, thereby proving or disproving the hypothesis and laying the groundwork for the next level of hypothesis. This cycle never ends and is the essence of research.

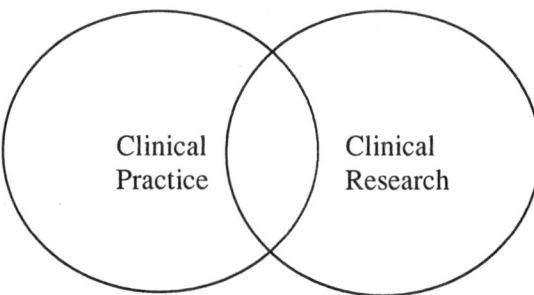

Figure 2. Clinical practice is often different from clinical research. It is important to differentiate the two. Although there is an area of common ground, when a PI is engaged in clinical research, he or she should be rigidly applying and following the regulations of the clinical trial. In contrast, clinical practice is more judgmental and as long as the clinician can defend the rationale of his or her action and judgment, with respect to the level of standard of care, he or she will be in conformity with the practice of medicine. The PI should be keenly aware of him or herself as being a clinical researcher and may be also a sponsor for the FDA with respect to investigation of a new drug. Although there is no formal training to become a PI, many training options exist; The PI must be familiar with all the components of conducting clinical research. The challenges and potential pitfalls are discussed in this chapter.

Table 1. PI's Responsibilities in Conducting Clinical Research *

- Have appropriate qualifications and resources
- Provide adequate medical care for any adverse experiences
- Provide IRB with appropriate documents and obtain IRB approval
- Comply with the protocol, deviating only with IRB approval, except in case of emergency
- Ensure the appropriate storage and use of the investigational product at the trial site
- Follow randomization and blinding procedures
- Obtain and document informed consent
- Inform subjects, IRB, sponsor, and the institution of premature termination
- Keep case report forms (CRF) and allow access to the IRB, monitors, auditors, and the FDA
- Maintain appropriate trial related documents
- Document financial arrangements with the sponsor
- Provide progress reports to the IRB at least annually

*Reproduced from a presentation by Jay Siegal, M.D., Director, Office of Therapeutics Research and Review (OTRR), Center of Biologics Evaluation and Research, Food and Drug Administration.
(http://www.nihtraining.com/crtpub_508/index.html)

Table 2. Sponsor's Responsibilities in Conducting Clinical Research *

- Maintain quality control and standard operating procedures
- Trial conduct, documentation, reporting, handling data
- Manage clinical trial, consider establishing a data monitoring committee
- Follow appropriate procedures for handling data and for document retention
- Define trial related functions and allocate responsibilities
- Provide and update an investigator's brochure
- Oversee the investigational product
- Quality, characterization, storage, packaging, blinding, supply, disposition, stability, samples and records
- Ensure access to records by monitors, auditors, IRB and FDA
- Evaluate safety as trial proceeds – notify investigators, IRB and FDA of important new findings
- Select and train monitors and ensure that the trial is adequately monitored

*Reproduced from a presentation by Jay Siegal, M.D., Director, Office of Therapeutics Research and Review (OTRR), Center of Biologics Evaluation and Research, Food and Drug Administration
(http://www.nihtraining.com/crtpub_508/index.html).

3. CHALLENGES TO THE PI

In this section, I will discuss the challenges faced by PIs in clinical trials. These challenges fall into seven main areas: 1) individual; 2) collegial; 3) academic environment; 4) institutional; 5) ethical, regulatory, and legal; 6) funding; and 7) audits.

3.1 Individual challenges

The major motivating force for the PI to conduct clinical trials is twofold. First, he or she may be morally compelled to develop a better treatment to alleviate the suffering patient. Second, he or she may be motivated to be the first to find a solution for a difficult clinical problem or a cure for an incurable disease, such as cancer. Although the second motivation is important, the overriding reason for designing and conducting a trial should be to alleviate human suffering. In clinical trials, the PI should always take the high moral ground and remember to do no harm to the patient. In fact, this is the ethical basis upon which a protocol is approved by the IRB. To ensure that there are no other motives, a PI should be totally detached with respect to the outcome of the clinical trial. The PI's main goal is to achieve the highest degree of integrity in the conduct of clinical trials. In the process, the PI's journey is truly arduous because there are so many responsibilities, committees, and agencies to deal with (Figure 3). Unless the PI is fully committed to taking on these responsibilities, he or she should not launch a clinical trial.

It is important to develop a sense of total detachment with respect to the outcome of clinical trials because several emotional factors may potentially influence the outcome of the trial in a biased and non-scientific way. These factors include the desire for recognition, the feeling of control, stubbornness about proving one's hypothesis to be correct, and monetary gain. Any of these factors will cloud the outcome of a clinical trial if a true sense of detachment is not developed. Therefore, a PI should develop the qualities listed in Table 3. Equally important is honesty to oneself, from which the truth comes.

The role of the principal investigator in cancer clinical trials

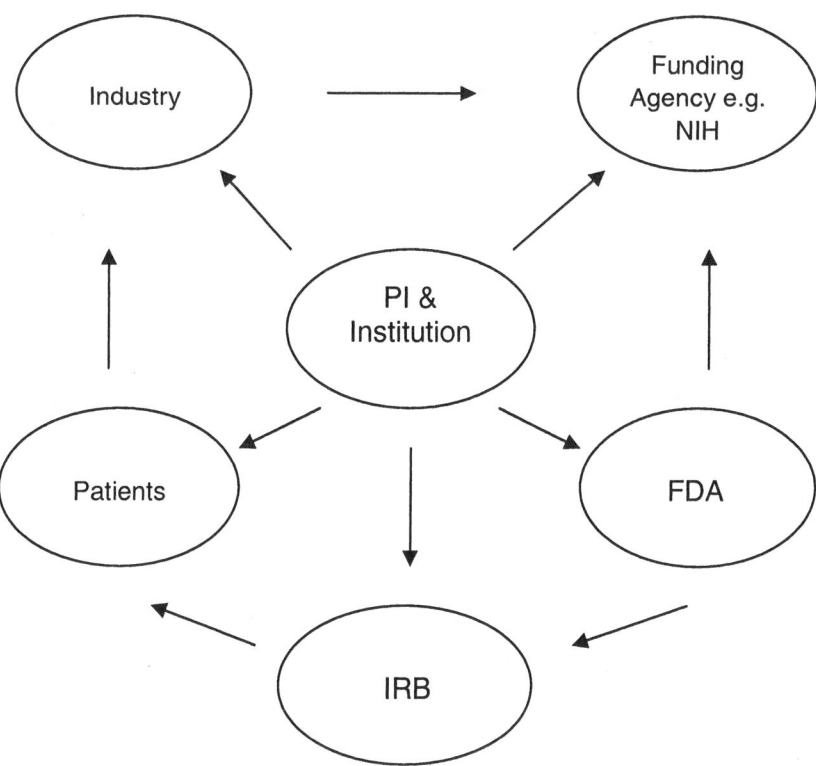

Figure 3. The PI interacts closely with his or her home institutions, the internal review board (IRB), the patients who are being enrolled in the protocol, the FDA, and the funding agency (e.g., the NIH), and at times with industry when it is a sponsor of a new drug or when it provides funding for a PI.

The goal of clinical research, or any research for that matter, is to gain knowledge for humanity by developing a hypothesis based on a keen observation. The process itself is noble, but the result should be obtained in an impartial and emotionless way. Whether the result of a trial is positive or negative, it sets up a new cycle of observation and hypothesizing. Thus, new protocols are developed with appropriate methods and statistical approaches to reach the next conclusion. This cycle never ends and is the very essence of research (Figure 1).

Table 3. Characteristics to be developed by the PI *

1. Focus
2. Preparedness
3. Conviction
4. Perseverance
5. Creativity
6. Curiosity
7. Resilience
8. Risk-taking
9. Independence
10. Sense of higher purpose

*Reproduced from Profiles from the World's 100 Greatest People, Inteliquest Media Corporation, Salt Lake City, Utah.

3.2 Collegial challenges

Throughout the planning and conduct of a cancer clinical trial, the PI is involved with many different committees, organizations, and personnel (Figure 3). He or she is the leader of the team within the institution. The team may consist of co-investigators, nursing staff, cancer registrars, secretarial staff, residents, students, and volunteers. The PI represents the team when dealing with different institutions outside his or her own institution. These agencies are further discussed in Chapters 2 (IRB), 3 (NCI), 4 (FDA), and 5 (Cooperative Research Groups). Therefore, as the team leader, the PI is required to develop leadership, competence, and charisma. The PI must set a good example in running a proper clinical trial, developing personnel management skills, and having the ability to work well with different people on the team.

It is the PI's responsibility to ensure that all participating faculty and research staff observe pertinent laws, regulations, and institutional policies and guidelines. It is also the PI's responsibility to ensure that members of the team responsible for performing the study are qualified, appropriately trained, and adhere to the provisions of the IRB-approved protocol. Honesty and transparency are key so that every team member understands the goal of the trial. The PI must remember that every member of the team deserves respect and understanding. The PI must also remember that his or her own conduct is being scrutinized by all the members of the team and may be reported to the IRB or other committees within the institution or outside if the conduct is deemed to be inappropriate. A complaint may also be made by the patient. Loyalty from team members is a result of respect, not abuse of power. Although exercise of power may transiently solve a temporary problem, in the long run, such a behavior will be brought to light and the program will fall into pieces. Most, if not all institutions that receive federal funding for research have a channel specifically designated for "whistle blowing," through which a subordinate may report inappropriate behavior or misconduct of a superior.

In summary, the PI should leave his or her office each day with a sense that the research program is in total compliance with the rules and regulations of the institution and federal law. In this way, if an audit (Chapter 9) is required the next day, the PI and his or her team will be ready to present all the documents to the auditors. The ethical integrity of the PI and the team should always be the foundation upon which all daily activities are conducted. Although whistle-blower accusations may be well-founded, certain situations may result from misunderstanding, overreaction, or wrongful accusation. Therefore, the PI should be vigilant about acting appropriately at all times and resolving misunderstandings quickly.

3.3 Challenges from the academic environment

Academic medicine is currently at a profoundly low ebb. Reduced reimbursement, increased workloads, decreased resident help, limited donations, and tight NIH budgets have resulted in a significant squeeze on financial and personnel support for academic medicine. Only those clinician scientists who have great passion and tenacity will survive in these trying times.

Unless the NIH substantially increases its support for clinical scientists to conduct research and clinical trials, this negative trend will continue and will adversely affect academic medicine. It has already negatively affected the morale and motivation of young clinicians who aspire to be clinical scientists. This important issue needs to be addressed at the departmental, institutional, national, and perhaps international level. For example, the predominance of surgery in medicine in the past century was accompanied by major discoveries in an environment with robust reimbursement and grant support, which resulted in surgeons becoming leaders in academic medicine. Currently, restricted funding and lower reimbursement due to managed care have significantly decreased the financial revenue of academic departments, especially surgery, slowing the pace of their research and threatening their academic goals.[1,2] Academic physicians in general, and academic surgeons in particular, need innovative approaches in order to restore their prominence and leadership in academic medicine.[3] In many institutions, academic pursuits that do not generate revenue for the department are not valued.

The leadership in academic departments is being replaced by more pragmatic business-minded people, making the situation even worse. Unless there is a new breed of creative leaders who value both research and clinical practices, clinical scientists will become an endangered species. In the meantime, the PI must be creative to apply funds from donations, private foundations, industry, and government in order to carry out clinical research or trials.

3.4 Institutional challenges

The current healthcare environment is such that reimbursement for a medical service is at its lowest in the last ten years. Therefore, it is incumbent upon hospital administrators to make sure they are in the black with respect to the operation of the medical center. For academic institutions with medical schools, the operations of the medical school and medical practices must be in the black as well. Over the past 10-15 years, medical practice has evolved significantly from relatively simple third- party payers to a complex variety of third-party payers. The complex issues of reimbursement will not be discussed in this chapter, but the message for clinical researchers is that because medical expenses are enormous and every effort from every direction is to curb further costs, any research and particularly research that does not bring in direct money from funding agencies, is discouraged by hospital administrators. A sharp dichotomy, therefore, exists between medical care and research mission of an academic institution. This dichotomy has not been resolved and not a single good solution has been instituted.

Although clinical researchers in an academic institution are not only interested in the practice of medicine but also in clinical research to gain new knowledge to advance medicine, the emphasis on generating more revenues from clinical practice predominates over the pursuit of clinical research. The actual funding to conduct clinical trials is relatively limited and at times grants from the NIH may not even cover the actual expenses. Thus, for the PI to have adequate support to conduct clinical research, a commitment from the institution is needed in the form of protected time and an infrastructure that will provide funds, facilities, and expertise to help the PI conduct clinical trials (Chapters 12, 14 and 15).

Research is a slow process. Most of the time, the results are negative and advancement in the field is minimally incremental. Significant breakthroughs and discoveries do not happen every day, and when they do, they are the result of months or years of hard work. A great deal of patience is needed to complete oftentimes very laborious studies. If institutional support is lacking, clinical trials should not be conducted because such trials are bound to result in failure, with a concomitant waste of time for both the PI and his or her team, as well as for the research subjects.

For an academic institution to make an ongoing commitment to both enhance the mission of clinical research and increase revenues, administrators need long-term vision that balances revenue-generating operations with infrastructure and programs to support clinical trials. The cost-benefit ratio for these programs needs to be calculated not only on a daily basis, but perhaps 5-10 years after the infrastructure and programs are established. In fact, major medical institutions that excel in both grant support and clinical activities have successfully struck such a balance. Once the balance is established, the vicious cycle is broken, and clinical research can generate new findings and knowledge that will offer new ways to solve clinical problems. The cost-benefit ratio then significantly increases as new discoveries are made. Thus, it is important for administrators to realize that money should be invested in research.

3.5 ETHICAL, REGULATORY AND LEGAL ISSUES

3.5a Ethical issues

There are no absolute standards for every ethical issue that comes up during the course of a clinical trial. It is in the discussion, the weighing of risks and benefits for an individual patient who is a research subject, that a balanced decision to enter a patient into a clinical trial is made. Such a decision should not be made by the PI alone, but should become the responsibility of the institutional Ethics Committee. Therefore, the Ethics Committee and the IRB should work together in a congenial and harmonious fashion to help the cancer patients or research subjects, and the PI. The PI should be considered a valued partner by the Ethics Committee and IRB. While it is important to protect the rights of patients, it is also the responsibility of the Ethics Committee and IRB to help the PI to navigate through the maze of ethical dilemmas. It is important for them to provide proactive strategies that will help educate PIs about ethical issues, instead of penalizing them severely when they get caught in an ethical dilemma. Current training requirements are inadequate. The FDA, NIH, and local IRB should all emphasize proactive education because conducting clinical trials without proper training is like traveling in uncharted waters. Any clinician or scientist who wishes to become a PI for clinical trials should, at a minimum, be familiar with several of the following online training modules from the NIH:

- http://www.nihtraining.com/

- http://cancer.gov/clinicaltrials/learning/page3

- http://cancer.gov/clinicaltrials/resources/basicworkbook

- http://cancer.gov/clinicaltrials/learning/clinical-trials-education-series

It is important to develop a simulation program to test the PI in difficult clinical situations. Some of the programs listed have limited simulations. More comprehensive simulation programs dealing with day-to-day ethical challenges of clinical trials should be developed.

As mentioned earlier, the PI should have no conflicts of interest, including a desire for recognition and monetary gain. Therefore, to be an ethical PI in clinical trials, one has to have the sole goal of conducting a trial to address a scientific question and bring the study to a fruitful conclusion relating to the hypothesis (Figure 1). On the basis of the major laws, regulations, and guidance relating to clinical trials with human subjects, Emanuel, et al., have proposed at least 7 ethical requirements for making a decision regarding clinical trial involving human subjects. They are 1) social value; 2) scientific validity; 3) fair subject selection; 4) favorable risk-benefit ratio; 5) independent review; 6) informed consent; and 7) respect for enrolled subjects.[4] In addition, collaborative partnership between the PI and the human subject should also be emphasized. PIs are encouraged to visit the NIH ethics website:
http://www.bioethics.nih.gov/resources/index.html.

3.5b   Regulatory issues

Regulations for conducting clinical trials are made to ensure that all the institutional and governmental rules or laws are being followed. The overriding reason for having regulations is to have conformity, homogeneity, and an exact approach to accomplish a previously agreed upon set of rules written in a protocol, so that there is a sense of integrity to the project once it

The role of the principal investigator in cancer clinical trials 169

is accomplished. Without regulations there would be no accountability. Therefore, it is important for the PI to be in compliance with regulations.

To ensure compliance, the PI is subjected to audit (Chapter 9). The consequences of an unsatisfactory audit can sometimes be serious, severely hampering the progress of the project as well as the career of the PI. The goal of the auditors is to make sure that any noncompliant acts will be revealed. The agency conducting the audit ensures that noncompliant acts are penalized appropriately. The ultimate pain inflicted on the PI can be minimal or extensive to the point of prosecuting the PI if the noncompliant act has legal and criminal implications. Because of the potential danger of facing such a penalty, it is intuitive and wise for the PI to understand both why the regulations exist and that there is no compromise but to be compliant with them. This should be understood when the PI signs the dotted line of each protocol before beginning a clinical trial. Before submitting an NIH grant, the PI is asked to sign off on the following statements:

> *By signing this application, I certify (1) to the statements contained in the list of certifications * and (2) that the statements herein are true, complete and accurate to the best of my knowledge. I also provide the required assurances* and agree to comply with any resulting terms if I accept an award. I am aware that any false, fictitious or fraudulent statements or claims may subject me to criminal, civil, or administrative penalties. (U.S. Code, Title 18, Section 1001)*
>
> ☑ ** I agree*
>
> ** The list of certifications and assurances, or an Internet site where you may obtain this list, is contained in the announcement or agency specific instructions.*

It is mandatory that the PI should read every line and make sure absolute compliance is achieved. Otherwise, the PI may be subjected to criminal, civil, or administrative penalties.

Although PIs may find that they have an innate resistance to the rules and regulations for conducting a trial, particularly when they consider themselves experts in the field, they must understand that it is not their prerogative to change the protocol without letting the local IRB or appropriate federal agency know. Therefore, even if the PI has only good intentions, any change of a protocol without appropriate notification constitutes a major violation of the regulations and will have a severe consequence.

Regulations impose restrictions regarding the creativity of research, and since cancer clinical trials are research, these restrictions may be in direct confrontation with the very premise of research creativity. Therefore, the PI should be proactive in discussing these restrictions with their local IRB, Ethics Committee, and the governmental agencies overseeing the research so that these restrictions may be officially lifted from the protocol. Healthy communication should be established so issues relating to the regulations can be voiced quickly and discussed. Any changes can then be made if it turns out that the regulations do not meet the intention of the original creators, hamper the progress of the clinical trials, or are potentially having negative effects on the research subjects. This type of healthy communication is best demonstrated by the American College of Surgeons, working with the government to modify HIPAA regulations (Chapter 11). The current regulatory requirement is to inform the IRB and FDA of any change in the protocol. Such a requirement, therefore, needs to be incorporated into the planning for cancer clinical trials, and the budget should reflect the need to attend to these regulatory details when running a trial.

The PI must adhere to the rigid rules of the protocol while conducting the cancer clinical trial. Clearly, each patient should be considered as a subject and not as a patient. Any deviation from the protocol will constitute noncompliance and a violation. The PI should be aware that when a complaint about the conduct of a trial is brought up, the institution must conduct an investigation. World-wide release of the investigation will be issued to all the parties involved, including co-investigators and all the agencies, as shown in Figure 3, through the Federal Wide Assurance that is granted to an investigator's home institution. When a negative judgment is rendered or misconduct is found, it will be published on the FDA's website: http://www.fda.gov/ora/compliance_ref/bimo/dis_res_assur.htm

If misconduct is found to be intentional fraud (Chapter 13), the PI will be barred from receiving any NIH funding for five years. The PI's institution may also be affected by any serious occurrences or violations with temporary suspension of all clinical trials, as was the case in two notable, recent examples at Johns Hopkins[5] and Duke.[6, 7] Potentially, the medical staff board of a PI's institution may submit such a misconduct finding to the State's Medical Licensure Board for consideration of disciplinary action.

While it is important to emphasize the issue of sanctity of scientific integrity within the context of clinical trials, it is not only counterproductive, but destructive when scientific integrity is used to haunt and lynch the PIs who may be noncompliant due to technical errors. Auditors, or those involved with the evaluation of a study should not automatically assert that any violation of the protocol is a violation of scientific integrity. They should give the PI the benefit of the doubt. Every regulation should not and cannot be considered an absolute law cast in stone as it may not apply in certain situations. Therefore, there should be room for appeal or consultation with the PI. Nonetheless, the PI must appreciate the importance of conducting clinical trials in accordance with the laws and regulations, and if he or she disagrees with them, the PI should make every attempt to change them through the proper channels.

Regulatory violations may occur for several reasons: 1) lack of knowledge, 2) negligence, and 3) bypassing regulations out of compassion to make an exception for an individual patient. Therefore, the PI should not act alone, but always in consultation with the Ethics Committee and the IRB. In view of the potential pitfalls and complex ethical issues of conducting cancer clinical trials, it is important for any institution to formulate clinical trial bylaws for PIs and to describe penalties associated with violations, just like bylaws of the medical staff for practicing clinicians in any licensed hospital.

3.5c Legal issues

In the practice of medicine, any deviation from established standards of care or negligence may be brought up by patients in the form of litigation. Such cases will be processed through the legal malpractice system. Medical malpractice law is a specialty within the legal system. Therefore, when a patient decides to sue, he or she will be represented by a plaintiff malpractice lawyer and the notification to the physician will be made. Upon receipt of such notification, a defense malpractice lawyer will usually be hired by the physician. Depositions, arbitration, or an eventual court case to be decided by a jury may follow. Malpractice may result in further criminal charges.

In contrast, in the context of a clinical research trial, no established legal system is available. Oftentimes, a violation may be reported by a patient, a subordinate such as a nurse, or a colleague. In such situations, the complaint will be reviewed by an ad hoc committee and if the complaint is deemed valid, an investigation will be forthcoming, and the final decisions will be made by the committee. Because of potential implications for the PI's medical career and possibly criminal charges, lawyers may be involved. In general, issues about research conduct are somewhat new to lawyers. There is not an established legal subspecialty like malpractice law. When a

PI is being investigated by a university committee, he or she must hire a malpractice defense attorney.

3.6 Funding

Before the PI begins a study, funding should be secured. In general, NIH is the major source of funding. According to the NIH, the definition of PI is as follows:

Principal Investigator: *The principal investigator (PI) (also may be known as "program director" or "project director") is the individual, designated by the grantee, responsible for the scientific or technical aspects of the grant and for day-to-day management of the project or program. The PI is not required to be an employee of the grantee. However, since the grant, if awarded, is made to the organization, the applicant organization must have a formal written agreement with the PI that specifies an official relationship between the parties, but need not involve a salary or other form of remuneration. If the PI is not an employee of the applicant organization, NIH will assess whether the arrangement will result in the organization being able to fulfill its responsibilities under the grant, if awarded.*

The PI is a member of the grantee team responsible for ensuring compliance with the financial and administrative aspects of the award. He or she works closely with designated officials within the grantee organization to create and maintain necessary documentation, including both technical and administrative reports; prepare justifications; ensure that Federal support of research findings is appropriately acknowledged in publications, announcements, news programs, etc., and comply with organizational as well as Federal requirements. NIH encourages the PI to maintain contact with the NIH Program Official with respect to the scientific aspects of the project and the designated GMO concerning the business and administrative aspects of the award.

(http://grants.nih.gov/grants/policy/nihgps_2001/part_i_1.htm#_Toc504811751)

There are many good resources that discuss how to write and obtain a grant.[8,9] Additional websites are listed below:

www.training.nih.gov/careers/careercenter/grants.html#prop

www.niaid.nih.gov/ncn/grants/app/default.htm

http://www.survival.pitt.edu/library/documents.asp

http://www.facs.org/cqi/src/youngbroch.html

When the PI wishes to conduct one's own study, he or she may submit an R01 grant or a response to a specific request from the National Cancer Institute soliciting proposals within a certain area of clinical research. The PI will then write a grant that follows the usual format, including a protocol, hypothesis, rationale, specific aims, preliminary data and research methods. If the grant is funded, there will be money to conduct a clinical trial. Some types of studies are frequently sponsored by pharmaceutical companies. Since pharmaceutical studies require appropriate patients for the study, the PI will match his or her interests with the pharmaceutical company's and will collaborate on a research project. In the process of doing so, the project is usually quite well-structured and the primary function of the PI is to rewrite the protocol into the institutional format and submit it to his or her institution's IRB for approval. Once approved, the protocol can begin, patients can be enrolled, and the PI should conduct the study in compliance with all the requirements of the protocol. Oftentimes, with pharmaceutical companies, legal contracts will be signed, which requires the legal counsel for both the institution and the company. NIH or other grants will be processed through the office of contracts and grants within the institution.

3.7 AUDITS

Audit is a process to assure the integrity of the clinical trial and the PI (Chapter 9). Oftentimes after an audit, either the auditing committee or the FDA points out the PI's deficiencies and noncompliant acts relating to the conduct of the clinical trial as outlined in the original protocol. Violations may be classified as minor or major. Sometimes, the conclusion for the auditors may be quite harsh, including phrases like, "violation of the integrity of the study" and "may be harmful to patients." It is a good idea for each PI to be briefed about the auditing process before the study begins. In the early part of the trial, a mock audit may be helpful to the PI. To be human is to err. A more compassionate and forgiving spirit should be adopted[10] by the auditing committee.

4. HOW TO TURN CHALLENGES INTO USER-FRIENDLY STRATEGIES

The PI must be familiar with all of the issues and challenges presented in this chapter. After a thorough review of these issues, the hope is that the PI will develop a strategy and infrastructure to deal with these challenges, while remembering that it is noble to conduct cancer clinical trials in order to help cancer patients. PIs should constantly remind themselves of the characteristics they should possess if they wish to be involved with clinical trials (Table 3). These personal values are essential for building character for physicians in general, and, in particular, for clinician scientists who have keen observational skills and a determination to advance the field, so that new frontiers can be reached and innovative therapies can be established.

The responsibilities and modus operandi of a PI are summarized in Table 5. To avoid serious pitfalls in conducting clinical trials, the PI should adhere to the ten rules enumerated in Table 4. Although the rules may expand as the PI becomes more involved with clinical trials, they serve as important initial guidelines to keep the PI out of trouble. To start with, the PI should develop a well thought out protocol to tackle an important clinical observation and hypothesis (Figure 1). The simpler the protocol, the more focused the trial will be. The PI should distinguish between caring for the patient and treating the research subject (Figure 2), and understand the complicated infrastructure of a clinical trial from within and without (Figure 3). The PI is the captain of the team, but also a member. Rules and regulations apply to this team. Communication within the team is critical for it to function well and be successful. The clinical trial must be well-funded and carefully monitored to ensure that it is properly conducted. At any time, the PI should be ready for both an internal audit by an institutional committee and an external audit by the FDA. He or she has to "survive" the audit, otherwise the trial will be terminated. The PI needs to know the significance of any violation or noncompliance in carrying out the protocol. In general, when one major violation is made, it is quickly assumed by the auditing committee and others that the PI may be prone to make other major violations. Therefore, on the basis of these assumptions, the IRB, or the FDA will in general put all the PI's protocols on hold, particularly if a violation is a major one. The PI needs to understand that auditors look for strict adherence to the protocol, even when issues of compassion and ethics are the reason for noncompliance or violation. Only when such a violation is explained to the appropriate committee before the audit will it not be considered a violation or noncompliance, but an exemption.

Table 4. Ten rules not to be broken by the PI.

1. Do not initiate a clinical trial for the sake of running it, but rather a burning desire to solve a clinical dilemma.
2. Do not write a lengthy and complicated protocol, because it will be difficult to achieve compliance.
3. Do not deviate from whatever is written in the protocol, as the protocol is the regulatory document of compliance.
4. Do not initiate the protocol unless it is truly funded.
5. Do not commit yourself beyond the financial and time commitment.
6. Do not forget your deadlines.
7. Do not cover up your mistakes. Report immediately that they are not intentional and that you anticipate immediate remedy and resolution.
8. Do not make any statements in your chart without supporting sources of evidence.
9. Do not report anything that you are not sure of and report only what you know to be true.
10. Do not commit plagiarism. Always paraphrase someone's writings and reference them.

Table 5. Summary of the Essential Modus Operandi of the PI

- You must be qualified to be a Principal Investigator.
- As the PI, the buck stops with you.
- The PI is responsible for protocol design and implementation, subject selection and treatment and data collection and verification.
- Documentation is essential.
- Clearly articulated informed consent is critical. It must be signed and dated before patient enrollment begins.
- Clinical research must meet standards. These standards require adequate infrastructure.
- Implement and document your study as though it might be audited by an internal or external team.

Reproduced from presentation by Gregory Curt, MD, Clinical Director, National Cancer Institute, National Institutes of Health (http://www.nihtraining.com/crtpub_508/index.html).

The PI must ensure that all steps of the protocol are conducted in compliance with the regulations and should read the regulations in detail before launching a clinical trial. It is equally important for the institution to have experts for the PI to consult with regarding all compliance issues and regulations. Whenever an adverse event occurs, the PI should automatically and quickly summarize the adverse event and report it to the IRB and the FDA, no matter what and how minor it is. It is also important to write in the consent form that adverse reactions may occur that are not included in the consent form so that subjects understand that certain unforeseen adverse reactions may occur during a clinical trial. To follow all of the regulations and be compliant, each study requires an adequate number of clinical coordinators and nurses available to 1) register these adverse reactions, and 2) to report them appropriately, using a previously designed format. Because PIs are often quite busy, a clinical trial should not be conducted without adequate personnel simply because the PI may not have the time to register these adverse reactions in a timely manner.

A PI does not want to break the rules intentionally, but at times, a rule may be so impractical that a change is needed. In such cases, the PI should express his or her concerns to the local IRB and perhaps even the FDA and NIH. Although it may take some time to change the rules governing a protocol, once these rules are formally changed, everyone benefits, especially our patients, or rather subjects.

5. SUMMARY

In summary, cancer clinical trials are not easy to run. Every PI should be well prepared to meet the complex challenges inherent in conducting clinical trials and be proud to be engaged in the search for a "cure" for cancer patients.

ACKNOWLEDGEMENTS

I would like to thank Pamela Derish of the UCSF Department of Surgery for her editorial review of the manuscript. Also, I appreciate the effort of Jorge Arteaga and Regina Hopkins of the UCSF Department of Surgery in the preparation of the manuscript.

REFERENCES

1. Debas HT. Impact of the health care crisis on surgery: perspective of the dean. *Arch Surg.* Feb 2001;136(2):158-160.
2. Chang AE. Protecting an Endangered Species: the Surgeon-Scientist. *Contemporary Surgery.* Vol 62,; 2006:102-104.
3. Jones RS. Requiem and renewal. *Ann Surg.* Sep 2004;240(3):395-404.
4. Emanuel EJ, Wendler D, Grady C. What makes clinical research ethical? *Jama.* May 24-31 2000;283(20):2701-2711.
5. Steinbrook R. Protecting research subjects--the crisis at Johns Hopkins. *N Engl J Med.* Feb 28 2002;346(9):716-720.
6. Kaplan S, Brownlee S. Duke's hazards. Did medical experiments put patients needlessly at risk? *US News World Rep.* May 24 1999;126(20):66-68, 70.
7. Marshall E. Shutdown of research at Duke sends a message. *Science.* May 21 1999;284(5418):1246.
8. Inouye SK, Fiellin DA. An evidence-based guide to writing grant proposals for clinical research. *Ann Intern Med.* Feb 15 2005;142(4):274-282.
9. Zeiger M. *Essentials of Writing Biomedical Research Papers.* 2nd Ed. ed. New York: McGraw Hill; 2000.
10. Bosk CL. *Forgive and Remember.* Chicago: The University of Chicago Press; 1979.

Chapter 9

THE AUDIT PROCESS AND HOW TO ENSURE A SUCCESSFUL AUDIT

Y. Nancy You, MD [1,4]; Lisa Jacobs, MD [2,4]; Elizabeth Martinez, LPN, BS [4] David M. Ota, MD [3,4]

[1] *Department of Surgery, Mayo Clinic, Rochester, MN* [2] *Deparment of Surgery, John Hopkins University, Baltimore, MD* [3]*Department of Surgery, Duke University Medical Center, Durham, NC* [4] *American College of Surgeons Oncology Group, Durham, NC, USA*

Supported by the Ruth L. Kirschstein National Research Service Awards Training Grant T32CA101695 and the American College of Surgeons Oncology Group Grant U10CA76001, both from the National Cancer Institute.

Key words: Audit, quality assurance, clinical trials

1. INTRODUCTION

Over the past several decades, there has been increasing emphasis on evidence-based clinical practice. Prospective randomized multi-institutional clinical trials have emerged at the pinnacle of evidence-based medicine. The integrity and dependability of this gold standard must be assured if results from clinical trials are to define the optimal care for patients afflicted by malignancies.

Since the early 1980's, formal policies for monitoring clinical trials have been instituted by the National Cancer Institute (NCI), the world's largest sponsor of clinical trials involving anti-neoplastic therapies. *Quality assurance* may be defined as "any method or procedure for collecting, processing, or analyzing study data that is aimed at maintaining or enhancing their reliability and validity."[1] Quality control of clinical trials requires supervision of the entire trial process. Key elements to monitor include: adherence to the protocol, absence of bias in treatment assignment, confirmation of subject eligibility, protection of human research subjects, accountability of the study medications, accuracy and timeliness of data submission, and honesty in data analysis and reporting.

This chapter aims to summarize the purpose, the federal requirements, the processes and the outcomes of quality assurance audit programs, particularly in regards to clinical trials sponsored by cooperative groups.

2. WHY AUDIT?

Clinical trials have played pivotal roles in the care of cancer patients. Randomized comparisons of therapies have defined the optimal treatment strategy; early-phase investigations involving novel agents have stimulated and advanced cancer care; and multi-institutional trial participation has propagated promising new treatments to many patients. As scientists and care providers, clinical trialists must assure and protect the integrity of clinical trials. A *quality assurance audit* is a formal process by which the quality and completeness of the reported trial data are independently appraised in relation to the raw clinical data and the actual conduct of the trial. Detecting both systematic errors as well as deliberate falsifications of data is important for ensuring that trial outcomes are valid. Indeed, quality control represents both an ethical obligation to the human subjects who voluntarily participate in the clinical trials, as well as a scientific obligation to the trial investigators who contribute to the collective results of the trial.

The NCI has defined several goals for the quality assurance program of cooperative groups.[2]

1. Auditing aims to *prevent* problems by fostering the development of a responsible research team. Investigators who understand the importance of faithful adherence to the trial protocol will likely recruit and train support staff who are careful and honest in data collection and reporting.[3] Building such a research team guards against noncompliance with the protocol or the regulatory requirements.
2. The audit program aims to *detect* problems through periodic monitors and checks. Random errors and systemic errors may result in data that are missing, incorrect or variable beyond expected ranges. These errors may be detected by statistical methods. Auditing, as defined above, is a process where reported data are checked against the original medical records or source documents, constitutes a more detailed and rigorous method of error detection.[1]
3. The third goal of the audit process is to ensure timely and effective *correction* of detected errors. Indeed, deficiencies identified in an audit

require responses from enrolling institutions within a pre-defined time frame.
4. Finally, the quality assurance audit has been increasingly recognized as a valuable *educational* opportunity. Through on-site visits, the audit staff not only evaluates the trial support structure at individual institutions, but also compares and shares sound research practices from other member institutions. Additionally, as identified deficiencies are communicated and plans for corrective action are developed, the investigators and the institution have the opportunity to learn and improve their research practices in the future.

3. WHAT ARE THE FEDERAL INFRASTRUCTURE AND REQUIREMENTS FOR AUDITING?

Since the inception of the Clinical Trials Cooperative Group Program in the mid 1950's, the peer-review quality assurance program has been a key and required component of the National Cancer Institute funding process. Over the ensuing decades, the federal requirements became formalized. In 1977, the Food and Drug Administration (FDA), in their responsibility of overseeing the use of Investigational New Drug (IND) in human subjects, proposed a system of annual site visits to each investigator. This was soon adopted and practiced by many of the individual cooperative groups. In 1982, the NCI formally required the presence of an on-site monitoring program for all clinical trials cooperative groups.[4] Subsequently, the Clinical Trials Monitoring Branch (CTMB) of the Cancer Therapy Evaluation Program (CTEP) was established at the NCI. The jurisdiction of CTMB applies to all clinical trials sponsored by the Cooperative groups, the Community Clinical Oncology Program (CCOP) as well as the Cancer Trials Support Unit (CTSU).

The responsibilities of the CTMB include the following:

3.1 Establish federal requirements and guidelines for auditing programs

The primary responsibility of the CTMB is to establish federal guidelines for the monitoring of clinical trials, including those for quality assurance audits specifically.

According to the CTMB, an audit program accomplishes the following objectives:
1. to verify the study data relevant to the primary endpoints of the clinical trial through independent verification against source documents;
2. to verify investigator compliance with the protocol; and
3. to verify investigator and site compliance with regulatory requirements.[2]

Additionally, the federal guidelines specify a minimum frequency for on-site audits. All institutions are required to be audited at least once every 36 months. Any institution that 1) has an Institutional Review Board (IRB) that reviews and approves trial protocols from cooperative groups (or holds an IRB agreement approved by the Office for Human Research Protections (OHRP)); and 2) consents and enrolls patients for clinical trials sponsored by the cooperative groups, is eligible for audits. All such institutions are thus bound by this requirement.

Furthermore, these institutions ought to formally belong to the membership of the cooperative group. While the definitions of membership categories vary among individual cooperative groups, three broad groups are recognized by the CTMB:
- *Main member institutions* are comprised of largely academic or major medical centers. These institutions typically tend to be high-volume accruers, and have devoted significant institutional resources such as research or regulatory personnel to clinical trials.
- *Affiliates* typically include community-based institutions, which may share certain institutional research infrastructure with Main member institutions.
- *CCOPs* are comprised of community physicians working in groups, clinics, hospitals, or health maintenance organizations (HMOs).

It is important to realize that when institutions terminate or withdraw their membership from a cooperative group, they must discontinue consenting or enrolling new patients to trials sponsored by that cooperative group. However, these institutions remain eligible for on-site audits as long as extended follow-up and data collection are being conducted for any of the patients enrolled prior to membership termination.

3.2 Oversee the conduct of audits

Additional responsibilities of the CTMB relate to overseeing the conduct of on-site audits and reviewing compliance with federal guidelines. Specific roles of the CTMB include:
1. The CTMB staff reviews the scheduling of all audits. In order for CTMB to assess compliance with the required frequency of audits, all cooperative groups must maintain a comprehensive and updated

tabulation of its member institutions. Such a roster must include the following details: 1) dates on which the institution are affiliated with or terminated from the cooperative group; 2) accrual of patients to trials sponsored by the cooperative group during the preceding 36 months divided by year; 3) projected patient accrual for the upcoming year; 4) the date of the most recent audit; and 5) the projected date for the next proposed audit.
2. The CTMB reviews audit reports and findings. When individual cooperative groups identify data irregularities or other deficiencies suggestive of intentional misconduct, cooperative groups are required to report their findings immediately to the CTMB. The CTMB may subsequently alert other federal agencies such as the Food and Drug Administration (FDA), the Office of Research Integrity (ORI) and the Office for Human Research Protections (OHRP). Additionally, the CTMB may coordinate and conduct special audits for further investigation. The audit staff participating in such special audits is jointly selected from the cooperative group, the CTMB, as well as other federal agencies. The final composition of the audit team remains at the discretion of the CTMB.[2]
3. The CTMB monitors for consistency in the conduct of on-site audits within and across the cooperative groups. Thus, CTMB representatives may elect to attend any routine on-site audits. The presence of CTMB is essential for maintaining uniformity in the conduct of clinical trials auditing programs among all the cooperative groups. The consequence of not having a central agency setting rules and standards for conducting clinical research is that different rules and standards would be created among cooperative groups.

3.3 Serve as an educational resource

Finally, the CTMB is responsible for serving as the educational resource for issues and questions regarding quality assurance, monitoring and audit processes from the oncology clinical trials community.

4. WHAT PREPARATIONS ARE NEEDED PRIOR TO AN ON-SITE AUDIT?

The majority of the audits conducted by a cooperative group are routine audits which occur at a minimum frequency of once every 36 months or 3 years for a given institution. In addition, cooperative groups may choose to audit those institutions that have newly initiated patient enrollment. These "*initial treatment audits*" typically occur within a certain period (e.g. 18 months) of the first patient registration at an enrolling site. Individual cooperative group may also decide to audit an institution more frequently. These "*off-cycle audits*" are considered when data quality is questionable, when trials involving investigational agents are active, and when a substantial increase occurs in patient accrual or reported adverse events.[5] Each cooperative group should establish its policies and standard operating procedures for on-site audits, and clearly communicate them to their member institutions.

In general, the planning and arrangements for an on-site audit begin several months in advance of the anticipated audit date. Pre-audit arrangements include: scheduling of the time and place of the audit, selection of the protocols and patient cases to be audited, and selection of the audit team.

4.1 Scheduling of the on-site audit

The CTMB requires that the date of the scheduled audit be entered into the CTMB Audit Information System (AIS) at least six to ten weeks prior to the audit date. Therefore, institutions that are due for audits in the upcoming months are identified from the group membership roster several months ahead. The cooperative group audit team staff then contacts the responsible physician leader or main research staff at the institution to schedule a date for the audit. The date of the anticipated audit should be chosen ensuring that the research staff will be available to assist the visiting audit team throughout the day, and the physician leader or his/her designee will be available for the final exit interview where audit findings are reviewed. Once an agreed-upon date is identified, written confirmation is exchanged between the audit team and the institution. It is the responsibility of the cooperative group to provide the confirmed date of the audit to the CTMB AIS within the required time frame.

4.2 Selection of the protocols and patient cases to be audited

All active protocols being conducted at the institution are eligible to be selected for review. A minimum of 3 protocols should be selected for audit according to guidelines from the CTMB. When more than 3 protocols are active at the institution being audited, priorities may be given to those protocols involving investigational agents, complex multimodality interventions, and high accrual.[2] For institutions with fewer than 3 active protocols, all protocols may be reviewed. The list of protocols to be audited is typically chosen by the statistical and the data management office of the cooperative groups.

Patient cases to be reviewed include announced cases and unannounced cases. The CTMB requires that the cooperative group supply the institution with the list of announced cases to be reviewed at least 2 weeks but not more than 4 weeks prior to the date of the scheduled audit. The site is notified of the unannounced case at the time of the audit. All announced cases receive a complete review. Unannounced cases may receive only a limited review concentrating on verification of protocol compliance and regulatory requirements.

According to CTMB requirements, the minimum number of cases to receive a complete audit review should be 10% of all patients accrued since the previous institutional audit.[1,2] A complete review achieves all three objectives of an audit discussed in 5.1, namely compliance with regulatory requirements, accountability of pharmacological agents, and adherence to the trial protocol. When the medical records of an announced case are not available for review on the day of the audit, another patient case should be selected for complete review. It is important to note that unannounced cases which may have received only a limited review do not count toward the minimum of 10% as required by the CTMB.

4.3 Selection of the on-site audit team

The audit team should be composed of staff who are familiar with the federal requirements of the audit process, the conduct and regulations of clinical trials, and the protocols being audited. The CTMB guidelines specify that at least one member of the audit team should have sufficient medical background as to verify patient eligibility, assess protocol compliance and review medical interventions. It is also important to recall that members of the CTMB or any other federal agency may choose to attend any audit conduced by the cooperative groups.[2,5]

5. HOW IS AN ON-SITE AUDIT CONDUCTED AND HOW TO PREPARE FOR IT?

5.1 Components of an on-site audit

The objectives of an audit are to verify the study data submitted to the cooperative groups, and to verify compliance with the protocol as well as the regulatory requirements. Accordingly, the key components of an audit include:

1. Assess compliance with research regulations by reviewing the Institutional Review Board (IRB) documentations and the informed consents of each protocol;
2. verify accountability of investigational agents by reviewing pharmacy operations and records;
3. evaluate protocol compliance through patient case review; and
4. conduct an exit interview where preliminary findings of the audit are discussed.

5.2 Institutional preparation for an on-site audit

The best preparation for an audit is performed prospectively. As protocols are activated and patients are enrolled, records should be meticulously kept, tracked and stored. Participating physician investigators should periodically review the performance of the research team, identify any problems and correct them internally. [3, 6]

Prior to the scheduled audit, during the weeks after the institution is notified of the protocols and the patient cases to be audited, the institution should ensure that all relevant materials would be available. Relevant materials include any and all source documents which would enable verification of submitted data. *Source documentation* is defined as the first recording of any observation made or data generated about a patient while the patient is enrolled in a clinical trial. Examples include original IRB documents, informed consents, NCI Drug Accountability Record Forms (DARFs), medical records (notes, diagnostic test reports, laboratory data, procedural reports, etc.), research records signed and dated by the study personnel prospectively while evaluating a patient for the protocol, and subject diaries or calendars. All source documents should include patient identifiers as well as dates and signatures of their authors. Therefore, protocol-specific Case Report Forms (CRFs) which include data transcribed from primary records and documents cannot serve as source documents.[2]

In order to expedite the on-site audit, the IRB documentation, the informed consents and the NCI DARFs may be requested and reviewed by the audit team prior to arrival on-site. Therefore, it is prudent for institutions to keep IRB approval letters in a separate binder filed under each specific protocol. Furthermore, to facilitate the audit team's navigation through the institution's medical records on the day of the audit, the research team should locate and centralize needed source documents as much as possible. Dividers and tags to flag relevant sections are highly recommended.[6] Organized notebooks are essential for auditors to link source documents with data recorded on a CRF and to track revised informed consents with protocol amendments. The absence of such organized documents can result in a problematic audit and outcome. For those institutions utilizing electronic medical records only, they may be required by the cooperative group to produce paper versions of the relevant records. They should also disclose information regarding the security of the electronic records to the auditors. Specifically, procedures regarding eligibility for access, protection (e.g. password), electronic signature and the tracking of record changes may be discussed.[5]

In the process of preparing for an audit, institutions may recognize delinquencies in the upkeep of their research records or other deficiencies in their research practices. Corrective actions may be initiated as soon as these deficiencies are recognized, and may include: correcting mistakes on submitted CRFs, completing and updating IRB documentations, reporting adverse events, and streamlining certain institutional procedures. At the time of the audit, although the original deficiencies will still be considered as deficiencies, they will generally be rated less severely because of the corrective action plan already instituted by the site prior to the date of the audit.

5.3 Assessments and findings of an audit

During an audit, evaluations of each of the three key components (i.e. the IRB and informed consent, the pharmacy and the patient cases) are conducted independently of each other. Each component is assessed and rated as either Acceptable, Acceptable needing follow-up, or Unacceptable. While these ratings are difficult to define precisely, the CTMB has established a set of major or lesser deficiencies that is used commonly by all cooperative groups. A complete set of ratings as defined by the CTMB can be found at http://ctep.cancer.gov/monitoring, and are outlined below.

5.3.1 Review of IRB documentation and informed consent contents

Source documents from the IRB should identify the specific protocols being audited, the type of IRB review (e.g. full board, or expedited), the reason for review (e.g. initial, renewal, or amendment), and the dates of approval and approval expiration. The CTMB requires that the following items be reviewed at the minimum:
1. Documentation of the initial approval of each protocol and informed consent by a full IRB;
2. Documentation of annual re-approval of each protocol and informed consent by a full IRB;
3. Documentation of IRB approval of all protocol amendments and consent form revisions;

4. Documentation that IRB approvals are dated prior to the first patient registration.

While continuing re-approval of the protocols must be completed in a timely manner, patient registration must be suspended if re-approval is delayed for any reason. Re-approval is termed *"Delayed"* when previous approval has ended for more than 30 days but less than 1 year; termed *"Expired"* when previous approval has ended for more than 1 year; and *"Missed"* when re-approval documentation are missing.

Informed consents from each of the selected protocols must be reviewed for inclusion of all required elements as well as of the risks and benefits listed in the protocol model informed consent approved by the NCI. An informed consent must describe the purpose, duration, experimental procedures, risks, benefits, alternatives of the proposed study; it must explain the extent of the confidentiality of medical records while noting that the cooperative group and federal agencies may inspect records; it must address compensation, research-related injuries, and voluntary participation; and finally it must provide contact information for further questions.[7] For protocols with specific components such as specimen banking or correlative basic science studies, the informed consent must include sub-sections delineating each component with separate signature lines.

Common examples of major deficiencies in IRB documentation and informed consent include: initial approval of the protocol and consent were never received, missing, or improperly conducted via an expedited review; re-approval was delayed, expired or missing; patients were registered or treated prior to initial approval, or during a period of delayed re-approval; Serious Adverse Events (SAEs) are not reported to the IRB; and required elements are omitted from the informed consent.

5.3.2 Review of Accountability of Investigational agents and pharmacy operations

For all audited institutions, a tour of the pharmacy and/or drug storage facility may be requested. Drug accountability practices and drug storage and handling procedures are discussed. The shelf inventory records are compared to the drug inventory logs, and the drug accountability records are compared with patient administration records. For those institutions participating in protocols involving the use of investigational agents supplied by Pharmaceutical Management Branch (PMB), the Division of Cancer Treatment and Diagnosis (DCTD) at the NCI, particular emphasis is placed on pharmacy review.[8]

The audit process and how to ensure a successful audit 189

In lieu of defined deficiencies, the CTMB has defined criteria for compliant and non-compliant practices with regards to several specific areas:
1. The NCI Drug Accountability Report Forms (DARFs) are correctly and completely filed;
2. Drugs are accounted for specifically for each protocol, each patient, and each dose administration;
3. DARFs are kept at each satellite location where the drugs are stored or dispensed;
4. DARFs serve as the primary transaction record, accounting for all agent orders, agent returns, inter-institutional transfers, etc. and result in a balance that matches with the amount of the drug supplied from NCI;
5. Outdated, damaged, discontinued agents, and drugs related to completed or closed protocols, are promptly returned to the NCI;
6. Storage is separated by protocols;
7. Storage area is secure with restricted access only.

Detailed listings of other examples of compliant and non-compliant practices are found at http://ctep.cancer.gov/monitoring. The most common errors found during a pharmacy review involve inaccurate record keeping on the DARFs and the lack of restricted access to the storage area.

5.3.3 Review of patient records

Patient record review constitutes the main component of on-site audits. Data submitted via CRFs to the cooperative groups are checked against the source documentation. Six areas will be reviewed according to guidelines from the CTMB:
1. Informed consent

The original informed consent document should be a complete document (no missing pages), contain patient and/or witness signatures dated prior to participation in any protocol-related activities, and kept current when protocol amendments require patient re-consent.
2. Eligibility

Elements of the inclusion and exclusion criteria are verified to ensure that the enrolled patient was eligible for the specific protocol. Enrolling investigators may consider including specific statements in the original medical records which verify each of the specific conditions of the eligibility criteria.
3. Treatment

Treatment interventions including operations, sample acquisition procedures, and other medical therapies are reviewed for dates of initiation and completion, schedule of administration, and the agents and dosages administered. Any adjustment, delay or deviation from the protocol must be justified. An unjustified dose deviation of >10% constitutes a major deficiency. For studies including operative interventions, the operative report will be reviewed to confirm adherence to the protocol requirements.

4. Disease outcome and response

Tumor response should be assigned according to the response criteria outlined in the protocols.

5. Toxicity

An adverse event (AE) may be any unintended or unfavorable sign, symptom or disease occurring during or for a pre-defined period after the protocol intervention. However, toxicity refers specifically to an AE which has been determined to have a causal relationship to the protocol intervention.[9] Both AEs and toxicities must be carefully identified, assessed and substantiated in the medical records. The determination of grade and causality attribution must be performed by the investigator or other medical personnel. Any repetitive failure to report or incorrect reporting of the toxicities is noted as a deficiency.

6. General data quality

The quality of submitted data is assessed for completeness, accuracy and timeliness. Medical records are checked for protocol-specified laboratory tests and diagnostic studies.

Common examples of deficiencies in each of the six areas are provided by the CTMB guidelines at http://ctep.cancer.gov/monitoring.

6. HOW ARE AUDIT FINDINGS REPORTED AND HOW TO RESPOND TO THEM?

6.1 Assessments of audit findings

After all relevant information is reviewed; the audit team makes an overall assessment of the research performance at the audited institution. Each of the three components (IRB/informed consent, pharmacy and patient case review) is independently assessed and assigned a rating of Acceptable, Acceptable needing follow-up or Unacceptable. Standardized criteria for each rating are defined by the CTMB for use by all cooperative groups.

Table 1. Rating criteria for IRB/Informed consent and for Patient Case Review

Acceptable	• No deficiencies • Few lesser deficiencies • Major deficiencies identified during the audit that have been corrected prior to on-site audit (documented) and requires no further action
Acceptable needs follow-up	• Multiple lesser deficiencies • Major deficiencies not corrected prior to on-site audit
Unacceptable	• Excessive number of or recurring lesser deficiencies • Flagrant major deficiency • Multiple major deficiencies

Table 2. Rating criteria for Pharmacy

Acceptable	• No noncompliance • Non-compliant items identified during the audit that have been corrected prior to on-site audit (documented) and requires no further action
Acceptable needs follow-up	• Non-compliant items not corrected prior to on-site audit
Unacceptable	• Multiple non-compliant items • Unable to track the disposition of NCI-supplied investigational agents

6.2 Communication of audit assessments

The initial communication of audit assessments takes place during the exit interview at the conclusion of the on-site audit. This is typically conducted by the audit team with enrolling investigators, research staff, and possibly the research regulatory personnel from the institution. As preliminary findings are discussed, the exit interview serves as a forum for face-to-face discussion, information exchange and education.

A preliminary report of audit findings must be completed by the cooperative group audit staff and faxed to the CTMB within one working day of the on-site audit. Major deficiencies in any component must be delineated. Any findings suspicious for intentional misrepresentation of data must be reported to the CTMB immediately by phone. The CTMB must be involved in subsequent actions taken towards such behaviors.[2]

A final report of audit findings is filed by the cooperative group with the CTMB Audit Information System within 70 working days of the on-site audit. This report includes detailed information regarding the institution, the protocols reviewed, the number of patient cases reviewed, names of the investigational agents and treatment modalities, and the average accrual per year. The institutional staff, the audit team staff, and other investigators present at the on-site audit and the exit interview should be noted. All deficiencies and audit assessments are detailed and separated into each of the three components. Recommendations made at the exit interview as well as any plans for possible re-audit are recorded in the final report.

6.3 Follow-up and expected responses from institutions

After the submission of the final audit report to the CTMB, the institution is expected to submit a written response. This plan of action must address each specific area of major deficiency and non-compliance, covering each and every component rated as Acceptable Needing Follow-up or Unacceptable. Prior to submission, the proposed plan is typically communicated with the cooperative group within a few days for review. A finalized plan of action must be filed with the CTMB within 45 days after the final audit report. Proposed corrective actions may include correction of errors detected on CRFs, re-submission of CRFs with corrected clinical information, completion of all regulatory documentation, plans to obtain extra training in the conduct of clinical trials, and others. All corrective action plans should provide a statement as to the changes at the institution that will prevent similar errors in the futures. Failure of an institution to file a written response may result in suspension of patient enrollment at the given institution.[5]

When any one of the audited components was found to be Unacceptable at a given institution, a re-audit must be conducted if the institution remains an active site. Re-audits are typically conducted within 12-18 months of the original audit, and may be conducted on-site or off-site. As re-audits are mandated by the CTMB, they must be reported to the AIS as soon as they have been scheduled.

In rare incidences of very poor trial performance, unresponsiveness to audit findings, and failure to develop or follow a corrective plan of action, the cooperative group may suspend patient registration privileges at an institution or even recommend termination of membership.[5, 10]

6.4 Scientific misconduct

Fraud or misconduct is difficult to define. According to the Policy on Responsible Conduct of Research (RCR) from the Office of Research Integrity, scientific misconduct encompasses the following elements: 1) a significant departure from accepted practices of the relevant research community; 2) the misconduct is committed intentionally, knowingly, or recklessly; and 3) the allegation is proven by a preponderance of evidence.[1]

The reported frequency of scientific misconduct has been low. In 1993, the Cancer and Leukemia Group B reviewed their audit outcomes over a ten-year period from 1982 to 1992 and identified only two instances of scientific impropriety, constituting a rate of only 0.28%.[11] Both instances occurred within the first few years of establishing a formal audit program and included one case of scientific fraud and another of gross scientific error where an excessive number of ineligible patients were enrolled in a trial. Similarly, the Southwestern Oncology Group detected no instance of scientific misconduct during a review of their audit experience.[12]

Despite its low incidence, scientific misconduct often takes on a high public profile when discovered. When occurring in association with clinical trials, cases of misconduct or fraud can have great and immediate consequences to the public welfare as well as the academic community.[10] Therefore, any suspected misconduct should be reported to the CTMB as soon as possible. This allows direct oversight and guidance in proceeding to necessary investigations as well as to proposed disciplinary actions.[1] Perhaps the most highly publicized case of scientific misconduct in recent years is that of the Poisson case, affecting several studies of the National Surgical Adjuvant Breast and Bowel Project (NSABP).[13] Discrepancies noted in data submitted to the coordinating office prompted two successive on-site audits led by members of the cooperative group. During these audits, it was discovered that some data had been altered to allow otherwise ineligible patients to be enrolled onto clinical trials. The NSABP immediately suspended the accrual privileges of the investigator and notified the NCI. All subsequent investigations were led and directed by the Office of Scientific Integrity (OSI) and kept in a confidential manner to the fullest extent possible. During a subsequent on-site audit conducted by a team of both OSI and NSABP staff, the findings of the initial audit conducted by the

NSABP staff were confirmed. Re-verification of all submitted data against source documentation identified evidence of data fabrication in 7% of all patients enrolled by the investigator.[14] Subsequently, the investigator was replaced, and a thorough re-analysis of the trial outcomes eliminating patients in question was carried out and published.[14] This case illustrates the crucial roles of the audit program in identifying and correcting problems, as well as in reassuring the public of the validity of reported results.

7. THE IMPACT OF QUALITY ASSURANCE AUDIT PROGRAMS ON SITE CONDUCT OF CLINICAL TRIALS

The educational benefits of an audit program are multifold. The audit experience emphasizes to the investigators the need for meticulous trial conduct and record-keeping. Through audits, the investigators become familiar with the standards of documentation as well as with the regulatory requirements of human subject research. Additionally, most cooperative groups allow investigators to participate as audit team members and actually conduct on-site audits. This peer-review process gives participants a chance to both learn and disseminate optimal methods of clinical research.[6]

While audit experiences of cooperative groups have only been scarcely reported, available literature suggests that the site performance improves in conjunction with increased experience with monitoring programs. In 1985, three years after NCI mandated that auditing programs be established among cooperative groups, a summary report of the audit data from the 17 then active cooperative groups was published.[4] This report revealed an overall satisfactory level of performance. More impressively, dramatic improvements were observed in the performance of smaller affiliated institutions over the three years, where ineligible cases declined from 16% to 8%, treatment deficiencies declined from 62% to 19%, and unsupported response assessments decreased from 17% to 10%. Additionally, only 6% of the institutions had deficiencies in the regulatory elements in 1984 compared to 45% in 1982. These data demonstrated that educational efforts over time can improve site performances as reflected in audit outcomes. Similar trends in improvement were subsequently reported by both the Southwestern Oncology Group (SWOG)[12] and the Cancer and Leukemia Group B (CALGB).[11] Over a 10-year period (1982-1992), deficiency rates significantly improved from 28% to 13.3%, and 49.6% to 28.2% for main and affiliated institutions respectively at the CALGB. Therefore, on-site peer review of investigator performance has stimulated quality improvement over time.

While colleagues in medical oncology and pharmaceutical industries have conducted clinical trials since the 1950's, the collective participation in the clinical trials program by surgeons has only become a national priority recently.[15] In Europe, the European Organization for Research and Treatment of Cancer (EORTC) has long recognized the importance of quality control in surgical trials. A large quality assurance program was initiated in 1987. When their experience with surgical melanoma trials was reviewed, the frequency of protocol violations was found to have decreased from 28% to 11% over a 3-year period from 1988 to 1992. These findings led the European researchers to conclude that quality assurance audits are not only feasible but also beneficial for surgical clinical trials.[16, 17]

In 1996, the American College of Surgeons Oncology Group (ACOSOG) was established as a cooperative group dedicated to evaluating the multidisciplinary management of patients with malignant solid tumors. As the formative years of surgical training have traditionally emphasized basic science research in the laboratory, most practicing surgeons are unfamiliar with clinical trials. During the initial years after the inception of ACOSOG, educational programs regarding clinical trials methodology as well as the quality assurance audit process were delivered during six ACOSOG semiannual meetings, a dedicated post-graduate course at the American College of Surgeons Clinical Congress, and two training seminars. Additionally, a robust audit program with clearly defined guidelines was established. Surgical investigators are encouraged to participate as audit team members, peer-review other institutions and exchange experiences with other investigators. A recent review of the audit outcomes over time revealed the dramatic effects of these educational efforts. From 2001-2004, initial treatment audits were conducted at 217 enrolling sites: 125 (58%) academic (or teaching affiliated), 78 (36%) community, and 14 (6%) other (VA, army, etc). Over these 4 years, the overall audit outcomes significantly improved, with overall Acceptable rates of 64%, 64%, 80%, and 93% respectively. Remarkable improvements were observed in patient case review, where rates of acceptable outcomes increased from 47% to 94%. Therefore, despite a substantial Unacceptable rate (36%) during the initial years, the conduct of clinical trials by surgeons has improved significantly through robust educational programs. In our experience, we did not detect any difference between the performances of academic vs. community institutions in both regulatory requirements or in patient case review, although experiences from a few other investigators have demonstrated more dramatic improvements for community institutions in particular.[4, 18] Many other factors including the type of institution, investigator training or experience with clinical research, number of support staff, and presence of a dedicated research office may contribute to site performance in an audit.

Although the impact of these factors has not been elucidated, available literature clearly indicate that quality assurance audits can stimulate improvements in the conduct of clinical trials. They also serve as benchmarks for measuring the impact of educational programs.

8. CONCLUSION

Clinical trials are valuable in both advancing the scientific knowledge of surgical oncology and defining the very best care for patients afflicted by malignancies. As an obligation to both the scientific community and the general public, the cooperative audit programs and the CTMB collaborate to ensure that the conduct of clinical trials are meticulous and the data are validated. However, audit programs should be viewed not merely as a surveillance mechanism. It serves as a stimulus for performance improvement by providing opportunities for peer-review and education.

REFERENCES

1. Knatterud, G.L., F.W. Rockhold, S.L. George, et al., Guidelines for quality assurance in multicenter trials: a position paper. *Control Clin Trials.* **19**(5), 477-93 (1998).
2. *CTEP NCI Guidelines: Monitoring of clinical trials.* http://ctep.cancer.gov/monitoring.
3. Califf, R.M., S.L. Karnash, and L.H. Woodlief, *Developing systems for cost-effective auditing of clinical trials.* Control Clin Trials. **18**(6), 651-60; discussion 661-6 (1997).
4. Mauer, J.K., D.F. Hoth, D.K. MacFarlane, et al., *Site visit monitoring program of the clinical cooperative groups: results of the first 3 years.* Cancer Treat Rep. **69**(10), 1177-87 (1985).
5. The American College of Surgeons Oncology Group (ACOSOG). *The audit manual.* 2004.
6. Ota, D., *The audit program of the American College of Surgeons Oncology Group.* American College of Surgeons 89th Clinical Congress post graduate course. 2003.
7. Morse, M.A., R.M. Califf, and J. Sugarman, Monitoring and ensuring safety during clinical research. *JAMA.* **285**(9), 1201-5 (2001).
8. Siden, R., R.M. Tankanow, and H.R. Tamer, Understanding and preparing for clinical drug trial audits. *Am J Health-Syst Pharm.* **59**(25), 2305-6 (2002).
9. *CTEP NCI guidelines: Adverse event reporting requirements.* http://ctep.cancer.gov/reporting/newadverse_2005.pdf.
10. Mason, S., J. Nicholl, and R. Lilford, What to do about poor clinical performance in clinical trials. *BMJ.* **324**(7334), 419-20 (2002).
11. Weiss, R.B., N.J. Vogelzang, B.A. Peterson, et al., A successful system of scientific data audits for clinical trials. A report from the Cancer and Leukemia Group B. *JAMA.* **270**(4), 459-64 (1993).

12. Sunderland, M., S Kuebler, G Weiss, et al., Compliance with protocol: quality assurance (QA) data from the Southwestern Oncology Group (SWOG). *Proc Am Soc Clin Oncol.* **9**, 60 (1990).
13. Fisher, B. and C.K. Redmond, Fraud in breast-cancer trials. *N Engl J Med.* **330**(20), 1458-60 (1994).
14. Christian, M.C., M.S. McCabe, E.L. Korn, et al., The National Cancer Institute audit of the National Surgical Adjuvant Breast and Bowel Project Protocol B-06. *N Engl J Med.* **333**(22), 1469-74 (1995).
15. McCulloch, P., I Taylor, M Sasako, et al., Randomised trials in surgery: problems and possible solutions. *BMJ.* **324**(7351), 1448-51 (2002).
16. Therasse, P. and A.M. Eggermont, Research and quality control in surgical oncology. *Surg Oncol Clin N Am.* **10**(4), 763-72, viii (2001).
17. Bourez, R.L. and E.J. Rutgers, The European Organization for Research and Treatment of Cancer (EORTC) Breast Cancer Group: quality control of surgical trials. *Surg Oncol Clin N Am.* **10**(4), 807-19, ix (2001).
18. Hjorth, M., E. Holmberg, S. Rodjer, et al., Patient accrual and quality of participation in a multicentre study on myeloma: a comparison between major and minor participating centres. *Br J Haematol,* **91**(1), 109-15 (1995).

Chapter 10

THE PRIVACY RULE (HIPAA) AS IT RELATES TO CLINICAL RESEARCH

John M. Harrelson, MD and John M. Falletta, MD
Duke University Health System, Durham, NC, USA

1. INTRODUCTION

The U.S. Congress passed the Health Insurance Portability and Accountability Act (HIPAA) in 1996 to protect a worker's health insurance coverage as the worker changes employment, to reduce fraud, and to establish national standards for electronic healthcare transactions. Also reflected in HIPAA is a concern for the privacy of a person and the confidentiality of his/her health information. The increase in computerized medical records and electronic transfer of information by e-mail, fax and the Internet has led to a heightened concern that the confidentiality of health information could be compromised. Federal privacy regulations implemented as a result of HIPAA (Title 45 CFR parts 160 & 164, referred to as the Privacy Rule)[1] apply to "covered entities", which are defined as health plans, health care clearinghouses or health care providers who transmit any health information electronically. Individual investigators involved in research with human subjects must comply with the regulations if they are also health care providers who electronically transmit health information or if they are employees or members of a covered entity.

With the implementation of the Privacy Rule, research involving humans as research subjects must be conducted according to three sets of regulations. Investigators doing research involving a product regulated by the Food and Drug Administration (FDA) are required to meet all relevant FDA regulations. Such research ordinarily involves the use of a drug, device or biological product, whether the regulated product has received FDA approval for marketing or remains an investigational product. If the investigator receives U.S. federal funds to support his/her research, or if the investigator is a faculty or staff member of an academic institution that has made a commitment to the U.S. Department of Health and Human Services (DHHS) to follow all federal regulations governing research involving humans subjects, the investigator is required to comply with regulations found at 45 CFR 46, including subparts A-D.[2] Subpart A, titled "Federal Policy for the Protections of Human Subjects," is referred to as the Common Rule. These regulations, while very similar to the FDA regulations, differ in part because their scope includes research not involving a drug, device or biological product, such as behavioral research, epidemiological research and educational research. A description of how the FDA regulations and 45 CFR 46 differ is available.[3]

Both the Common Rule and the FDA regulations require that research involving human subjects be reviewed and approved by an Institutional Review Board (IRB) that is duly constituted and registered with the Office for Human Research Protections (OHRP) (for the Common Rule) and with the FDA. The criteria for IRB approval of such research are found at 45 CFR 46.111 (Common Rule) and 21 CFR 56.111 (FDA regulations).[4] The criteria are essentially the same.

These regulations are unchanged by the Privacy Rule. While they provide for protection of the research subject's privacy and for the confidentiality of his/her research data, such protections are enhanced by the Privacy Rule. It adds a layer of privacy protections for subjects by defining the ways in which individually identifiable health information may be used in research. This chapter will explore the ways in which these three sets of regulations must be combined while the investigator is conducting clinical research.

2. WHAT NEW CONSIDERATIONS DOES THE PRIVACY RULE ADD TO RESEARCH?

PHI:

The Privacy Rule defines individually identifiable health information transmitted or maintained by a covered entity in any form (electronic, written or oral) as "protected health information" (PHI) and establishes the conditions under which investigators may access and use this information in the conduct of research. PHI is any information that relates to the past, present or future physical or mental health or condition of an individual who can be identified by any of eighteen specific identifiers [name, geographic location smaller than a State or the first three digits of a zip code, dates except year, telephone number, fax number, e-mail address, social security number, medical record number, health plan beneficiary numbers, account numbers, certificate or license numbers, vehicle identifiers and serial numbers, device identifiers and serial numbers, URLs, Internet protocol (IP) address numbers, biometric identifiers, full face photographs, any other unique identifying number, characteristic or code (45 CFR 164.514(b)(2)(i)]. Health information in this context includes biological specimens if they can be individually identified.

Authorization:
Except as otherwise permitted, the Privacy Rule requires that a research subject "authorize" the use or disclosure of the PHI to be utilized in the research. This authorization is distinct from the subject's consent to participate in research, which is required under the Common Rule and FDA regulations. Just as a valid consent under Common Rule and FDA regulations must meet certain requirements, a valid authorization must contain certain core elements [45 CFR 164.508(c)(1-2)]. The subject must specifically authorize what research information may be shared by whom, and who may receive the information, must acknowledge the expiration of the authorization and have the right to revoke the authorization, and must be informed that further disclosure by recipients of the information may not be covered by the federal privacy rules. This authorization may be incorporated in the informed consent document or be a stand-alone document.

Privacy Board:
The Privacy Rule [45 CFR 164.512)(i)(1)(i)(B)] describes a new board, constituted in a manner similar to an IRB, that has authority to implement the Rule as it relates to alteration of authorization or waiver of authorization.[6] Those alteration/waiver criteria are described below. Note that the Privacy Board has no authority to implement either the Common Rule or FDA regulations.

Review Preparatory to Research:
The Privacy Rule makes clear that some action to satisfy the Rule is required by the investigator if he/she wants to use PHI for research purposes. This action may be as simple as notifying the relevant covered entity of the research plan, or as complex as obtaining IRB or Privacy Board approval for waiving authorization to use PHI for research. If an investigator wishes to review PHI in order to determine the feasibility of a research project, he/she may do so by notifying the covered entity, usually through the IRB or Privacy Board, of a planned "Review Preparatory to Research" [45 CFR

164.512(i)(1)(ii)]. By this notification the investigator declares that he/she will use the PHI solely as needed to prepare a research protocol or for similar purposes preparatory to research, that the PHI will not be reused or re-disclosed for another purpose or leave the investigator's institution (covered entity), and that the PHI is necessary in order to develop the protocol. Note that a Review Preparatory to Research may be used by an investigator, prior to IRB approval of the entire research protocol, in order to review the PHI of potential research subjects; however, the investigator may not contact potential subjects to ask for their participation in the research without first obtaining IRB approval of the research. Likewise, the investigator may wish to record PHI or other identifiable private information obtained from a Review Preparatory to Research; however, the investigator may not do so without first obtaining IRB approval of the research and either consent of the research subject or IRB-approved waiver of consent.

Decedent Research:

The Common Rule defines a human research subject as a living individual. The Privacy Rule recognizes both living and deceased humans as individuals whose privacy must be protected. If an investigator wishes to do a research project using PHI of deceased individuals, he/she may do so without concern for Common Rule considerations. But since Privacy Rule considerations must also be met, first the covered entity must be notified, usually by notifying the IRB or Privacy Board, in order for the investigator to attest that the use of PHI is solely for research using the PHI of decedents, and that the PHI sought is necessary in order to perform the research. The covered entity (IRB or Privacy Board) may request documentation of death [45 CFR 164.512(i)(1)(iii)].

Databases and Repositories:

The Privacy Rule recognizes the creation of a research database or a specimen repository to be a research activity if the data stored contain PHI.[7] Similarly, each use or disclosure of PHI from a database or repository for research purposes is considered a separate research activity. The Privacy Rule does not permit authorization to be given for unspecified future research.[7,8] Thus the authorization to include PHI in a database and/or specimen repository must specify the research purpose for which the use or disclosure will occur. As with any authorization, this may either be combined with an IRB approved consent for research or obtained as a separate document. As noted below, all future research uses and disclosures of PHI from a database or repository require IRB +/- Privacy Board approval. The IRB may require re-consent/authorization if the intended purpose of the future research is outside the original intent of the database/repository. Or, alternatively, the IRB may waive consent and authorization. Anonymization and de-identification of the data or release as a limited data set with a data use agreement (discussed below) are alternate considerations that may be useful in certain circumstances.

3. OTHER INTERACTIONS BETWEEN THE PRIVACY RULE AND THE COMMON RULE

As described above (Review Preparatory to Research), DHHS has provided guidance that it considers research to be occurring if the investigator records PHI or other identifiable private information during the search for potential subjects (during the ascertainment/recruitment process). The investigator must therefore first obtain IRB approval of the research, and then obtain either consent and authorization of the subjects or IRB +/- Privacy Board approval of a waiver of consent and authorization to conduct the study.

To approve a waiver of consent under the Common Rule [45 CFR 46.116(d)], the IRB must find that:

a) The research involves no more than minimal risk.
b) The waiver does not adversely affect the rights and welfare of the subject.
c) The research could not be practicably carried out without the waiver.
d) Whenever appropriate, the subjects will be informed of any pertinent information.

In order for the IRB or Privacy Board also to approve an alteration or waiver of authorization, the Privacy Rule [45 CFR 164.512(i)(2)(ii)) requires the IRB or Privacy Board to find that:

a) Disclosure of the PHI involves no more than minimal risk to the privacy of individuals.
b) The waiver will not adversely affect the privacy rights or welfare of the subject.
c) The research could not practicably be carried out without the waiver.
d) The research could not practicably be carried out without access to the PHI.
e) The privacy risks are reasonable in relation to the information to be gained.

f) There is an adequate plan to protect the identifiers from improper use and disclosure.
g) There is an adequate plan to destroy the identifiers at the earliest opportunity.
h) There is written assurance that the PHI will not be further disclosed.

3.1 How can the investigator reduce the impact of the Common Rule and the Privacy Rule on his/her research that utilizes data/sample repositories?

Both the Common Rule and the Privacy Rule contain provisions that, if met, permit research to proceed without further restrictions from either Rule. For example, a research activity does not prompt Common Rule or Privacy Rule considerations if the research does not involve a "human subject", as defined by 45 CFR 46.102(f), and the research does not involve the use or disclosure of PHI, as defined by 45 CFR 160.103. More precisely stated for our purposes, if the information associated with the research data and/or samples is modified so it does not relate, either directly or indirectly, to an identifiable living person, and the information either does not involve PHI, or includes only a few specific indirect identifiers linked to the person (limited data set) and is accompanied by a data use agreement, then research with those data/samples can be declared not to involve a human subject and thus not to be subject to the Common Rule, and either not be subject to or be in compliance with the Privacy Rule.

By far the most common use of these approaches relates to research with a database and/or a sample repository.[7] By meeting the following conditions, the investigator is able to reduce the impact of both Rules on his/her research activity.

1) Modify information associated with the data/samples so the information does not relate to a "human subject", thereby permitting the research not to be subject to the Common Rule. (9)

This can be achieved either by anonymizing (unlinking) the data/samples or by establishing the conditions whereby the subject's identity cannot readily be ascertained. Either approach satisfies Common Rule considerations. In many circumstances, anonymization also satisfies the Privacy Rule.

a) Anonymizing (unlinking) the data/samples involves removing all identifiers and codes that directly or indirectly link a particular data point or sample to an identifiable person. These data/samples then become irreversibly unlinked from any subject identifiers.

b) Establishing the conditions whereby the subject's private information or specimens cannot be individually identifiable either directly or indirectly through a coding system:

(i) Confirmation that the private information or specimens were not collected specifically for the currently proposed research project through an interaction or intervention with living individuals; and

(ii) The investigator cannot readily ascertain the identity of the individual(s) to whom the coded private information or specimens pertain because, for example:
   (a) the key to decipher the code is destroyed before the research begins;
   (b) the investigator and the holder of the key enter into an agreement prohibiting the release of the key to the investigator under any circumstances, until the individuals are deceased;
   (c) there are IRB-approved written policies and operating procedures for a repository or data management center that prohibit the release of the key to the investigators under any circumstances, until the individuals are deceased; or
   (d) there are other legal requirements prohibiting the release of the key to the investigators, until the individuals are deceased.

2) Modify information associated with the data/samples so the information does not contain PHI, rendering the data not subject to the Privacy Rule, or presenting the PHI as a limited data set with a data use agreement, thereby fulfilling Privacy Rule requirements.

a) The information will not contain PHI if the information does not include health information (45 CFR 160.103), or the health information linked to the data/samples has been de-identified (45 CFR 164.514(b)). Note that the Privacy Rule describes two methods for de-identification: the "statistical method" (45 CFR 164.514(b)(1)) and the "safe harbor" method (45 CFR 164.514(b)(2)). While the latter is by far more commonly used than the former, the "statistical method" has the virtue of permitting more identifiers, including selected direct identifiers, to be retained with the de-identified data as long as a person such as a statistician, using generally accepted statistical and scientific principles, determines that the risk of data/sample re-identification is very small.

b) The PHI can be presented as a limited data set (45 CFR 164.514(e)) by removing all direct personal identifiers, and removing postal address information except for town or city, State and zip code (nine digit zip code is permitted). Event dates, the subject's age (without restriction) and an identifying code derived from the subject's PHI (such as subject initials) may be included in the limited data set. Therefore data in a limited data set are not de-identified data.

A data use agreement must be in place to ensure that the limited data set recipient will only use or disclose the protected health information for limited purposes. This agreement must establish the proposed uses of the data and who is permitted to have access to the data, and must ensure that no other use will be made of the data, no attempt will be made to contact individuals whose data are included in the limited data set, and appropriate safeguards are in place to protect the data from unauthorized use.

In summary, note that a research use of anonymized (unlinked) data is not subject to the Common Rule, and likewise, a research use of de-identified data is not subject to the Privacy Rule.

The only setting where anonymization (unlinking) of data/samples does not also confer the status of de-identification is when the anonymized (unlinked) health information contains an event date more specific than the year, a geocode (such as the subject's home address) more specific than State or 3 digit zip code, or a subject's specific age if over 89 years (instead record as age 90+ years).

The only setting where de-identification does not also confer the status of anonymization (unlinking) is when a code with a link back to the subject's identity is retained with the de-identified data.

4. CONCLUSION

The Privacy Rule has increased the complexity of life for an investigator engaged in research with human subjects. However, contrary to the fears of many and the claims of some, the Privacy Rule need not stifle such research.

By understanding all of the regulations that govern research with human subjects, including the Common Rule, FDA regulations and the Privacy Rule, investigators are able to perform scientifically sound and ethical research. The IRB with which the investigator works can be a valuable resource to guide the research team as the study is designed and submitted for approval.

REFERENCES

1. August 2003 Complete Privacy, Security, and Enforcement (Procedural) Regulations Text (45 CFR Parts 160 and 164) http://www.hhs.gov/ocr/combinedregtext.pdf/, Sponsor: DHHS Office for Civil Rights, Accessed: 23 January 2006.
2. Code of Federal Regulations Title 45 Part 46 http://www.hhs.gov/ohrp/humansubjects/guidance/45cfr46.htm/, Sponsor: DHHS Office for Human Research Protections, Accessed: 23 January 2006.
3. Guidance for Institutional Review Boards and Clinical Investigators, 1998 Update, Appendix E: Significant Differences in FDA and HHS Regulations http://www.fda.gov/oc/ohrt/irbs/appendixe.html/, Sponsor: FDA, Accessed 23 January 2006.
4. Code of Federal Regulations Title 21 Part 56 http://www.cfsan.fda.gov/~lrd/cfr56.html/, Sponsor: FDA, Accessed 23 January 2006.
5. HIPAA Privacy Rule – Information for Researchers http://privacyruleandresearch.nih.gov/, Sponsor: NIH, Accessed 23 January 2006.
6. Privacy Boards and the HIPAA Privacy Rule http://privacyruleandresearch.nih.gov/pdf/privacy_boards_hipaa_privacy_rule.pdf/, Sponsor: NIH, Accessed 23 January 2006.
7. Research Repositories, Databases and the HIPAA Privacy Rule http://privacyruleandresearch.nih.gov/research_repositories.asp/, Sponsor: NIH, Accessed 23 January 2006.
8. Institutional Review Boards and the HIPAA Privacy Rule http://privacyruleandresearch.nih.gov/pdf/IRB_Factsheet.pdf/, Sponsor: NIH, Accessed 23 January 2006.
9. Guidance on Research Involving Coded Private Information or Biological Specimens, August 10, 2004 http://www.hhs.gov/ohrp/humansubjects/guidance/cdebiol.pdf/, Sponsor: DHHS Office for Human Research Protections, Accessed 23 January 2006.

Chapter 11

THE COMMISSION ON CANCER, AMERICAN COLLEGE OF SURGEONS' RESPONSE TO HIPAA

E. Greer Gay, RN, PhD, MPH

American College of Surgeons, Chicago, IL, USA

Abstract: The Commission on Cancer is able to continue serving the CoC-Approved Cancer Programs following enactment of a business associate agreement between each of the programs and the ACoS. Worrisome unintended consequences, potentially threatening the value of the products that the CoC provides cancer patients, providers, and families, were not realized because of the Business Associate role that the CoC assumes with each of the CoC-Approved programs.

Key words: Health Insurance Portability and Accountability Act, Business Associate Agreement (BAA), Electronic Medical Record (EMR), Administrative Simplification Act, Quality Improvement, Approvals, Standards

1. INTRODUCTION

The Health Insurance Portability and Accountability Act of 1996 (HIPAA) has many laudable components, in that it improves health insurance portability, promotes standardization of electronic medical records (EMRs) and simplifies administration while *maintaining the privacy* of individual patients. Sections 261 through 264 of that Act, the *Administrative Simplification* provisions, required the Department of Health and Human Services (DHHS) to release standards for electronic exchange, privacy and security of health information. The goal was to provide patients more control over the privacy of their personal health information (PHI), permitting them the right to know how, why, and to whom personal health information would be released by "covered entities."[1]

Under the aegis of the Clinton Administration final regulations for HIPAA, published December 28, 2000, would have had a negative impact upon the relationship of the Commission on Cancer (CoC) and the CoC-approved cancer programs and their patients. The CoC is a consortium of professional organizations dedicated to reducing the morbidity and mortality of cancer through education, standard setting, and the monitoring of quality care.[2] At risk was the continuation of a rich resource available to cancer patients, providers, and families provided through the National Cancer Data Base (NCDB) as well as the recognized process whereby cancer programs in the US are approved.

Public outcry was significant. Some felt the rules were not stringent enough. Others felt the rules essentially shackled health care operations to the point that health care was compromised. Faced with this objection, the Bush administration suspended the enactment of the regulations, opting for a review of the impact on the health care delivery system.[3]

After considerable input from the public, modifications were made to the Privacy Rule in August 2002. The changes essential struck a balance, assuring "individuals' health information is properly protected while allowing the flow of health information needed to provide and promote high quality health care...."[4] The changes in the regulations were welcome relief to the Commission on Cancer (CoC) for the language in the regulations provided a means whereby the CoC could continue to work with their approved programs.[5] The purpose of this chapter is to review what and how the Privacy Rule affects the American College of Surgeons' (ACoS) relationship with the CoC-approved programs and the efforts taken to assure compliance for the participating programs.

2. BACKGROUND AND ROLES OF THE COMMISSION ON CANCER

Established by the ACoS in 1922, the multi-disciplinary CoC sets standards for quality multidisciplinary cancer care delivered primarily in hospital settings, surveys hospitals to assess compliance with those standards, collects standardized and quality data from approved hospitals to measure treatment patterns and outcomes, uses the data to evaluate hospital provider performance, and develops effective educational interventions to improve cancer care outcomes at the national and local level.[6]

The CoC goals reflect the mission of the Commission, i.e., to provide the best cancer care for the patient through establishing standards for cancer programs, surveying and approving cancer programs, overseeing and coordinating national site-specific studies on patterns of care and outcomes of patient management through annual data collection and analysis and dissemination of data for 60 cancer sites, coordinating a network of 1,800 physicians, collaborating in community cancer control activities.[7]

Commission membership is comprised of more than 100 individuals, either surgeons representing the ACoS or representatives from the 37 national, professional organizations affiliated with the CoC. These individuals serve on one of the standing committees and/or one of the Disease Site Teams (DSTs) in order to accomplish the CoC goals by:[8]

- Establishing standards for 1,438 Commission-approved cancer programs and evaluating and approving programs according to those standards.
- Overseeing a nationwide network of around 1,800 physician-volunteers who provide state and local support for Commission and American Cancer Society cancer control initiatives.
- Providing oversight and coordination for educational programs of the Commission, which are geared towards surgeons, physicians, cancer registrars, cancer program leadership, and others.
- Providing clinical oversight and expertise for Commission standard-setting activities and for the development, review, and dissemination of patient care guidelines.
- Overseeing and coordinating national site-specific studies of patterns of care and outcomes of patient management through the annual collection, analysis, and dissemination of data for all cancer sites.

These activities are coordinated through the Approvals Committee, Cancer Liaison Physician (CLP), and Quality Integration Committee (QIC), in conjunction with input to and through the Disease-Site Teams (DSTs), on which sit nationally recognized leaders in the care of the cancers associated with each disease site.[9]

3. THE NATIONAL CANCER DATA BASE

The NCDB, established in 1989 as a comprehensive clinical surveillance information repository resource about cancer care in the United States, serves as a resource for analysis and feedback to more than 1,400 CoC-approved programs.[10] Though in the past, participation was voluntary. However, with the new Cancer Program Standards, participation is mandated as a means to track and improve cancer care at the local level. The NCDB was the first national, institutionally based, database to routinely track and compare the treatment of all types of cancers. The NCDB currently captures 75 percent of all newly diagnosed cancer cases in the United States annually and holds information on over 15 million cases of reported cancer diagnoses for the period 1985 through 2002. This longitudinal depth allows for the systematic evaluation of changing patterns of diagnosis and disease presentation and first course therapy by diagnosis year. Data collected include tumor characteristics, staging information, type of first course treatment administered, and disease recurrence and survival information. These data elements are submitted to the NCDB using nationally standardized data transmission formats.[11]

The NCDB resides in and is operated by the ACoS. The basic framework for much of the analytic work and report generation conducted by the NCDB is based on the overarching commitment of the CoC; i.e., to reduce the morbidity and mortality of cancer through education, standard setting and the monitory of quality of care.[12] The information gleaned from analyses of the NCDB is returned to the local hospitals' Cancer Committees for their review and direction. The benchmark reports provide a hospital's cancer program the tools to compare practice with similar types of hospitals. This type feedback to the local facility provides approved programs direction for quality improvement, an expectation for maintaining an approved status.[13]

Data confidentiality has always been of prime importance to the CoC and the ACoS, but even more so since the passage of HIPAA. Case records reported to the NCDB are maintained in the CoC data warehouse in such a way as to maximize confidentiality, while at the same time foster the analytic utility of the data, whether this be for aggregate analytic purposes or for generating hospital-based benchmark reports.

4. WHAT IMPACT WILL HIPAA HAVE ON THE COC'S ROLE?

HIPAA standards apply only to health care providers who transmit any health information electronically, health plans, and health care clearing houses, i.e., 'covered entities' (HHA/OCR, Feb./Mar. 2003). Hospitals, i.e., 'covered entities' could maintain their relationship with the CoC as long as a Business Associate agreement that met federally mandated requisites existed between the covered entity and the business associate (45 CFR Section 160.103). By definition a Business Associate (BA) is an organization or a person who performs a function or activity on behalf of, or provides services to the core functions of a Covered Entity and involves individually identifiable health information.[14]

The CoC serves approved cancer programs (covered entities) in the capacity of a "business associate" through providing assistance to health care operations, defined as core functions.[15] These functions include assistance with quality improvement and accrediting through the Approvals Program. CoC staff analyzes submitted data and provide feedback to these programs on their current practices. The CoC also supplies benchmarks, based on aggregate NCDB data, to the facilities, so that each one can compare their practices to similar cancer program practices at regional and national levels.

Given the added responsibilities of the covered entities, the ACoS engaged an external review of the security of the ACoS data storage activities.[16] A separate server was installed to assure adequate firewall protection for accessing and transmitting PHI from the CoC-approved programs. Passwords requirements were strengthened. Policies and procedures with regard to access to and use of the data were clarified. Further, the American College of Surgeons provided appropriate technical training of staff and surveyors addressing security standards and College responsibilities to clients served. College staff were encouraged to maintain open lines of communication with constituent programs.

5. THE COC'S ROLE AS A FACILITATOR OF QUALITY IMPROVEMENT ACTIVITIES

Critical to the BA functions provided by the College to CoC-approved cancer programs is the ability to receive a limited data set that defines cancer care practices at each local facility. Analysis of these data sets becomes the basis for the feedback the College provides the programs about quality cancer care practices and how each facility compares to similar facilities at the aggregate level.

The August 2002 final regulations permitted use of a limited data set for research, public health, or health care operations purposes if the covered entity uses or discloses only a "limited data set as defined in 45 C.F.R.§ 164.514(e)(2) and a "data use agreement," as defined in 45 C.F.R.§ 164.514(e)(4), is in place between the covered entity and the business associate.[17] The rule specifies the removal of the following direct identifiers for a data set to qualify as being limited: name, street address, phone/fax numbers, e-mail address, Social Security number, certificate/license numbers, vehicle identifiers, URLs and IP addresses, full face photographs, etc., medical record numbers, health beneficiary numbers, other account numbers, device identification/serial numbers, and biometric identifiers. The CoC does not collect any of these variables; hence by definition the ACoS collects a "limited data set".[18]

Once data are received at the NCDB, technical staff provides analysis of the data. Highly experienced clinicians provide direction to the feedback provided the CoC-approved programs. Also, aggregated data tabulations by type of hospital, region of the country, and division of the American Cancer Society from all disease sites are available on a secure web site with access limited to designated representatives of each cancer program. These programs are expected to use this feedback for quality improvement efforts.

6. CHALLENGES FACING THE APPROVALS PROGRAM

The Commission on Cancer (CoC) Approvals Program serves as the nationally recognized body to approve cancer programs nationwide. Expectations for approval are described in the manual *CoC Cancer Program Standards 2004*. These standards define what is expected relative to each cancer program's prevention, early diagnosis, pretreatment evaluation, staging, optimal treatment, rehabilitation, surveillance for recurrent disease, support services, and end-of-life care. Among the requirements are cancer conferences, quality improvement activities, patient follow-up, and an on-site survey by a physician surveyor. With the publication of the December 2001 regulations, cancer programs expressed concern about their ability to complete selected activities required by the CoC Cancer Program Standards.

6.1 Cancer Conferences

Recognizing that cancer is a complex group of diseases, the CoC Cancer Program Standards (2.6 through 2.9) promote consultation among surgeons, medical and radiation oncologists, diagnostic radiologists, pathologists, and other cancer specialists. This multidisciplinary cooperation results in improved patient care. Cancer conferences are "an essential forum to provide multidisciplinary consultative, services to cancer patients," "encourage multidisciplinary involvement prospectively," and are "integral to improving the care of cancer patients by contributing to the patient management process and outcomes."[19] In light of the HIPAA regulations, given the Clinton administration's read on the regulations, these conferences would have been impossible to continue in the format envisioned and for the purposes they serve. Nonetheless, the August 2002 final HIPAA regulations "Accommodate the various circumstances of any covered entity - particularly so in the definition of the relationship with the B.A."[20] Cancer conferences are critical to a cancer program's approval. Those same regulations state that "A covered entity's policies and procedures should allow appropriate individuals within an entity to have access to PHI as necessary to perform their jobs with respect to the entity's covered functions."[21]

6.2 Surveys

Cancer program surveys are a comprehensive evaluation of the entire scope, organization, and performance of a cancer program. A cancer program survey is performed every three years by a physician surveyor, specially trained to evaluate compliance with the 36 standards that are required for approval. Surveyors, representing the ACoS, have the most opportunity to be affected by the regulations. They actually enter each facility and have access to PHI through the survey process itself (e.g., attending Cancer Conference, auditing randomly a selection of actual patient charts).

The ruling under the Clinton administration would not have permitted the survey to be conducted as comprehensively as need be to assure the quality of cancer care at the cancer program level. The August 2002 regulations, however, saw these activities as part of accreditation, or official approval. The regulations permitted this type activity within the scope of the business associate role. Nonetheless, to assure HIPAA compliance, the CoC, ACoS requires each surveyor to enter into a Surveyor Agreement, which essentially assures that the Surveyor is acting as an agent of the College and will abide by the Business Associate Agreement between the Cancer Program and the ACoS. No PHI is shared outside the survey process itself.

6.3 Treatment Outside the Facility and Follow-Up

Follow-up is critical to the evaluation of cancer care, the value of which is recognized to the extent that programs are required to do so for attaining Approval status (Standards 3.4 and 3.5). Tracking patients over time is critical to the evaluation of treatment effectiveness, a critical element in facility quality improvement efforts. Prior to the August 2002 rulings, uncertainty regarding whether or not this would be allowed existed, making cancer program registrars and HIPAA compliance officers nervous. Once again, the August 2002 Federal Register's rules gave the Approval's Program far more leeway than would have been the initially proposed rules. The latter regulations allowed health-covered entities to use or disclose individually PHI to other covered entities for purposes of health care operations as long as each *had or has* a client relationship with the patient. The registrar, as an agent of the covered entity and in light of promoting quality of cancer care, could and should follow up on patients who have been in their facility.[22]

7. CONCLUSIONS

The CoC is able to continue serving the CoC-Approved Cancer Programs following enactment of a business associate agreement between each of the programs and the ACoS. Those worrisome unintended consequences, potentially threatening the value of a rich resource available to cancer patients, providers, and families, did not occur. The changes in the regulations, published in August 2002, were welcome relief to the CoC. Both the Approvals Program and the National Cancer Data Base (NCDB) were no longer at risk. The CoC can continue its work to set standards for quality multidisciplinary cancer care delivered primarily in hospital settings; survey hospitals to assess compliance with those standards; collect standardized and quality data from approved hospitals to measure treatment patterns and outcomes; and use the data to evaluate hospital provider performance and develop effective educational interventions to improve cancer care outcomes at the national and local level.

ACKNOWLEDGEMENTS

The chapter could not have been written without the contributions of Andrew Stewart, Jerri Linn Phillips, Asa Carter, and Connie Bura, The American College of Surgeons, Division of Research and Optimal Care, Cancer Programs.

REFERENCES

[1] Office of Civil Rights (OCR) 2003.
[2] (http://www.facs.org/cancer/coc/cocar.html).
[3] OCR 2003
[4] OCR 2003
[5] (USDHHS 2003).
[6] (http://www.facs.org/cancer/coc/cocar.html).
[7] Ibid.
[8] Ibid.
[9] Ibid.
[10] (http://www.facs.org/cancer/ncdb/ncdbabout.html).
[11] (Stewart 2004).

[12] (http://www.facs.org/cancer/coc/cocar.html).
[13] (CoC Standards 2004).
[14] Aug. 2002
[15] Ibid.
[16] (NSAG 2003).
[17] (Federal Register, Vol. 67 (157), 8/14/2002).
[18] NAACCR
[19] (CoC Cancer Program Standards 2004).
[20] (45 C.F.R. § 160.103; p. 53248)
[21] (Federal Register, Aug. 14, 2002, p. 53197).
[22] (45 C.F.R. §164.506 (c) (4)).

Chapter 12

ETHICAL AND LEGAL ISSUES IN THE CONDUCT OF CANCER CLINICAL TRIALS

Gerianne J. Sands* and Peggy A. Means**

Fred Hutchinson Cancer Research Center, Seattle, Washington, USA

NOTE: *Gerianne Sands is the Associate General Counsel at Fred Hutchinson Cancer Research Center. The views expressed here are those of the author and not that of Fred Hutchinson Cancer Research Center. Ms. Sands can be contacted by writing to the Office of the General Counsel, Fred Hutchinson Cancer Research Center, POB 19024, MS J6-205, Seattle, Washington 98109-1024 or by e-mail at gjsands@fhcrc.org. **Peggy Means is currently a consultant whose familiarity with the issues relating to the conduct of cancer clinical trials derived from her work at Fred Hutchinson Cancer Research Center in Seattle, Washington. Ms. Means recently concluded a 16-year tenure at Fred Hutchinson in which she held positions as the Chief Operating Officer and Senior Vice President for Strategic Planning. The views expressed here are those of the author and not that of Fred Hutchinson Cancer Research Center.

INTRODUCTION

Cancer clinical trials like most research involving human participants are conducted within a complex regulatory environment. Much of that regulatory framework is designed to resolve the many ethical and legal issues that arise in the conduct of research involving humans. As discussed in other chapters of this book, the physician who elects to engage in cancer clinical trials research must become familiar with this complex regulatory environment to the fullest extent possible. But a familiarity with the regulations alone is not enough. To be a fully informed and actively engaged researcher in cancer clinical trials, it is crucial that the physician investigator also become familiar with the ethical and legal principles embraced in these regulations.

Equally important to the physician investigator is the ability to make an informed decision as to the "right" cancer clinical trial(s) to select for the cancer patients being treated. The "right" cancer clinical trial is the one that will both best serve the interest of the patients under the physician's care and will match the physician investigator's capacity to meet (or exceed) the ethical and legal requirements imposed by the trial. The physician investigator must conduct the cancer clinical trial with a risk averse approach that is responsive to the heightened expectations and rigorous scrutiny of scientific and peer review bodies, ethical committees, patients and their families, as well as the public at large. To accomplish this, the physician investigator should seek assistance from resources provided by their home institutions and should participate in educational and training programs.

As those who have experienced the rigorous scrutiny of regulatory agencies, courts of law and the sting of public and media critics can attest, it is crucial that physician investigators and their supporting institutions embrace an anticipatory and proactive approach to the conduct of cancer clinical trials. For physician investigators who choose to initiate studies involving investigational new drug applications, it is important for them to understand that they will be held to a standard historically applied to pharmaceutical and biotech companies. If the supporting infrastructure is not available to the physician investigator to meet or exceed the regulatory standards, pressure should be applied to senior leadership and governing bodies to elevate these requirements in the institution's list of priorities. For investigator-initiated studies, if the institution is unwilling to invest the necessary resources, the investigator should consider collaboration with investigators at institutions or companies with access to these resources or consider hiring outside groups, such as clinical research organizations or consultants, to monitor their studies.

2. COMPLEX REGULATORY ENVIRONMENT

The regulatory framework in which cancer clinical trials are conducted today is complex and pervasive. Physician investigators at a minimum are required to complete a training program that provides a basic understanding of this regulatory environment. The majority of regulations affecting the conduct of cancer clinical trials are at the federal level in the United States. The U.S. Department of Health and Human Services' Office of Human Research Protections ("OHRP") is the principle regulatory oversight body for most research involving human participants. The Food and Drug Administration ("FDA") is also authorized to regulate research related to the drugs or devices that it approves for use in cancer treatment. Although there are similarities between these two regulatory schemes, they are not identical and physician investigators must be familiar with both.

In cases in which the physician investigator elects to act as a sponsor for an "investigator initiated" investigational new drug application ("IND"), additional requirements are imposed on that physician investigator[1] as "sponsor." The assumption of responsibility for these demanding "sponsor" obligations should be carefully considered. Physician investigators engaged in cancer clinical trials involving devices not yet approved by the FDA must also become familiar with Investigational Device Exemption regulations.[2] With increasing regularity, commercial sponsors of cancer clinical trials are also requiring adherence to international standards known as the "ICH Guidelines."[3]

Federal regulations and policies imposed as a condition of funding for cancer clinical trials by agencies such as the National Institutes of Health ("NIH") must also be observed.[4] The Centers for Medicare and Medicaid Services ("CMS") impose restrictions on the extent to which the costs of participation in certain "qualifying" clinical trials can be recovered and define a key role for the physician investigator in the determination of which clinical trials are "qualifying."[5]

The physician investigator also plays a key role in ensuring compliance with federal regulations that require that any financial conflicts of interest held by physician investigators be managed, reduced or eliminated as a condition of support.[6] As will be discussed later in this chapter, many comprehensive cancer centers and academic medical centers conducting cancer clinical trials have established conflict of interest policies that go well beyond the requirements imposed by federal law and state policies.

Another important federal law that affects cancer clinical trials is the Health Insurance Portability and Accountability Act ("HIPAA") and its implementing regulations.[7] Also, as discussed more fully in other chapters of this book, all federally funded research is expected to conform with the highest standards for research integrity expressed in federal research misconduct regulations.[8] There are additional laws and regulations regarding research involving research, licensure and privacy that vary by state and investigators should request information from their institutional representatives about these rules because in some cases they vary substantially from federal requirements.

Clinical trial registration requirements have been imposed as a prerequisite for publication of research findings by many scholarly journals[9] and public access to clinical trial results may be required either by research sponsors or more broadly as a result of Congressional action.[10]

3. SUPPORT SYSTEMS FOR REGULATORY COMPLIANCE

The task of navigating through this regulatory maze can be daunting to any physician investigator considering whether or not to initiate or participate in a cancer clinical trial. The issues confronting the physician investigator will vary depending on the type of cancer clinical trial involved. Those that arise as part of the complex and well-established "cooperative group" structure nurtured by the National Cancer Institute ("NCI") of the U.S. National Institutes of Health ("NIH") will be accompanied by a supporting network of resources, collaborators and coordinating centers to assist the physician investigator.[11] Industry-sponsored clinical trials in which a drug company holds the IND and contracts with performance sites and investigators to conduct the clinical trial is also an example of a setting in which much of the regulatory compliance infrastructure is established and monitored by the company in its FDA-regulated role as the trial sponsor.[12]

It is when physician investigators elect to initiate a cancer clinical trial based on their own protocol and when they further elect to hold the IND that they must establish themselves and/or rely on their own institution's support system to address the regulatory compliance issues. It is important that physician investigators seek out the institutional support systems in place to assist them. To the extent these support systems are not in place or are not adequate, the physician investigator should urge institutional officials to take reasonable steps to establish and/or improve them, or to agree to have the institution hold the IND so the investigator is not as vulnerable in an FDA audit.

With the assistance of experienced institutional review board ("IRB") members and with the help of regulatory affairs managers and legal counsel, the physician investigator can succeed in the conduct of cancer clinical trials within this restrictive regulatory environment.

4. GENERAL ETHICAL AND LEGAL PRINCIPLES

The physician investigator conducting cancer clinical trials must be cognizant of the ethical and legal principles that form the basis for the regulatory environment described above. The general ethical principles applied in research involving human participants identified in <u>The Belmont Report</u>[13] are summarized by Dr. Robert J. Levine in his important work entitled <u>Ethics and Regulation of Clinical Research</u>.[14] These ethical principles include respect for persons, beneficence and justice.

The "respect for persons" principle requires that the physician investigator embrace two interrelated ethical considerations. The first is that all potential trial participants in cancer clinical trials must be approached and treated as autonomous beings who are entitled to make independent decisions about whether they want to enroll in a clinical trial. The second is that extra care must be given to ensure that those individuals whose decision-making capacity is compromised by illness, condition, age or circumstance receive the assistance necessary to make an independent decision. This principle has contributed much of the basis for the requirement of a carefully constructed informed consent process.

The "beneficence" principle focuses on the critical need to ensure that any decision to conduct a cancer clinical trial at all or to enroll individuals into any cancer clinical trial is wholly supported by a finding that the benefits to the participant (and in some cases to society) outweigh the risks. This principle has provided the basis for the regulatory framework that requires that proposed clinical trials be independently reviewed to determine, among other things, whether the trial is well-designed and scientifically sound. The informed consent process requirements focus on a comprehensive risk and benefits explanation for the participant. Additionally, the data and safety monitoring and continuing review requirements have been established to ensure that ongoing reconsideration of the risk-benefit ratio is ensured.

The "justice" principle emphasizes the importance of enrolling clinical trial participants in a fair manner that does not burden more vulnerable participants with greater exposure to risks of a cancer clinical trial. It also requires that the physician investigator make reasonable efforts to afford fair and equitable access to more vulnerable populations to extend the benefits of participation in the trial. This principle is embodied in the independent review by institutional review boards and ethical committees of the recruitment and outreach procedures to be used in the conduct of cancer clinical trials.

5. UNIQUE ETHICAL AND LEGAL CONSIDERATIONS

In addition to these general ethical and legal principles that are faced by all researchers involved in research involving human participants, the physician investigator involved in cancer clinical trials must also consider the unique ethical issues that arise in a setting in which the research participants are patients suffering from a disease for which the standard treatment available is not suitable to either effectively treat the patient's condition or to improve the patient's quality of life. Volumes have been and will continue to be written about these unique ethical and legal considerations. This overview will simply highlight a few significant examples.

5.1 Physician as Researcher

Dr. Levine describes one of these unique ethical considerations in his discussion of the different standards that apply for clinical vs. research consent in his review of the informed consent process.[15] Cancer patients rely on the judgment of their treating physicians in making informed decisions about a course of treatment. When that same treating physician is also acting as the principle investigator or co-investigator of a cancer clinical trial, steps must be taken to ensure that the patient as a prospective clinical trial participant is exposed to and actively engages in a more complete and interactive informed consent process than might be typical in most clinical treatment settings. Prospective participants in cancer clinical trials are required to read and are encouraged to ask questions about all aspects of the cancer clinical trial described in lengthy and sometimes complicated informed consent forms. More documentation of the informed consent process is also required in the research context. In some cases, potential cancer clinical trial participants are offered an opportunity to ask questions of other physicians or health care professionals who are not involved in the conduct of the cancer clinical trial in order to ensure an enhanced degree of objectivity.

5.2 Therapeutic Misconception

A related ethical consideration that exists in the cancer clinical trial setting is a concept known as the "therapeutic misconception." The concept of "therapeutic misconception" was described by Dr. Paul Appelbaum and his colleagues in 1987[16] as the belief that some patients as research participants hold that the research study or clinical trial in which they are invited to participate is primarily intended to benefit them individually. Although some participants may benefit others may not. In fact, some participants may see their condition worsen or they may suffer side-effects that will threaten their very survival. Further in support of the conclusion that the belief of individual benefit is a misconception, Dr. Appelbaum, et al. explained that "the unique aspects of clinical research include the goal of creating generalizable knowledge; the techniques of randomization; and the use of a study protocol, control groups and double-blind procedures."[17]

One problem with the existence of a "therapeutic misconception" in the cancer clinical trial setting is that the participants who hold this belief may never fully and autonomously consider the "risks" associated with participation even if the informed consent process creates the ideal setting for that consideration. Another problem is that it exacerbates the already challenging task facing physician investigators of distinguishing between their roles as clinician and their roles as researchers in their interactions with the patient as a potential clinical trial participant. As summarized in related discussions in this book, the key solution to resolving the "therapeutic misconception" issue is to utilize an informed consent form and engage in an informed consent process that clearly describes to all potential cancer clinical trial participants the known and likely risks of participation and the non-research alternatives available to them.

5.3 Financial Conflicts of Interest

Finally, a critical ethical consideration that can pose serious legal risks for physician investigators and their institutions is the extent to which the cancer clinical trial is affected by financial conflicts of interest. These financial conflicts of interest can be either individual or institutional or both. An individual conflict of interest is one in which the physician investigator (or a spouse or household member) has a financial interest that could be significantly affected by the outcome of the cancer clinical trial. An example would be a physician investigator's ownership of shares of stock issued by a pharmaceutical company who is sponsoring the physician investigator's cancer clinical trial. An example of an institutional conflict of interest is where a research institution or academic medical center that is approving and conducting the cancer clinical trial has a financial interest in a company whose cancer treatment drug is being tested in the same trial. The interest could be stock ownership or ownership of a patent interest the values of which could be significantly affected by the outcome of the cancer clinical trial.

The claims asserted by the family of Jesse Gelsinger in their widely publicized lawsuit against the University of Pennsylvania following Mr. Gelsinger's death (while participating in a 1999 gene therapy trial) are illustrative of how ethical principles involving financial conflicts of interest can be transformed into a significant legal risk exposures for a physician investigators and their affiliate institutions under certain circumstances.

In the Gelsinger case, both the physician investigator and the University of Pennsylvania held financial interests in the company that financed the gene therapy trial being conducted by the University's Institute for Human Gene Therapy. It was alleged that these interests were intentionally not disclosed to Mr. Gelsinger. The Gelsinger lawsuit and U.S. Department of Justice investigations were both resolved through an initial settlement between and among the parties.[18] There was no judicial determination as to whether any non-disclosure was intentional or whether the decision to enroll Mr. Gelsinger in the trial was improper or motivated by a profit incentive on the part of the physician investigator and/or the University of Pennsylvania. Nevertheless, the events leading up to the Gelsinger incident and others that followed at other institutions catapulted the topics of individual and institutional financial conflicts of interest in human subjects research into the spotlight.

Numerous scholarly reviews, articles, journal articles and guidelines have been published and recommendations ranging from outright prohibition to careful management of financial conflicts of interest have been debated and discussed in recent years.[19] To improve the physician investigator's understanding of how to ethically resolve his/her potential for financial conflicts of interest in cancer clinical trials, it is helpful to understand how these financial conflicts may arise.

A variety of factors have produced an increasing level of cooperation between research institutions including academic medical centers and the pharmaceutical and biotechnology industries in the conduct of cancer clinical trials as well as the commercialization of technologies in the field of cancer diagnosis and treatment. One factor was the passage of the Bayh-Dole Act in 1980[20] which encouraged research institutions to retain ownership of inventions from federally supported research. This development promoted the practice of technology transfer through which commercially viable products and technologies would be licensed by research institutions to pharmaceutical, biomedical and biotechnology companies. Another factor is the increased reliance by physician investigators and research institutions on private funding for the conduct of cancer clinical trials, most notably from pharmaceutical and biotechnology companies.

As summarized by the "Policy and Guidelines for the Oversight of Individual Financial Interests in Human Subjects Research" adopted by the American Association of American Medical Colleges ("AAMC") in 2001, opportunities to profit from research may affect – or appear to affect – a researcher's judgments about which subjects to enroll, the clinical care provided to subjects, even the proper use of subjects' confidential health information. Financial interests also threaten scientific integrity when they foster real or apparent biases in study design, data collection and analysis, adverse event reporting, or the presentation and publication of research findings."[21]

Many research institutions and academic medical centers have elected to revise their individual financial conflict of interest policies that were established or refined in the mid 1990's in response to federal regulatory requirements.[22] In general these modifications have imposed stricter limitations on the financial interests that can be held by physician investigators when engaged in the conduct of human subjects research, including cancer clinical trials.

Some research institutions and academic medical centers have also established institutional conflict of interest policies that require careful review and consideration as to whether a clinical trial can be conducted at an institution that holds a potentially significant financial interest in the outcome. Those institutions who have established policies for institutional conflict of interest reviews have been guided by the 2002 AAMC Task Force Report recommendations[23] and the earlier work of the Association of American Universities ("AAU").[24]

The fundamental ethical and legal principle that serves as the foundation for individual and institutional financial conflict of interest polices is that of full disclosure. Full disclosure by physician investigators of the existence of current or future individual financial interests to their research institutions or academic medical centers is crucial. Depending on the policies and procedures in place at each research institution or academic medical center, the physician investigator may need to engage in a conflict management or mitigation process with institutional representatives.

Depending on the nature of the individual financial interest, it may also be necessary for the physician investigator to decide whether to simply eliminate the financial conflict of interest by electing to withdraw from participation in the cancer clinical trial or to dispose the interest. In most cases, physician investigators will be required to disclose to potential cancer clinical trial participants the existence of certain individual financial interests that are deemed by the institutional review board as significant. This participant disclosure process is usually incorporated into the informed consent process described earlier.

Since the policies and procedures at research institutions and academic medical centers vary widely, physician investigators interested in initiating or participating in a cancer clinical trial should thoroughly investigate the financial conflict of interest process at their own research institutions or academic medical centers. Diligent compliance with the financial conflict of interest policies and procedures is the best defense that a physician investigator can mount if faced with a legal challenge. In a high-visibility clinical trial, the investigator may want to eliminate any financial conflicts even if he or she is permitted by the institution to retain an interest, simply to avoid any appearance of a conflict.

6. CONCLUSION AND RECOMMENDATIONS

In conclusion, physician investigators who elect to participate in cancer clinical trials must be vigilant in their monitoring of the ever-changing regulatory compliance environment. It is important that they avail themselves and their staff of all opportunities for education, training and professional development in the courses focused on the ethical and responsible conduct of research involving human participants. Particular attention should be directed to the unique ethical and legal issues involved in the conduct investigator-initiated clinical trials or those that could involve individual or institutional conflicts of interest. If the conduct of cancer clinical trials is encouraged and supported by the physician investigators' research institution or academic medical center, the senior leadership at those institutions must demonstrate their commitment to establish and adequately fund regulatory compliance resources to assist and support physician investigators in this important and noble work.

REFERENCES

1. 21 Code of Federal Regulations Part 312
2. 21 Code of Federal Regulations Part 812
3. The International Conference on Harmonisation of Technical Requirements for the Registration of Pharmaceuticals for Human Use, commonly referred to as the International Conference on Harmonisation or "ICH" was adopted as guidance by the U.S. Food and Drug Administration in 1997. (See Federal Register, Vol. 62, No. 90, May 9, 1997, pages 25691-25709)
4. For an up-to-date listing, see http://grants.nih.gov/grants/oer.htm
5. See www.cms.hhs.gov/manuals/06_cim/ci30.asp
6. 42 Code of Federal Regulations Part 50
7. 45 Code of Federal Regulations Part 164
8. 42 Code of Federal Regulations Part 93
9. See http://www.cmaj.ca/cgi/content/full/171/6/606 and http://www.icmje.org/clin_trialup.htm
10. S.470 called the "Fair Access to Clinical Trials Act of 2005" or "FACT" was introduced into the Senate on 2/28/05. FACT would mandate the creation of a publicly accessible national data bank of clinical trial information comprised of a clinical trial registry and a clinical trial results database.
11. http://www.cancer.gov/cancertopics/factsheet/NCI/clinical-trials-cooperative-group
12. See FDA regulations describing "sponsor" obligations at 21 Code of Federal Regulations Subpart D, as amended.
13. The Belmont Report: Ethical Principles and Guidelines for the Protection of Human Subjects of Research by the National Commission for the Protection of Human Subjects of Biomedical and Behavioral Research (1979) also known as the "Belmont Report."

14. Levine, Robert J., Ethics and Regulation of Clinical Research (2d ed. 1988) New Haven, CT: Yale University Press.
15. Levine. Robert J., Ethics and Regulation of Clinical Research (2d ed. 1988), Chapter 5.
16. Appelbaum, Paul S., "False Hopes and Best Data: Consent to Research and the Therapeutic Misconception, 17 Hastings Center Rep., April 1987.
17. Appelbaum, Paul S., "False Hopes and Best Data: Consent to Research and the Therapeutic Misconception, 17 Hastings Center Rep., April 1987, at 20.
18. http://www.irbforum.com/forum/read/2/95/95 `
19. See Coleman, Carl, et al., The Ethics and Regulation of Research with Human Subjects (Matthew Bender & Company 2005), especially Chapter 5 for a thought-provoking review of these debates and discussion.
20. 35 U.S.C. § 200, Patents: Part II. Patentability of Inventions and Grant of Patents Chapter 18, Patent Rights in Inventions Made with Federal Assistance.
21. "Policy and Guidelines for the Oversight of Individual Financial Interests in Human Subjects Research" by the AAMC Task Force on Financial Conflicts of Interest in Clinical Research (December 2001) at p. 3.
22. See: http://grants.nih.gov/grants/policy/coifaq.htm for a discussion of investigator disclosure and institutional conflict of interest management requirements for institutions receiving funding support from the National Institutes of Health ("NIH") and the National Science Foundation ("NSF").
23. See: http://www.aamc.org/members/coitf/
24. http://www.aau.edu/research/COI.01.pdf

Chapter 13

THE ROLE OF THE OFFICE OF RESEARCH INTEGRITY IN CANCER CLINICAL TRIALS

Peter Abbrecht, MD, PhD, Nancy Davidian, PhD, Samuel Merrill, PhD and Alan R. Price, PhD

Office of Research Integrity, Department of Health and Human Services, Rockville, MD, USA

NOTE: The views expressed in this article are those of the authors and do not necessarily reflect those of the Office of Research Integrity, the United States Department of Health and Human Services, or any other Federal agency.

1. INTRODUCTION

This chapter stresses the importance of integrity in cancer clinical trials and provides examples of cases of research misconduct, handled by the Office of Research Integrity and its predecessor, the Office of Scientific Integrity, for the National Institutes of Health and the Department of Health and Human Services, in which clinical research coordinators, research nurses, and physicians did not maintain high standards of integrity in their research records.

2. BACKGROUND

In 1989, the National Institutes of Health (NIH) created the Office of Scientific Integrity (OSI), in response to Congressional concerns about public reports of fraud in biomedical and clinical research supported by NIH at major universities and research hospitals. Simultaneously, the Department of Health and Human Services (HHS) issued regulations for research institutions to deal with allegations of scientific misconduct (42 Code of Federal Regulations, Part 50, Subpart A). These regulations required institutions that receive NIH and other U.S. Public Health Service (PHS) research funds to conduct inquiries and investigations when warranted, and to provide reports to OSI on such investigations, whether they found scientific misconduct (for falsification, fabrication, or plagiarism in research) or no misconduct, for further review or investigation by OSI. In 1992, HHS moved OSI into the Office of the HHS Secretary, and OSI was renamed the Office of Research Integrity (ORI). In 2000, based on recommendations from NIH and an HHS Review Group on Research Integrity, ORI ceased under PHS policy to conduct independent investigations in the extramural or PHS intramural programs. Instead, ORI depended on receiving institutional investigation reports, followed by thorough oversight by ORI, which negotiated voluntary agreements with respondents who committed misconduct or recommended findings of scientific misconduct to the HHS Assistant Secretary for Health (ASH) for charge letters of proposed misconduct findings, which could be appealed to the Departmental Appeals Board (DAB) for a formal public hearing before a DAB tribunal. In 2005, HHS published a revised regulation on research misconduct (42 Code of Federal Regulations, Part 93), effective June 16, 2005, in which ORI negotiates with or makes findings of research misconduct against respondents, for falsification, fabrication, or plagiarism in proposing, performing, or reviewing research or in reporting research results. In the revised regulation, the former PHS term "scientific misconduct" was changed to "research misconduct" to be consistent with the Government-wide terminology developed by the Office of Science and Technology Policy. ORI's findings may be appealed to the DAB for a hearing before an administrative law judge, whose decision is provided to the ASH for decision and HHS action. ORI/HHS publishes formal notice of its findings of research misconduct, with the name of the respondent(s), his/her title, the institution at which he/she committed research misconduct, and the HHS administrative actions taken against the respondent(s), including requirements for requesting correction or retraction of falsified papers, in several Federal publications: *Federal Register*, GSA Debarment List online (for debarment), *NIH Guide for Grants and Contracts*, and ORI's Website (http://ori.hhs.gov), Newsletter, and Annual Report, all of which can be reached through Internet searches.

In the 16 years since 1989 under this system, over 700 formal case involving inquiries and investigations have been handled by OSI and ORI. OS made 25 findings through 1991, and ORI has made 164 findings of scientifi misconduct between 1992 and November 2005.

Of the ORI findings, 14 involved cancer-related clinical trials (see Table). Of these, 12 addressed either cancer treatment or prevention, while one (Ms. Conrad) was a case control study of radon-related lung cancer and another (Dr. Fossel) was a study of the possible use of nuclear magnetic resonance (NMR) spectroscopy on blood to detect the presence of malignant disease. Only four of the respondents found by ORI to have committed scientific misconduct in cancer clinical trials held degrees above the baccalaureate level, with three M.D. (Drs. Poisson, Tewari, and Herman) and one Ph.D. (Dr. Fossel) degrees. Except for the M.D.-Postdoctoral Fellow (Dr. Tewari), the remaining doctoral degree holders were all Principal Investigators (P.I.s) for the studies in which they committed misconduct. Three of the other respondents were registered nurses. The ten non-doctoral degree holders were all in positions of data manager, study coordinator, clinical research coordinator (CRA), or research program coordinator (one being designated a research assistant and another a research associate).

The majority of the trials listed in the Table (9 of 14) were sponsored by the National Cancer Institute (NCI), either through cooperative arrangements (National Surgical Adjuvant Breast and Bowel Project [NSABP] and the Southwest Oncology Group [SWOG]) or by individual NIH research project grants. In addition, significant clinical cancer trial support was provided by the National Eye Institute (NEI), through its Collaborative Ocular Melanoma Study (COMS); by the National Institute of Environmental Health Sciences (NIEHS); and by the NIH Division of Research Resources (DRR) (now the National Center for Research Resources, NCRR) through its General Clinical Research Centers (GCRC) funding.

The instances of falsification and or fabrication in these cancer trials occurred either in an effort to enroll patients who did not meet all of the eligibility requirements for a study, an attempt to improve the apparent outcome of the study, or to provide data required for the protocol for research work that was not actually done.

Some examples of such ORI clinical cancer research cases follow:

Roger Poisson, M.D., who was a surgeon at St. Luc Hospital in Montreal, Canada, had instructed his research staff to falsify or fabricate at least 177 records of laboratory tests and dates of procedures conducted between 1977 and 1990 for the NCI-supported mastectomy vs. lumpectomy cancer treatment trial of the NSABP. Instances of scientific misconduct included falsifying and failing to report conditions that would have disqualified a patient for trial entry (peau d'orange skin change in breast cancer, congestive heart failure in a patient enrolled in a trial with cardio-toxic drugs, inadequate white blood cell count for initiation of chemotherapy), misrepresentation of biopsy site for estrogen/progesterone receptor assays (primary tumor vs. axillary nodes), and fabrication of follow-up data, including continued reports of contacts with a patient who was deceased. Dr. Poisson gave various explanations for his actions, such as "Our cardiologists felt that she was a good candidate and we accepted their words" for the patient with congestive failure. In 1993 Dr. Poisson was debarred by ORI/HHS from Federal funding and prohibited from serving on PHS advisory groups for 8 years.

Vicki Hanneken, R.N., who was a CRA at Decatur Memorial Hospital in Illinois, falsified or fabricated clinical and study records in 60 instances for 35 patients in the Selenium and Vitamin E Cancer Prevention Trial (SELECT), funded by NCI/NIH through SWOG. Prior to being appointed to the CRA position, Ms. Hanneken had worked for a decade as an oncology home care and hospice nurse, receiving outstanding evaluations. However, in her work on the SELECT trial, Ms. Hanneken apparently had difficulty in collecting the required patient data. Her acts of scientific misconduct included fabrication and falsification of patients' laboratory values on original and source documents, falsification of information on patients' clinical progress records, and alteration of visit and laboratory report dates to fit the protocol time windows. The falsifications were done to make it appear that the trial was being conducted in such a manner that protocol requirements were met for patient eligibility and continuation in the study. Ms. Hanneken entered into a Voluntary Exclusion Agreement (VEA) in which she agreed to exclude herself from contracting or subcontracting with any U.S. Government agency and from serving in any advisory capacity for PHS for 3 years.

Eric Fossel, Ph.D., who was an Associate Professor of Radiology at Beth Israel Hospital and Harvard Medical School in Boston, altered NMR imaging data from a privately-funded Multi-Center Breast Trial and reported these falsified results in an NIH grant application, claiming a falsely high sensitivity for a diagnostic blood test for predisposition to malignancy or relapse. Although purportedly blinded to diagnoses, Dr. Fossel obtained the patients' diagnoses by reference to the patients' clinical records (through his wife, who was a co-investigator) and through access to the Hospital's electronic records. He then altered the line-width data to match the patients' diagnoses. In 1996, Dr. Fossel entered into a VEA with the PHS to exclude himself from contracting or subcontracting the Federal Government and from serving as a PHS advisor for 3 years.

Thomas Philpot, R.N., was an experienced research nurse who committed scientific misconduct while employed at two institutions, Rush-Presbyterian-St. Luke's Medical Center (RPSLMC) and MacNeal Cancer Center, an NSABP-affiliate of Northwestern University (NWU). According to the record, he developed an exceptional rapport with his research patients and trained new personnel in the collection, documentation, and reporting of clinical research data. Mr. Philpot committed misconduct by fabricating telephone contacts with NSABP protocol patients and fabricating data on patient survival, treatment failure, and morbidity that were submitted to the NSABP Biostatistical Center. One of Mr. Philpot's misconduct incidents at RPSLMC was discovered by a routine computer check. The incident at MacNeal was uncovered during a routine audit of NSABP records by NWU/NSABP staff. ORI charged Mr. Philpot with scientific misconduct and required a 3-year supervisory plan for him in any PHS-supported clinical research.

Vivian Tanner, who was designated as the Clinic Coordinator for COMS research at the Cleveland Clinic Foundation (CCF), had to be certified by COMS. Her specific responsibilities, as set forth in the COMS Manual of Procedures, included scheduling patient visits and surgical procedures, maintaining and reviewing all CCF study documentation, and reporting the data to the COMS Data Coordinating Center (DCC). Misconduct by Ms. Tanner was initially detected during a routine clinic monitoring visit at CCF by the COMS DCC. Over a number of years she falsified and fabricated research data (physical examination, blood test and chest X-ray results) for 21 of the 24 patients. HHS debarred her from participation in federal grants and contracts for a period of 3 years.

Terence Herman, M.D., was an Associate Professor of Radiation Therapy at Harvard Medical School (HMS), a staff member of the Joint Center for Radiation Therapy, and a member of the Division of Radiation Oncology at the Dana Farber Cancer Institute (DFCI). His misconduct occurred in a clinical trial of trimodality (cisplatin, hyperthermia, and radiation) treatment of superficial malignant tumors. The protocol called for the physician to make sequential measurements of two dimensions of each tumor during the course of treatment, and the response was to be assessed by the degree of measurable reduction in tumor size. However, Dr. Herman did not routinely measure tumors, by caliper, ruler, CT scan, or any other objective means, and he published fabricated or falsified measurements in a paper in the *International Journal of Radiation Oncology•Biology•Physics* in 1989, leading him to report a falsely large number and magnitude of positive responses to hyperthermia therapy. Suspicion of misconduct was raised by a co-worker and resulted in an internal audit of his protocol by the DFCI Quality Control Center, followed by a joint investigation by HMS and DFCI. Dr. Herman entered into a VEA with ORI to be supervised for a 3-year period for any PHS-sponsored research in which he was involved and to retract that portion of the questioned paper that dealt with tumor response.

As illustrated in the cases described above, the administrative actions imposed by ORI against respondents involve debarment from Federal funding, typically for 3 to 5 years; close supervision of their future research; and/or special certification of their research. All of the respondents in the Table were also prohibited from serving on PHS advisory groups for a certain period.

The proportion of doctoral degree holders (29%) among those who committed misconduct in the small ORI sample represented in the Table is markedly lower than that in the remainder of ORI's scientific misconduct findings cases (approximately 65%), reflecting the fact that the P.I.s on NIH grants (generally doctoral degree holders) tend to be the respondents more frequently involved in non-clinical cases involving laboratory research than involved in clinical trials.

Although most of the respondents who committed misconduct in the cancer clinical trials were relatively low ranking staff members, rather than P.I.s, several of the institutional reports to ORI noted that lack of supervision, training, oversight, and on-site presence by the P.I. may have contributed to the occurrence of or opportunity for misconduct.

In ORI's experience, most of the problems in clinical research, including cancer clinical trials, arise from overworked physicians/researchers who do not maintain careful oversight over trials; overloaded clinical research coordinators or research nurses, who did not have time to complete their work and paper requirements; poorly trained clinical research staff; pressure to enroll patients; other job-related problems; or personal/home problems. The problems with clinical data integrity are reported by internal quality control groups; external quality control groups, like data coordinating centers or external auditors; co-workers and colleagues; direct supervisors; and patients or their care-givers who contact the trial appointment desks.

These problems in clinical research go beyond the ORI issues of falsification and fabrication of clinical and study records and reports. They lead to other non-ORI matters, such as failing to report adverse events to the institutional review board (IRB), to the sponsor, or to the Food and Drug Administration (FDA); failing to obtain or to document informed consent; deviating from the clinical trial protocol, such as including a subject who was ineligible or administering another drug that was off-protocol, so long as the patient and research records were accurately reported; failing to obtain IRB or FDA approval for changes made in a formally approved protocol; forging a physician's signature on medical orders; or breaching a patient's or subject's confidentiality. While these are not ORI issues, they fall under FDA or HHS Office for Human Research Protections (OHRP) authority and are addressed by those offices.

In addition, NCI's Clinical Trials Monitoring Branch (CTMB) expects all cooperative clinical trial groups and individual institutions to report any data discrepancies or evidence of manipulation of clinical data or records. NCI/CTMB staff then notifies ORI about pending audits of such trials, and ORI staff often attend as observers, seeking to preserve any evidence of falsification or fabrication that may constitute research misconduct. ORI may then work with the research university or hospital to ensure an appropriate inquiry and/or investigation if the evidence of significant misconduct is sufficient (ORI does not expect or want cooperative clinical cancer groups themselves to try to investigate misconduct at their member institutions, where they generally lack administrative authority over the property or personnel in question).

ORI remains interested in working with clinical research investigators and their staffs, including the critically important CRAs, to detect early or prevent such problems in clinical research, which may lead to research misconduct and public exposure. To that end, ORI has sponsored several conferences (see http://ori.hhs.gov/conferences), including "Fostering Integrity in Clinical Research at Academic Medical Centers" in 2001 in Baltimore; "Enhancing Integrity in Clinical Research" in 2003 at the University of California at Los Angeles; "The Research Coordinator: Strategies for Promoting Integrity in Clinical Research" in 2005 at the University of Pennsylvania; and ""CSI" for Clinical Investigators: Making the Case for Integrity and Examining the Causes of Misconduct in Research," an ORI/Physicians for Responsibility in Medicine and Research pre-conference workshop for clinical researchers in 2005 in Boston. ORI welcomes expressions of interest from cancer clinical trials researchers and CRAs in further educational meetings.

3. CONCLUSION

This chapter stresses the importance of integrity in cancer clinical trials and provides examples of cases of research misconduct, handled by the Office of Research Integrity and its predecessor, the Office of Scientific Integrity, for the National Institutes of Health and the Department of Health and Human Services, in which clinical research coordinators, research nurses, and physicians did not maintain high standards of integrity in their research records.

Table. ORI findings of scientific misconduct in cancer-related clinical trial cases

Respondent's name	Rank/title of respondent	Institution	Sponsor/ funding agency	Clinical cancer trial type	Year ORI Closed
Roger Poisson,[1] MD	Staff Surgeon	St. Luc Hospital, Montreal	NIH-NCI	NSABP-multisite breast cancer treatment	1993
Anand Tewari,[2] MD	Postdoctoral Fellow, Surgery	Stanford University	NIH-DRR through the GCRC	Phase I interleukin-1β NSCLC treatment	1994
Denise R. Conrad[3]	Research Assistant, Preventive Medicine	University of Iowa	NIH-NIEHS	Radon exposure, as possible etiology of lung cancer	1995
Terence S. Herman,[4] MD	Associate Professor, Radiation Therapy	Harvard Medical School and Dana Farber Cancer Inst.	NIH-NCI	Hyperthermia, single site cancer treatment	1995
Barbara Jones[5]	Data Manager	St. Mary's Hospital, Montreal	NIH-NCI	NSABP multi-site breast cancer prevention	1995
Catherine Kerr[6]	Data Coordinator	St. Mary's Hospital, Montreal	NIH-NCI	NSABP multi-site breast cancer prevention	1995
Victoria Santa Cruz[7]	Program Coordinator	University of Arizona	NIH-NCI	Breast cancer self-care	1995
Vivian N. Tanner[8]	Clinic Coordinator	Cleveland Clinic Foundation	NIH-NEI	COMS multi-site ocular melanoma treatment	1995
Gail L. Daubert,[9] RN	Clinic Coordinator	Northwestern University	NIH-NEI	COMS multi-site ocular melanoma treatment	1995
Eric Fossel,[10] PhD	Associate Professor of Radiology	Harvard Medical School, Beth Israel Hosp.	Private foundation & NCI grant applications	NMR spectra use in cancer diagnosis and detection of recurrence	1996

Ann Marie Huelskamp[11]	Research Program Coordinator	John Hopkins School of Medicine	NIH-NCI	Metastatic breast cancer treatment and quality of patient life	1997
Maria Diaz[12]	Data Manager	Rush Presbyterian St. Luke's Hospital	NIH-NCI	NSABP (breast cancer) and ECOG (lung cancer) prevention	1999
Thomas Philpot,[13] RN, BSN	Data Manager	Rush Presbyterian, Northwestern University	NIH-NCI	NSABP – several multi-site breast cancer treatment protocols	1999
Vickie L. Hanneken,[14] RN	Clinical Research Associate	Decatur Memorial Hospital	NIH-NCI	SWOG SELECT prostate cancer prevention	2004

REFERENCES

1. Poisson notice: http://grants.nih.gov/grants/guide/notice-files/not93-177.html
2. Tewari notice: http://grants.nih.gov/grants/guide/notice-files/not94-244.html
3. Conrad notice: http://grants.nih.gov/grants/guide/notice-files/not95-138.html
4. Herman notice: http://grants.nih.gov/grants/guide/notice-files/not95-138.html
5. Jones notice: http://grants.nih.gov/grants/guide/notice-files/not95-178.html
6. Kerr notice: http://grants.nih.gov/grants/guide/notice-files/not95-233.html
7. Santa Cruz notice: http://grants.nih.gov/grants/guide/notice-files/not96-002.html
8. Tanner: http://ori.dhhs.gov/documents/newsletters/vol3_no3.pdf
9. Daubert notice: http://grants.nih.gov/grants/guide/notice-files/not96-080.html
10. Fossel notice: http://grants.nih.gov/grants/guide/notice-files/not96-160.html
11. Huelskamp notice: http://grants.nih.gov/grants/guide/notice-files/not97-097.html
12. Diaz notice: http://grants.nih.gov/grants/guide/notice-files/not99-057.html
13. Philpot notice, http://grants.nih.gov/grants/guide/notice-files/not99-028.html
14. Hanneken notice, http://grants.nih.gov/grants/guide/notice-files/NOT-OD-04-038.html

Chapter 14

STRATEGIES FOR THE ADMINISTRATION OF A CLINICAL TRIALS INFRASTRUCTURE: LESSONS FROM A COMPREHENSIVE CANCER CENTER

Leonard A. Zwelling, MD, MBA and Carleen A. Brunelli, PhD, MBA
Office of Research Administration, The University of Texas M.D. Anderson Cancer Center, Houston, Texas, USA

1. INTRODUCTION

Clinical research is really human subjects research. Research is defined as "a systematic investigation, including research development, testing and evaluation, designed to develop or contribute to generalizable knowledge" [45 CFR 46.102(d)].

Human subjects are "living individual(s) about whom an investigator (whether professional or student) conducting research obtains (1) data through intervention or interaction with the individual, or (2) identifiable private information" [45 CFR 46.102(f)]. The Food and Drug Administration (21 CFR 56.102(e)) identifies a human subject as an "individual who is or becomes a participant in research, either as a recipient of the test agent or as a control. A subject may be either a healthy individual or a patient".

What is immediately obvious from these definitions from the Code of Federal Regulations is that clinical or human subjects research is NOT clinical care.

Clinical care is a person-by-person endeavor. The physician can make independent judgments about a patient's care and initiate or alter that care. There is no required contract (i.e., an informed consent document) between the doctor and the patient with particular regard to the obligation of the doctor to the patient or to any outside monitoring body (i.e., an Institutional

Review Board). There is no need to draw any generalizable conclusions from the treatment. The only result that counts is the one experienced by the individual patient.

Human subjects research is the exact opposite. Physicians are not free to make judgments about what treatment individuals receive as that is determined by the protocol for which the subject has been recruited. That protocol has been approved by an outside body (an Institutional Review Board [IRB]). IRB has also approved an informed consent document that serves as a contract between the subject and both the investigator and the IRB. That document must describe how the patient will be treated and what that patient should expect in the way of benefits and potential risks. Perhaps, of greatest importance, the informed consent document must indicate that the patient (i.e., subject) can withdraw from the research at any time for any reason. It is virtually a unilateral contract which does, however, indicate that the investigator has fiduciary obligations to more than the patient. The investigator must follow the IRB-approved protocol. If the interests of the patient would be best served by deviating from the protocol treatment plan, the patient must be removed as a study subject before such a plan is initiated.

Clinical care is not subject to federal regulation, but rather is usually regulated by states through professional licensing procedures. Those performing clinical care really have fiduciary responsibilities to their patients only. Those performing clinical research have fiduciary responsibilities to boards (IRBs) that oversee human subjects research and the federal government as well as to the patients and subjects enrolled in clinical trials. Clinical investigators may even have competing fiduciary allegiances to the corporate sponsors of their clinical trials through contractual agreements. This has given birth to the concept of conflict of interest in clinical research and the development of methods to oversee, manage or eliminate such conflicts.

Finally, the record keeping and reporting necessary for clinical research far exceeds that of routine patient care.

In all of these ways, human subjects research is different and distinct from patient care. The summary of what "the pharmaceutical and medical device industries" consider "industry-accepted standards that govern clinical trials involving humans conducted to support applications and subsequent amendments for approval by the U.S. Food and Drug Administration (FDA)" is called Good Clinical Practice or GCP.[1] GCP is not at all like clinical practice. And, it is with an eye toward GCP that any clinical trials infrastructure should be developed.

To assist and support investigators performing clinical research requires infrastructure that differs dramatically from that which supports routine patient care. It is not intrinsically part of most hospitals or clinics. The personnel required to staff such an infrastructure require specialized training as the skills that they must bring to supporting clinical research are not those acquired in the routine training of most nurses, clerical staff, or even physicians.

The skilled personnel who make up a good clinical research infrastructure fill the gap between what personnel commonly learn in professional biomedical training and that which must be in place to fulfill the obligations to governmental agencies, commercial sponsors and human subjects. Means of filling this learning gap is what leaders of clinical research infrastructure must identify, develop and operationalize if the research institutions the infrastructure is to support are to remain in compliance with all of the regulations governing human subject research.

Most of the infrastructure we will describe in this chapter has been built by us in the free-standing, academic cancer center in which we work. However, the regulations we describe and the methods we have developed to fulfill the obligations placed on investigators by these regulations are widely applicable to all types of human subjects research.

In this chapter we will:

- Describe the players in human subjects research
- Describe the functions that must be in place to support good, compliant clinical research
- Describe our solutions to initiating and sustaining these functions with particular attention to the use of various electronic information system-based applications
- Describe two unique, but important aspects of modern clinical research that all research institutions must address—Scientific Misconduct and Conflict of Interest

2. THE PLAYERS

Investigators-There is no person more important to the proper and compliant performance of clinical research than the Principal Investigator. As noted in the Guide to Good Clinical Practice;[2] "Investigators can, and often do, delegate some of the work involved in the studies to their staffs. However, delegating the work does not relieve investigators of their responsibility. They have the ultimate responsibility for all work."

In particular, the GCP Guide refers to the responsibilities listed in the FDA Form 1572, the Investigator's Agreement. These include:
- Conducting any research study in accordance with the protocol
- Notifying a sponsor of any protocol changes
- Personally conducting the study or supervising others
- Informing subjects of the investigational nature of the drugs
- Insuring informed consent is obtained properly
- Reporting adverse events in accord with federal code
- Reading and understanding the investigator's brochure
- Informing all associates of their obligations under the study
- Maintaining accurate records. Making them available for inspection.
- Insuring that a regulatory compliant IRB is overseeing the research
- Reporting any changes in the research
- Making no changes in the protocol without IRB approval

This list is an excellent standard to which all principal investigators should be held, whether a trial is being conducted under FDA jurisdiction with an Investigational New Drug (IND) application, or with commercially-available agents. There is only one regulatory and ethical standard by which human subjects research should be conducted and will be judged. The commercial availability of the agent or device being tested does not affect the degree of regulatory oversight by the IRB or by the Office of Human Research Protections (OHRP). Investigators must familiarize themselves with the appropriate parts of the Code of Federal Regulations for the sake of their research subjects, their institutions and themselves.

At The University of Texas M.D. Anderson Cancer Center (UTMDACC) we initiated a series of training sessions specifically geared toward clinical investigators (see Training). Much of the content of this ten-hour course was dictated by the demands and responsibilities placed on clinical investigators by the Code of Federal Regulations.

<u>Research Nurses</u>-Many clinical investigators depend on research nurses to perform a number of vital tasks during the course of a clinical trial. These include:
- Assistance with study design
- Interacting with sponsors
- Protocol co-authoring
- Assistance in shepherding the proposed research through the various steps in the review and approval process
- IND preparation
- Patient recruitment
- Assistance with explaining protocol details to and obtaining informed consent from perspective subjects

- Assistance with data acquisition, management and entry into case report forms or computerized data bases
- Interactions with regulatory bodies as well as industry or governmental sponsors
- Protocol revision for IRB review and approval
- Continuing review preparation for IRB review and approval
- Adverse event reporting to the IRB and to sponsors
- Participation in monitoring and auditing
- Preparation of final reports and manuscripts for publication

A good research nurse is a full partner with the principal investigator and co-investigators. The research nurse can also be a quality control and regulatory compliance resource within the research team doing human subjects research. As such, training, specifically for research nurses is an essential part of the infrastructure needed to support high quality clinical research.

Data Managers-The list of tasks that research nurses may perform is long. In most cases, however, research nurses do not perform all of the functions listed above. The Clinical Research Associate (CRA) or data manager is usually uniquely positioned to focus on clinical trial data acquisition, tabulation and management. In many centers, data managers are centralized within the "protocol office". Investigators must, in essence, purchase their services either through the use of funds from industry sponsorship (sponsored research agreements or contracts) or through competitive grant funding (e.g., from a National Cancer Institute investigator-initiated award or an NCI Cancer Center Support Grant, CCSG or "core" grant).

One of the benefits of this centralization is that, unlike the research nurses who usually work with one investigator or a small team of investigators, data managers do not report long-term to the investigator for whom they may be working at any given time. In a sense, they are independent of the sphere of influence of the investigator and, thus may serve as a check against any bias.

Data managers functioning in this way provide a valuable service to the study, the investigator and to the research institution. They are uniquely positioned to independently judge the quality of the data they are compiling and whether the trial is being performed in accord with the IRB-approved protocol, GCP, and federal regulations.

They too, like research nurses, deserve special education in the rules and regulations governing clinical research.

Biostatisticians-The review of the biostatistical methods proposed to analyze the results of and draw conclusions from clinical trials is usually viewed as a scientific issue. And, it is. Under-powered trials (insufficient numbers of subjects to draw unambiguous and statistically-significant conclusions from trial data) are scientifically invalid and should never be approved by any scientific review committee or IRB.

However, the adequacy of the biostatistics associated with any trial is also a human subjects protection issue. No subject should be enrolled in any trial whose very design precludes the ability to draw significant inferences from the trial data. Inadequately powered trials are unethical.

It is wise then, that biostatisticians trained in the design and performance of clinical trials and the analysis of the data from such trials be involved with every step in the process of trial authoring and review. Each protocol should have a thorough biostatistics section which uses appropriate methodology to demonstrate how the design and number of subjects required will fulfill the objectives of the trial. Both the scientific review and human subjects protection review committees should have qualified clinical trial biostatisticians as members.

Pharmacists-As a critical link in the chain from orders written to drug administered, the pharmacist can provide another check and balance to the system supporting clinical research. The specially-trained research pharmacists who are schooled in the constitution and administration of novel agents often detect errors or protocol deviations that can not only save the integrity of the research data, but avoid mistakes in ordering that can be harmful to patients.

During the writing and review of any clinical study, the pharmacists should be included as the study design is created and the routes and vehicles by which a drug is to be administered are reviewed and discussed.

Protocol or Research Administration Office-This office has different names at different institutions. It performs a host of functions that are absolutely essential for a successful human subjects research program. At UTMDACC these include:

- Staffing the IRB
- Staffing the committees that review the scientific merit of protocols prior to IRB review
- Quality Assurance, auditing, and monitoring
- Clinical research and regulatory affairs training
- Information systems for regulatory support and data management
- Sponsor interactions and contracting
- FDA interactions and sponsorship of INDs
- Staffing the Conflict of Interest Committee
- Office of the Institutional Official for Human Subjects Research

- Office of the Research Integrity Officer
- Office of the Chief Research and Regulatory Affairs Officer

It is essential that this office have strong and knowledgeable leadership. We have found that the knowledge needed to oversee such an office can be embodied in a number of different types of administrators. However, the credibility of the office with the research faculty may well depend upon this office being led by a fellow faculty member.

If possible, an M.D. with experience in clinical trial-based research and a track record of accomplishment in clinical research is the ideal candidate. Unfortunately, such individuals are hard to find for these jobs, as people with such backgrounds are often unlikely to forego their own research and patient care efforts to become the full-time administrator most protocol offices need.

Any institution wishing to perform human subjects research would do well to invest in identifying, training and supporting the designated leader of this office. That person may well be the one who will be called upon to secure the integrity of the entire research enterprise should an individual investigator, trial or research group violate the tenets of research regulation or GCP during the course of a clinical trial. In such situations, a quick, focused and learned response by the office's leadership (along with that of the IRB and the institution as a whole) to federal regulatory agencies can be the difference between a protracted external investigation with possible institutional sanctions and open communications with the federal government that lead to a resolution of a difficult situation.

The Office of Human Research Protections-Formerly known as the Office for Protection from Research Risks (OPRR) under the National Institutes of Health, this office rose in the federal hierarchy to be housed in the office of the Secretary of the Department of Health and Human Services in 2000.[3] It retains many of the functions of OPRR (although not the oversight of vertebrate animal research). The most important of these functions is that all IRBs overseeing federally-funded human subjects research report to OHRP. In many research institutions including our own, all human subjects research, regardless of funding source, is overseen by IRBs. Thus, this critical element of the infrastructure supporting clinical research, the IRB, really reports to no one at the home institution, but to the federal government itself.

An institution's commitment to the IRB system and to OHRP is embodied in its Federal-Wide Assurance (FWA) document. This document formalizes the institution's agreement to conduct its human subjects research in accord with all federal statutes.[4] This document is signed by the IRB chair(s) and the institutional official for human subjects research, the individual with primary oversight for the human subjects program at the institution. There are also special educational requirements of each of those signatories.

The National Cancer Institute-Charged with overseeing the cancer research enterprise funded by federal tax dollars, the NCI has both intramural and extramural programs in clinical research. While the bulk of NCI research grant funds support laboratory-based research, there are programs supporting clinical trials both at the NIH Clinical Center in Bethesda, MD and throughout the country.

The most prominent of these programs involve cooperative group trials having large numbers of investigators from all over the country. The focus of the cooperative groups is the performance of large trials requiring significant numbers of patients to be accrued to answer research questions. Many (but not all) of these trials are randomized Phase III trials. However, Phase I and pre-clinical work is also supported by NCI.

From the infrastructure point of view, there are several key NCI-related issues that must be addressed by any center wishing to work with NCI or its funds.

First, these are tax payer dollars. Any institution successfully competing for these funds will be subject to a host of rules and regulations from those of reporting expenditures to those governing the processing of allegations of scientific misconduct (see below).

Second, data reporting to NCI can be onerous. It must be done in a rigorous, electronic format that changes frequently.

Third, NCI-sponsored trials are audited frequently and adherence to the highest standards of GCP is expected.

Fourth, infrastructure support is available on Cancer Center Support Grants (CCSG). These are large allocations of NCI funds aimed at the infrastructure supporting science already supported by other NCI and NIH grants. It is a way for NCI to leverage its investment in the cancer-related science occurring at major academic centers. The majority of CCSG dollars fund laboratory research support cores for the general use of NCI-funded investigators (e.g., DNA sequencing facilities, transgenic mouse colonies). However, clinical trials support infrastructure and a core called the Protocol Review and Monitoring System (PRMS), which serves as a quality assurance core, directly support clinical research and should be accessible to cancer centers with a CCSG in place.

Fifth, all institutions that receive NCI support for their clinical trials programs must have a comprehensive Data and Safety Monitoring Plan (DSMP) approved by and on file with NCI. In this plan, the manner by which data integrity and patient safety (human subjects protection) will be overseen by the institution must be described. This includes standard data and safety monitoring for typical treatment trials, as well as methods for trial oversight for large population-based studies or psychological, behavioral or quality- of-life studies. We found that using a matrix approach in our DSMP to facilitate the identification by principal investigators of the type of trial they are performing and the matching, required data and safety monitoring plan, was a satisfactory and user-friendly means of fulfilling this NCI mandate. Each type of trial was described in a table with the associated plan for data and safety monitoring which could be used when writing a clinical protocol by the PI.

The United States Food and Drug Administration-It is critical to remember that the FDA's major job is the regulation of the safety and efficacy of investigational new drugs and devices.[6] The FDA always has an eye on the well-being of those Americans who will be using the agents or devices whose approval the agency oversees. The FDA wants trials to progress toward the marketing of a useful product. While often mistakenly seen as a barrier to research progress, the agency is grounded in the commitment toward commercialization. Its standards must be high as the well-being of all Americans using a product approved by the FDA depends upon the rigor with which trials were performed and the diligence of the FDA in regulating the performance of the trials and analyzing the validity of the data coming from those trials.

Once an investigator or team of investigators decides that a drug or device is ready for human testing, an Investigational New Drug application (IND) or an Investigational Device Exemption (IDE) must be filed with the FDA. INDs (or IDEs) contain a large amount of manufacturing and animal testing results as well as an IRB-approved clinical protocol that describes the initial human testing to be done. A form called a 1572 must be signed by the principal investigator and submitted with the IND application. The form serves as a contract between the agency and the investigator concerning how the research team will conduct the research (see above).

INDs may also be required when commercially-available (and thus, FDA-approved) drugs or devices are being used in research if they are being tested in new ways, at a newer, potentially riskier dose, or via a new route of administration. (The FDA has published a guidance document advising institutions how to determine if protocols involving off-label use of anticancer drugs are exempt from IND requirements). Assuming research being performed with such agents or devices is IND-exempt is an error. If any doubt exists, the advice of the FDA or a formal request for an IND exemption should be sought.

The sponsor of an IND is "the person who assumes the ultimate responsibility for and initiates the investigation of the new drug, biologic, or device, including responsibility for compliance with provisions of the Federal, Food, Drug and Cosmetic Act and FDA regulations" [21 CFR 312.3]. Sponsors are often companies (e.g., a pharmaceutical company), but they can be individuals (e.g., a faculty member) or institutions.

The rigor and administrative support required of an IND sponsor are great. In our experience, few individual faculty members have the necessary training or access to resources needed to support an IND. At UTMDACC, the institution holds all such INDs and investigators are assisted in IND preparation by knowledgeable staff in the Office of Research Administration who also assists the PI with any communications with the FDA.

Periodically, FDA auditors may visit. They come to institutions with IRBs to audit the IRB's function, records, and policies. FDA auditors may come to audit a specific study or a specific investigator. It is imperative that those interacting with the FDA visitors understand the requirements of IND sponsors and treat the FDA visitor with the respect due any federal agent. In our experience, FDA visits can be the source of much learning and process improvement, if addressed as such. If handled in a confrontational fashion, these visits can be long, disrupting and have severe consequences.

It is very unlikely that the agency will find any program to be perfect. How an institution responds to the findings of the visit (given to the institution or investigator at an exit interview at the conclusion of the FDA visit as an FDA form 483), will determine the amount of cooperation the institution receives from the FDA after the visit as the institution or individual seeks to correct any identified deficiencies.

<u>The Drug, Biotechnology and Device Industries</u>-In the past, clinical research was performed in academic centers free from the need for regulatory oversight and financial support. OHRP did not exist. The Belmont Report that gave birth to the IRB system was produced in the late 1970's. The FDA only gained its regulatory responsibility for the oversight of the assessment of drug and device efficacy in 1962[5] (safety had been the FDA's only focus prior to 1962). Clinical research was often done without informed consent. And, the financial support needed for the work was relatively small and came from patient care revenues or occasionally from NIH grants.

The world of clinical investigation has changed. We have outlined why a modern clinical trials infrastructure must be built with any eye toward regulatory compliance. It must also be built to contend with the unique challenges that accompany doing business with the for-profit sector.

Companies, both closely-held and publicly-traded, are playing an ever-increasing role in the conduct of clinical research, particularly in clinical cancer research. In short, they have the molecules and they have the money.

With the molecular biology revolution, the primacy of the traditional pharmaceutical companies is being challenged by the Amgens and Genetechs of the world. Both the new biotechs and traditional "big pharma" are developing an array of new drugs and doing so at a rate that exceeds that of academia or the NCI. Furthermore, the stark delineation between academia and industry is breaking down. Academic faculty are working very closely with industry to develop drugs and get them ready for human testing. Some faculty are actually starting their own companies to commercialize their discoveries and profit from them. The Bayh-Dole Act of 1980 encourages this as it allows the intellectual property of inventions discovered on federal grants to be retained by the grant recipient.

The ivory tower is no more. This may be good for drug development, but it also may threaten the traditional role of academia in society as being the source of scientific truth untainted by commercial interests. This will be addressed in the section on conflict-of-interest (below).

Regardless, industry is a major player in clinical research. This is particularly true as the NIH does not support clinical research to the extent it supports laboratory-based research. Some 70% of clinical research in the United States is supported by the private sector.[6]

Any institution wishing to do clinical research needs to take into account the balance that must be struck between the desire for industry-developed compounds, devices, and financial support with the need to maintain the intellectual independence and objectivity that society looks to academia to embody. Squandering the unique role of academia (the unfettered pursuit of truth) by usurping the capitalistic corporate culture of for-profit industry may prove to be a high price to pay for both academia and the human subjects who look to the academic health care delivery institutions for the newest advances in medicine.

This entails awareness of a host of questions that each institution must answer and then develop a system to manage those answers to foster relationships with the private sector that do not compromise the institution's academic integrity:
- Are trials being supported by industry truly asking important research questions?
- Are they being asked with appropriate scientific and biostatistical rigor?
- Is the funding for the trial sufficient to support the trial's conduct?

- Are the contractual terms constraining in any way (publication rights, intellectual property, indemnification)?
- Will the results of the industry-sponsored trial be published in a timely and unbiased manner regardless of the trial's outcome?

Clinical research cannot be done without the support of the corporate sector. Furthermore, both the goals of the companies and those of the academic centers can be aligned with careful consideration of scientific, commercial, contractual and regulatory matters before a trial starts. However, to do this, the infrastructure for each of these functions must be in place.

3. THE FUNCTIONS

<u>Culture</u>-Nothing matters more to a clinical research infrastructure, yet nothing is more intangible than the culture of the institution in which a clinical research infrastructure is to operate. This culture is influenced by many things.[7,8]

History plays a unique role. How things have been done in the past is how they will be done in the future unless that way has been demonstrated to be outmoded, counter-productive, overly expensive, or risky—to patients or to the institution's reputation. Change in the way science is performed in the laboratory or clinical research arenas is hard to implement. Academic faculty members are skeptical and tend to require significant proof before implementing change in their belief systems or their actions. Implementing change in the systems supporting or regulating research, is even harder to implement.

The predominant attitude toward rules and regulations of all types can affect the atmosphere within which a clinical research infrastructure must operate. Do institutional and departmental leaders adhere to their policies or make exceptions based on political or personal considerations? Are local rules followed or broken? Is the IRB viewed as a "barrier or hurdle" to be overcome or a constructive body seeking to protect the interests of patients and investigators alike? Attitudes and behaviors reflecting those attitudes toward local rules will influence attitudes and behaviors toward federal rules and regulations.

Leadership is also crucial. The degree to which the executives of an academic organization support the clinical research infrastructure with space, positions, and funding is demonstrable and palpable to those in the infrastructure and to those research teams the infrastructure is to support.

But more important even than the tangible measures of support, the intangible advocacy of regulatory compliance by the institution's executives can set the tone for the entire endeavor. Emphasizing the need to adhere to GCP and not tolerating any deviation from it, as well as distancing the institution's administration from interceding in the decisions of the IRB are crucial ways for an institution's leadership to not only "talk the talk," but also to "walk the walk."

Scientific Review-Beyond the conceptual, an idea for a clinical research project finds its demonstrable beginnings in the clinical protocol document. While its format varies from sponsor to sponsor, critical elements must be included.

A protocol is essentially the research plan by which the safety and efficacy of a drug or device is to be tested. It is a recipe, but it is far more. All the scientific background supporting the proposed work is there. The exact scientific objectives of the study must be clearly stated. The precise description of the patients or subjects who may be included or excluded is in the protocol. Precisely what the test drugs or devices are should be described, as should the route of administration. What data will be collected, at what frequency and to whom it will be reported and with what consequences must be described. Particular attention to the need for independent data monitoring should be addressed in the protocol. How adverse events will be reported and to whom must be included. But, perhaps most importantly, the informed consent document that explains to prospective patients/subjects in lay terms what the research is, what alternative treatments might be, what risks they may be taking, and what their rights (e.g., withdrawing from the study without the need for justification) are has to be in the protocol.

This consent form is no substitute for the process by which consent is obtained from a prospective patient or subject. That is a dialogue between the research team and the subject in which the team completely informs and the patient elects whether or not to consent to participate in the proposed research. However, the document is the physical substantiation of that process. It is the record. At our institution, it is signed in triplicate—one copy for the patient, one for the medical record, and one for the investigator's files.

In academic centers, it is common for this protocol document to be heavily vetted within the departments of the principal investigator of the study and the departments of his/her collaborators. Each department should determine how important the new study is when compared to others already enrolling patients. Particularly, is the population proposed for the new research study already one being studied with another protocols? If so, how will it be determined who participates in which protocol? Having this critical decision being made based on which physician a new patient sees is unacceptable and unethical. Each unit in an academic center should determine, on a regular and on-going basis, its protocol priorities and make sure that all members of the department adhere to that prioritization plan.

Once a protocol is determined by the local department(s) or program(s) to be of sufficient merit and is likely to have sufficient numbers of subjects available to fulfill its objectives, the protocol is submitted to a central office to begin its journey through the review and approval process.

At UTMDACC, that office is the Office of Protocol Research (OPR). OPR registers the new protocol on our computerized data system which tracks the entire life of the protocol from this initial submission to its termination from IRB oversight.

In OPR, the protocol is assigned to a series of reviewers for scientific evaluation. Two medical reviewers (with no conflicts with the department from which the protocol emanated), as well as reviewers with expertise in biostatistics, nursing, pharmacy, diagnostic imaging, and pathology write an evaluation of the scientific methods and merit of the proposed research. As many protocols use our Protocol Document On-Line (PDOL) computer system (see below), these documents can be sent to the reviewers via secure, intra-institutional e-mail and the reviews returned in the same manner. The PDOL system maintains all communications related to a specific protocol in single electronic protocol folders. This has accelerated the review process. Furthermore, OPR encourages a dialogue between the reviewers and the principal investigator to work out any deficiencies with a proposed protocol before it is reviewed in the institutional scientific review committee.

The institutional scientific review committees (called the Clinical Research Committee or CRC or the Psychosocial, Behavioral and Health Services Research Committee or PBHSRC for survey, behavioral or other similar types of research) are open forums where each proposed protocol is discussed. Each PI presents the proposed objectives and methods. The reviewers discuss its strengths and weaknesses. Following an open discussion, the PI is asked to leave the deliberations and a vote is taken to determine the fitness of the protocol to move from the scientific review stage to the human subjects protection evaluation performed by the IRB. Often CRC or PBHSRC approval is with contingencies that must be met prior to the protocol moving to the IRB for evaluation (although the IRBs have recently decided that protocols with minor contingencies can go to the IRB without correction, if all contingencies are corrected prior to protocol Activation and patient accrual). A key part of any such discussion is the review of the protocol priority lists of the department from which the protocol under discussion originated. This is to determine that the new study does not compete for patients with a study already in progress.

Many major cancer centers employ a model similar to ours. It is usually supported in part by funds for the "Protocol Review and Monitoring System" on the Cancer Center Support Grants. The PRMS serves these institutions with a rigorous scientific review.

Institutional Review Board-The hallmark of clinical research in the United States is its oversight by a local institutional review board or IRB. The IRB is "any board, committee, or other group formally designated by an institution to review, to approve the initiation of, and to conduct periodic review of, biomedical research involving human subjects" [21 CFR 56.102]. Even though IRBs are federally-mandated, the federal government counts on a system of local control to fulfill the oversight mandates of the Code of Federal Regulations.

An IRB must have at least 5 members. One member's primary concern must be in a scientific area and at least one member's primary concern must be in a non-scientific area [45 CFR 46.207]. The board must have the expertise to review the research put before it and to promote "respect in their community" [45 CFR 46.207]. At least one person on the IRB must be unaffiliated with the institution. An IRB must reflect the sensitivity of the community in which it operates.

The IRB must be independent of the typical political pressure extant in most academic institutions. It must not be a rubber stamp for the research agendas of the academic department chairs or powerful members of the faculty. It must also be free from interference by the administrative leadership of the institution.

That is a tall order in complex institutions where the financial pressures brought about by ever-lower NIH grant pay lines, managed care and caring for a large uninsured population have a negative impact on research budgets. Studies sponsored by industry are often used as sources of support for themselves and for unsponsored trials by the same research team. For example, a research nurse whose salary is funded by a drug company trial may also support an unsponsored trial led by the same PI. Thus, trials may come to an IRB for review and approval where the major reason they are proposed is as a source of financial support for another, far more worthy, but unsupported investigation. The IRB may be the final line of defense to prevent an institution from agreeing to perform a trial whose outcome will be of little consequence to the future care of cancer patients, or one which could put potential subjects at increased risk.

There are several keys to establishing an IRB support infrastructure that assists with regulatory compliance, promotes the best research ideas, and is accessible to the research personnel who count upon the IRB's wise deliberations.

First and foremost, the IRB chair must be an experienced clinical investigator, knowledgeable in regulatory matters, willing to say no and sufficiently steadfast to withstand pressure to reverse IRB decisions. This individual would do well to be a regular attendee at annual meetings of the group called the Public Responsibility in Medicine and Research or PRIM & R and the Applied Research Ethics National Association or ARENA. These meetings are the major forums for ideas surrounding human subjects protection and changes in the regulatory environment.

Second, dividing the many IRB tasks among a group of Vice Chairs each of whom has expertise in specific IRB duties (e.g., continuing reviews, adverse event review, review of grant applications to determine if they need an IRB-approved protocol, etc.) is another efficient way to support the multiple tasks of the IRB.

Third, IRB membership and leadership should be rotated in some reasonable fashion to be inclusive of as many faculty as possible, while maintaining sufficient expertise to assure continuous oversight excellence.

Fourth, the office supporting the IRB must be sufficiently staffed with skilled professionals and led by knowledgeable administrators.

Fifth, we highly recommend an editor be retained by the protocol office to review all informed consent documents prior to IRB review. These consent documents should be written at the 8th grade reading level or lower and contain a host of vital components to be compliant with federal code and understandable to prospective trial participants. Also, having access to translation services allows research teams to offer trial participation to subjects who are not English speaking as consent documents must be understandable to prospective participants.

Sixth, the use of a modern information system to track the lives of all protocols, continuing reviews (the federally-mandated annual IRB protocol review), and internal and external adverse event reports is a must (see below).

Finally, the Institutional Official for human research protection must possess a willingness to take on the administration of the institution in defense of the IRB's autonomy. Sooner or later, a well-functioning IRB will make a difficult call. It may close a study for poor compliance with federal code. It may remove the clinical research privileges of an investigator who has not heeded regulatory standards. This can become a public matter and prove embarrassing to an institution. It is natural to try to prevent any such matter from going beyond the walls of the institution. Unfortunately, there are certain reporting requirements to sponsors and to the government when untoward actions must be taken by an IRB. The Institutional Official must make certain that any regulatory requirements triggered by IRB actions are met, regardless of the adverse external publicity or internal political strife.

These are difficult matters. However, not addressing them is not an option. It is best to address them in the dispassionate period prior to a crisis. This can be achieved by writing clear IRB policies and procedures that specifically describe what constitutes serious non-compliance, how the IRB will address incidents of serious non-compliance, and what the potential actions of the IRB in response to serious non-compliance can be.

Quality Assurance-Intentions and plans are important. But, actually checking to see how the infrastructure is working and whether or not that infrastructure is helping investigators produce a quality research product is part of the proper oversight of the conduct of clinical research.

We established an Office of Clinical Research Quality Assurance early in the history of our office. Its functions have expanded over time. These are:

- Auditing clinical trials
- Monitoring on-going trials, especially those for which UTMDACC serves as the IND holder
- Educating faculty and research personnel on all aspects of GCP and the CFR
- Serving an ombudsman function for research personnel to resolve concerns about the conduct of clinical research

The most basic of functions for any QA office is auditing. In our manuals we define auditing as:

"...a retrospective evaluation of the outcomes and conduct of a clinical trial. An audit usually occurs only once during the course of a protocol and identifies issues that have occurred in subjects who have completed or are nearing completion of therapy".

The major goals of audits are to measure the conduct of a clinical trial against the description of that conduct in the IRB-approved protocol document and whether the research was conducted in accord with GCP. In essence, did the investigators do what they said they were going to do? Were all consented subjects eligible? Was that eligibility documented in the primary source document, the medical record? Were drugs or devices used in accordance with the methods described in the protocol document? Were doses adjusted in accord with the protocol? Were adverse events properly recorded? Were records of responses and toxicities well-documented? Were all consent forms appropriately signed and dated?

These audits can be random or focused on particular trials (e.g., those not otherwise audited by industry sponsors or the NCI). They can be triggered by a complaint or request from a patient, a sponsor, the IRB or a federal agency.

It is best to have a standard procedure for performing these audits which should include a written description of the procedure, sufficient time to allow research teams to gather the primary source data, and an open atmosphere of information exchange before, during and after the audit. (The FDA is not so concerned about the latter issue when it audits a trial. Thus, internal procedures that aim at preparing research teams for external regulatory audits and raising awareness of the requirements of GCP and the possible consequences of a poor FDA audit, ought not be so concerned with giving teams enough time to do the data gathering that should be occurring as a trial progresses. Assembling charts and x-rays for audits should require a few days at most, which may be far more lead time than FDA auditors are likely to offer). These procedures should be widely publicized and a physician with no connection to the study should work with the QA staff in assessing the quality of the study during the audit.

The audit process should be more educational than punitive. However, if shortcomings found during audits are sufficiently egregious (and this should be defined in the audit policies and procedures), the findings may need to be reported to the IRB which may have to take action against a research team or investigator if GCP and/or CFR standards have been breached. Unfortunately, even if patient risk is never increased, poor documentation alone is sufficient grounds for IRB action. This is obviously because poor documentation leaves an unauditable record where actual risk to patients (or future patients) or actual efficacy cannot be assessed.

Even more critical, if audits adduce that patient risk was in excess of that which is reasonable and in excess of that which the IRB approved for that study, the IRB may need to take action. This could vary from requiring additional education of the research team prior to that team participating in any further clinical research to actually removing the clinical research privileges of faculty members for a lack of compliance with research and human subjects protection standards.

Monitoring is not the same as auditing. We define monitoring as:

"...an evaluation of the clinical research process which occurs throughout the life of the protocol. This ongoing review allows problems and solutions to be identified early in the course of the research".

Monitoring is more like continuous process improvement. It is focused on process and aims to catch problems early and correct them. Auditing is like checking for product defects at the end of an assembly line. You may find the defects, but there is little that can be done to fix them at that point.

We employ monitoring most commonly in our oversight of those protocols for which we serve as sponsor on the IND. The role of "sponsor" with the FDA is so important that we have to be as sure as we can be, that a trial is proceeding as planned and that all documentation and reporting is in accord with descriptions in the IRB- and FDA-approved protocol document.

The best possible way to avert problems in clinical research compliance coming to light during audits and monitoring visits is to prevent them from happening at all. And the best way we have found for that to occur is to educate those performing the research. It is unfortunate but few physicians and research nurses have been fully trained in the required compliance standards of the CFR or GCP. Thus, when audits or monitoring visits unearth poor compliance, it is usually a lack of knowledge, not malevolence, which is at its root.

Most institutions have implemented one to two hour human subjects protection training for key personnel on federal grants. We deem this inadequate training for conducting clinical trials. Furthermore, the various web sites professing to provide this education, can never address the unique institutional peculiarities inherent in any clinical research oversight program. Therefore, first with the research nurses and then with the faculty, we developed programs of detailed education for clinical research professionals.

The curriculum for the 10-hour, 5-part course for faculty and fellows is below (this description was authored by Ms. Kristin Bialobok, Manager of the Office of Clinical Research Quality Assurance):

Day 1: -History of Human Subjects Research
  -Evolution of Good Clinical Practice
  -Scientific Integrity/Conflict of Interest
  -The Office of Research Administration-Org Chart and Functions
  -MDACC Research Support and Office of Research Administration Databases

Day 2: -Responsibilities of an Investigator
  -MDACC Clinical Trials Review and Approval Process

Day 3: -The Informed Consent Process
-Introduction to MDACC Clinical Trials Information Systems

- Protocol Data Management System (PDMS)
- Protocol Document On-Line (PDOL)
  -Compassionate Use Process

Day 4: -Elements of a Protocol
-Source Documentation
-Adverse Events

Day 5: -FDA Inspections
-Institutional Audit Policies and Process
-MDACC Investigational New Drug Application (IND) Policy

In order to ensure a uniform clinical research knowledge base among the established faculty/fellows, with the least intrusion upon the limited time of a busy academic schedule, two different methods were developed by which clinical researchers could establish or develop expertise in this area.

Option 1: The experienced researcher could choose to attend the course offered to new faculty. Following each module a 20 question multiple-choice test was administered to all participants. A passing score of 85% or more on each module was considered established competency.

Option 2: The experienced researcher could choose to test out of the training sessions by successfully completing a competency test that corresponded to each of the five modules. The subject material covered on this examination was made available through several institutional Lotus Notes databases. Those choosing this option were instructed that all testing must be completed in the computer testing center in the Research Administration Department. A computerized software program was developed to administer the tests and assist in tracking statistics for each question on the test.

Faculty who chose to attempt to test out of the course and did not achieve a grade of 85% or higher were required to attend the class session that corresponded to the low scoring module. If after attending the class the faculty member was still unable to achieve a grade of 85% or higher, he/she was required to attend a one-on-one educational session with an instructor to review the failed module.

A time frame of one year was granted to the faculty in order to comply with this new requirement. Any faculty member not fulfilling his/her obligation by the established deadline had his/her clinical research privileges revoked until successful completion of the training and competency tests.

This has been a remarkably successful program. Over 800 people have completed it. We will be scrutinizing the quality of the monitoring and audit reports done since the course offering to see if they improve when compared with audits performed before the training was given. The process has already raised the consciousness of the faculty and fellows to the constraints imposed on their behavior, record keeping and latitude of judgment when performing clinical research. The basic message--that clinical research is a regulated activity that is not part of the continuum of clinical care, but qualitatively distinct from it—has been successfully conveyed.

A final function that should reside somewhere within the clinical research infrastructure is an ombudsman office. For the most part, research teams consist of PIs, usually physicians, with relatively great power in the political hierarchy, and everyone else from research nurses to data managers to pharmacists. These latter groups have great knowledge that may or may not be brought to bear in any situation dominated by the PI. If a trial is going amiss or is believed to be going amiss, these other research personnel, most of who depend directly on funds generated by the PI for their income, may be reticent to speak-up and head off a potential problem in GCP compliance.

We elected to create an ombudsman office to address complaints of non-compliance by research personnel in our QA office for a number of reasons.

The QA office is staffed by research nurses and certified clinical research associates. It is easier for a research nurse or data manager to discuss difficulties he/she is having with his/her PI with a fellow research nurse than with a vice president who is a part of the faculty.

Our QA staff has established relationships with the members of the various research teams through the QA auditing, monitoring, and educational activities. They are trusted by the research team personnel as sources of good advice and knowledge about federal code and GCP.

Finally, the QA staff has access to institutional leadership and IRB leadership who can assist in resolving these matters expeditiously and confidentially.

This is a program that really works and is a worthy investment in the clinical research infrastructure of any institution performing human subjects research.

Both the education and ombudsman programs are vital strategies that can prevent larger, more embarrassing problems by making sure they do not happen, or if they do, resolving them sooner rather than later.

4. INFORMATION SYSTEMS

Without the work capabilities gained through the use of modern computers, none of the functions described above could have been operationalized. Even the culture of an institution is altered when research teams have at their disposal, access to information about clinical research, the CFR, and IRB and institutional policies. What was once deemed impossible to track, now is readily at hand. That includes data and it also includes oversight of regulatory compliance. It is amazing how much better audits become when the research teams know that what they are doing is being monitored and their research records are going to be audited.

Whether an information system is designed to service a federal regulatory or local efficiency need, it is always best in an academic center to:
- Ask the faculty and their research teams what they
- need. Building a system no one will use or needs, wastes time and money.
- Once a need is identified, form an advisory committee of stakeholders to assist in the design, development and implementation of the system.
- Test, test, test! There is nothing more frustrating to faculty and research personnel alike than an over-promised, under-performing information system application. Let the users take test drives often at the earliest possible stage.
- Implement in stages and with plenty of warning
- Training, training, training. You cannot over-train. It must be continuous, even after an application has been successfully launched as new personnel are always in need of training.
- Support what you implement!

A Clinical Research Data Base-In 1984, under the direction of the then-Division Head of Medicine at M.D. Anderson, Dr. Irwin Krakoff, a novel seed was planted. Dr. Krakoff wanted a better way to track and report the results of NCI phase 1 clinical trials. Ms. (now Dr.) Susan Welch built the Protocol Data Management System on a MUMPS platform to perform that data management function for NCI trials.

Today that data base manages:
- The set-up in the data base of every new clinical trial as it begins the approval process. The trial's progress through the review and approval process is tracked in the data base.
- The registration of every patient on a clinical trial at M.D. Anderson (over 31,000 registrations in FY03). Eligibility criteria must be met or the patient cannot be registered. Without this registration, study drug will not be released from the pharmacy.
- On-study and off-study dates must be entered as must eligibility and evaluability information.
- Study data may be kept in the data base, but this is not

mandated. Laboratory results from the Division of Pathology and Laboratory Medicine automatically populate the data base for all patients on clinical trials.
- IRB information (continuing review dates, adverse event reports) are tracked with the data base
- Security and file back-up thus guaranteeing sponsors who use the data base that no one but the authorized research team has access to their proprietary information and that this information can be recovered should a disaster occur
- Electronic data transfer to both the NCI and to industry sponsors
- All meetings of the scientific review committees and the IRBs
- All communication to the faculty about the deliberations of those committees
- Auditing of accrual on clinical trials for reports on the scientific progress of the various studies.

It would be virtually impossible for the Office of Protocol Research to perform the work for the faculty and the regulatory agencies without this system. Over 900 treatment protocols are under IRB oversight. Over 12,000 adverse event reports must be reviewed by the IRB each year. All the protocols require at least annual continuing review by the IRB.

However, this is an old system by any standards of modern computing. We have begun the migration of this system to an Oracle data base called the Clinical Oncology Research data base. This has user-friendly graphic user interfaces and drop-down menus that make data and clinical trial management quick and easy. However, this migration is a slow process requiring much testing and slow roll out of the various units of the data base. This is taking several years as would any implementation of a data base of long-standing that must be used as it is changed.

Protocol Authoring-A well-written protocol has many required elements and IRB-mandated language in several places. Usually protocol-related information is collected as the protocol is submitted to the approval process. For example, questions must be answered to address the type of study being proposed, whether tissue is being used, whether there are any conflicts of interest, etc.

Having a template for faculty who are authoring trials would greatly decrease their work and create a uniformity to protocol documents. This would assist individual reviewers and the committees for which they review as well. Thus, we created the Protocol Document On-Line System.

This is a protocol authoring tool containing modular protocol sections with as much boiler-plate (IRB-mandated terms in consent document, adverse event reporting requirements, toxicity criteria, etc.) language as possible. It can even take imported or attached files into a protocol document to decrease the work of the author. It also creates very uniform and comprehensible informed consent documents in the format acceptable to the IRB.

Because the template is written in the Lotus Notes system that also supports our institutional e-mail, the documents can be submitted, reviewed and approved on-line. Without this innovation, we could not "move the paper" fast enough to satisfy the desire of the faculty or their sponsors to increase the pace of the approval process without compromising the quality of the scientific or human subjects protection review.

Web Sites-Everyone has got them and they all differ. If the protocol office is considering the development of a web site that will list protocols for the general public to view as a means of educating the public on the research agenda of the institution and potentially marketing these studies to recruit patients to them, the following should be considered:

- What is the goal of the web site? Is it educational or is it to find new patients for research?
- Has the IRB approved the content? It needs to as this can be construed as advertising for participation in a trial which requires IRB approval [9]
- If the trial to be posted to the web is industry-sponsored, has the sponsor approved the posting of the trial? We believe this is essential as sponsors may have their own reasons to have or not have information about their trial widely known
- What is the extent of the information which will be posted? We have not posted drug doses or schedules on our site www.clinicaltrials.org which predated the NCI's similarly-named site. The essential information about eligibility, contact names and numbers and a lay description (downloaded directly from the description in the consent document in the Protocol Document On-Line System) seem sufficient. Trials can be searched for by disease site, PI, or drug name.

Many commercial web sites have more or less information on the trials they list. Linking to these other sites may be of benefit. This is a decision that each institution must determine for itself with careful consideration of just what the web site is to do.

Integrity itself oversees the policies at NIH-funded institutions and can assist and guide the institutions in assessing misconduct allegations. While ORI can investigate an institution itself, for the most part, ORI leaves these matters in the hands of the institutions and their administrations.

What exactly must institutions do? Essentially, institutions need policies which are annually reviewed by ORI for approval. These policies need to address the following issues:

- Applicability-To whom does the policy apply
- Definition-What is the institution's definition of misconduct
- Mechanisms of reporting allegations-To whom and how
- Inquiries-the preliminary phase of allegation assessment (see below)
- Investigations-the more comprehensive assessment stage
- Data sequestration-protecting the participants (see below)

We will comment on how UTMDACC has chosen to address these six points. Each institution receiving federal funds must determine for itself how these matters will be addressed and codified in a policy.

Our policy applies to everyone who has anything to do with a research project at UTMDACC. It is not limited to faculty or to those supported by NIH funds.

We use the exact definition of scientific misconduct found in the CFR.

Allegations can come to department chairs or other academic leaders, the Research Integrity Officer (RIO) directly, the Institutional Compliance Officer, or, most likely, the Chief Academic Officer (CAO). We insist on a face-to-face meeting between the whistle blower and those to whom he or she is reporting the allegation.

In most instances, the CAO and RIO will be present at the meeting and confer to determine, given the facts before them, whether this is a good faith allegation of scientific misconduct. (If not, the President and CAO determine whether administrative action must be taken, but that has not occurred as of yet, as all such allegations are taken seriously and are assumed to be made that way).

Once the allegation has been determined to be in good faith, the CAO and RIO meet with the accused individual(s) (termed "the respondent") and his or her department chairman and delineate the allegation and review the steps that will be promptly initiated.

The first step is an inquiry. This is an "information-gathering and initial fact finding to determine whether an allegation or apparent instance of research misconduct warrants an investigation."[10] These are formal but tend to be less exhaustive than an investigation. All parties' rights are to be preserved, so confidentiality is critical. Evidence or findings developed in an inquiry may be used in a subsequent investigation.

At our institution, the inquiry is not done by either the CAO or RIO. Rather the CAO names a group of three senior level faculty members with experience in the scientific area of the respondent, but with no professional or personal conflicts of interest involving the respondent or the whistleblower. This panel reviews the associated supporting sequestered documents (see below) and writes a report to the President within 60 days. The work of the panel is staffed by the office of the RIO (at our institution that is the Vice President for Research Administration assisted by the Associate Vice President and Chief Research and Regulatory Affairs Officer).

This report is provided to the respondent by the President. The respondent has 10 days to comment upon it in writing. The President then determines if the allegations were unfounded or warrant a full investigation. If the allegations are determined to be unfounded, the process stops. If that is not the case, the investigation must start within 30 days.

An investigation is very formal. It is exhaustive. Usually, a new panel of three faculty experts is named by the CAO and RIO in consultation with the Chairperson of the Faculty Senate. This group is to finish its work and provide a new report to the President. While it is hoped that this process will be completed in 120 days, it can easily take longer to arduously sift through all appropriate data and interview all involved personnel. The guiding principles are fairness and confidentiality. The latter is most critical if the respondent is found to have not committed any scientific misconduct as efforts to restore or repair the reputation of the respondent can be very difficult if confidentiality is breached.

Finally, a word about data sequestration. Once the decision is made to begin the inquiry process, it is incumbent on the RIO to sequester all associated data and records. This includes notebooks, printouts, computers, hard drives, or case report forms for clinical research. It is essential that this be as thorough as possible as the reputation of the whistleblower and respondent depend upon the preservation of an accurate and intact data record as do the inquiry and investigation processes themselves. To avoid any allegations that the process was undermined by data tampering, these records need to be secured. The respondent may have access to the records

6. FINANCIAL CONFLICTS OF INTEREST

A professor learns of a novel prevention strategy for a lethal disease. He conducts a clinical trial that is 100% successful and now wants to charge a fee to use the information and prevent the disease's effects on the rest of his city's population.

While this may sound like a dilemma causing angst between administration and faculty at a modern medical school, this actually took place in 1799 at Harvard when one of its three professors, Benjamin Waterhouse, became familiar with Jenner's strategy to prevent smallpox.[11] As opposed to sanctioning their colleagues attempt to capitalize on his research, the school's two other professors were outraged.

Much has changed today and the subject of conflict of interest is guaranteed to create a varied response among faculty and administrators in academic medical centers. It is of particular importance for administrators overseeing the conduct of clinical investigation to consider conflict of interest and to have policies in place to address such conflicts or the appearance of such conflicts when they arise. This is because there is an inherent fiduciary relationship between a patient and a doctor. The patient assumes that what the doctor advises is in the patient's best interest. This is very different from the relationship between a clinical investigator and a research subject as we pointed out at the beginning of this chapter. Yet, many physicians offer their patients participation in research, the results of which may benefit the doctor and his/her academic career. This conflict, which derives from the dual role of physician and investigator played by some academic faculty members, is not new, nor are we suggesting this be changed. But, if that individual may personally benefit financially from the results of the research or if the physician's institution will benefit, there is a conflict that must be eliminated or managed.

So what is a conflict of interest?

Thompson defines it as, "a set of conditions in which professional judgment concerning a primary interest (such as a patient's welfare or the validity of research) tends to be unduly influenced by a secondary interest (such as financial gain)"[12]

In his new book, <u>Science in the Private Interest</u>, Sheldon Krimsky outlines the three stages of conflict of interest.[13]

- Antecedent acts-factors conditioning the state of

mind (e.g., gifts, equity, consultancies)
- States of Mind-sentiments and proclivities (e.g,, favoritism or bias)
- Outcome behavior (e.g., decisions)

Since we cannot do much to regulate the second nor can we easily link behavior to antecedent acts, the antecedent acts themselves are the focus of regulations to prevent conflicts of interest.

Why is this becoming the focus of such attention now?

- Academic medical centers are under far greater financial pressure than in the past as managed care, decreasing Medicare reimbursement, care of the uninsured and other factors decrease traditional sources of revenue.
- The Bayh-Dole act of 1980 in which academic centers were encouraged to "transfer technology" developed under federal grant support to the marketplace and retain the fruits of such commercialization has encouraged this activity which was never part of the activities of most academic centers in the past.
- The rise of faculty with companies and the new norm of the "entrepreneurial" faculty member has put pressure on administration to be more lenient in allowing faculty to do more financially rewarding and potentially conflicted forms of research.
- Greater demand on the part of Americans for the benefits of research to be garnered sooner in the form of newer treatments for serious illnesses has diminished the ivory tower's separation from the marketplace.

The private sector is an ever-larger supporter of clinical research. While the NIH provided $17.8B for research in 1999, most of this was for basic research. The top 10 pharmaceutical companies supported clinical research at the $22.7B level.[14]

But, of greatest importance is that several studies have shown that the results of trials supported by industry are more likely than those not supported by industry to favor the new therapy.[6] As Krimsky says in his book,[15] "university science becomes entangled with entrepreneurship; knowledge is pursued for its monetary value; and expertise with a point of view can be purchased." (Whether this is truly entrepreneurial can be questioned as few of these so-called 'academic entrepreneurs' risk their own money).[16]

The financial ties of concern include: consultancies, payments for service on advisory boards, payments for service on speakers' bureaus, royalties, licenses, promotion of sponsored symposia, gifts, trips, equity, options and food.[17] Many physicians deny that these affect their decision making, but a recent article in the <u>New York Times</u> indicates that the pervasive influence of drug companies on the prescribing practices of physicians.[18] No one should be considered immune from the power of detailing and advertising.

As Bodenheimer[6] and others[19,20] outline, companies:
- Opt not to do post-approval studies
- Design trials to favor their products
- Control data and can even elect not to publish unfavorable results
- "Ghost-write" articles for busy investigators
- Use CME meetings as a marketing arenas
- Inadequately disclose risk or benefits in informed consent documents
- Fail to report adverse events or suspend trials appropriately

No single event crystallized the issue of conflict of interest in academic medicine more than the death of Jesse Gelsinger during a gene therapy trial at the University of Pennsylvania in September, 1999.[21-23]

Jesse Gelsinger did not have cancer. Rather he had an inborn error of metabolism, ornithine transcarbamylase deficiency. He had volunteered to participate in an adenovirus-gene therapy protocol and died within days of being injected with the test agent. This was obviously a tragedy for the subject and for the research program. It was later learned that not only had there been inadequate reporting to the federal agencies overseeing this form of research with regard to previously observed adverse events, but the Director of the Institute for Human Gene Therapy owned stock in the sponsor of the research. The dean of the medical school and the university itself had conflicts of interest that should have precluded this trial's performance at this institution. These were blatant violations of human subject protection regulations. In addition, conflicts such as these should have been related to the subject and his family prior to his being asked to participate in the research. At our institution, this trial could not have occurred with conflicts of interest such as these in place.

Conflicts of interest have also been described in FDA review panels,[24] writers of medical guidelines,[25] sponsors of continuing medical education,[26] the billions of dollars spent each year on "free" drug samples for doctors' offices[27] and even inside the National Institutes of Health itself.[28,29]

It is generally acknowledged that work with the business sector, primarily pharmaceutical and biotechnology companies, is not only desirable, it is required if progress against cancer is to be made. Some of the most innovative and promising molecules have come from industry. In addition, industry is a far greater supporter of clinical research than is the federal government. So, it is not whether or not the potential for conflicts exist. It is managing or eliminating them to the greatest extent possible.

To that end, The University of Texas M.D. Anderson Cancer Center spent over a year reworking its conflict of interest policy. In September of 2003, the new policy was passed by the President's Advisory Board. Some of its most critical tenets are:

- Patient safety and the reputation and integrity of the institution are paramount
- Full disclosure of all relevant financial holdings and arrangements is required of all faculty and key institutional decision makers
- NO faculty member can serve on the Board of Directors or as an Officer of a for-profit company
- There are financial limits to consultant fees acceptable by the faculty
- No research is permitted in which payment is dependent on a specific outcome
- Time away to pursue outside financial interests is limited
- Faculty may hold equity in companies sponsoring their laboratory-base research, but a management plan must be in place to oversee this arrangement and there are limits to the faculty member's holdings
- In human subject research: no payment may be received (beyond costs of the research) for enrolling a patient in a clinical trail; no faculty with a significant financial interest can be a principal investigator of a trail sponsored by the company in which he/she has an interest; and members of the research team must have any potential conflicts disclosed to potential subjects in the informed consent document of the trial
- Conflicts in supervisory relationships and for institutional decision makers are also addressed in the policy

We believe that it is appropriate for institutions that have not recently reviewed their conflict of interest policies to do so after a vigorous discussion with all faculty and staff members who may be affected by such a policy. As the federal guidelines for the precepts in an institution's policy are not vague, each institution has to decide what the tenets of its policy will be.

However, one thing is clear, as indicated by Catherine D. DeAngelis in an editorial in JAMA in 2000:

"Without these policies and procedures, the academic institutions where most clinical research is based and their faculty members who perform the research are in grave danger of losing the support and respect of the public. Without this support and respect, trust in new medical discoveries and their applications will not be forthcoming. Without trust, medical research is doomed."[14]

7. ACKNOWLEDGEMENTS

The development of a portion of the program described in this chapter was supported by grants SO7 RR18240-01 and –02 from the National Institutes of Health.

We would like to acknowledge the continuous and continuing support of the administration of The University of Texas M.D. Anderson Cancer Center (Presidents Drs. John Mendelsohn and Charles A. LeMaistre, Chief Academic Officers Drs. Margaret L. Kripke and Andrew von Eschenbach, and Vice President for Patient Care Dr. David Hohn) without whose allotment of space, positions and funding, the infrastructure described in this chapter could not have been built. We would also like to acknowledge the many dedicated UTMDACC faculty members who have led and served on the committees we described with scant reward, other than the knowledge that they were assuring the continued excellence of our clinical science and guaranteeing the safety of all of the patients and subjects who have consented to participate in research here. Finally, we would like to acknowledge four very special people without whom we would never have been able to build the Office of Research Administration. First, we thank Ms. Martha Matza, Director of the Office of Protocol Research and leader of the Research Administration Information Systems team, without whom none of this would have happened, electronically or in real-time. Second, we thank Drs. Aman Buzdar and Richard Theriault, the chairmen of our IRBs who have been unflinching and courageous standard bearers for the Code of Federal Regulation, the three tenets of the Belmont Report, justice, beneficence, and respect for persons, and the protection of all patients and subjects involved in clinical research. Finally, we thank Mr. Dan Fontaine, Senior Vice President and Chief Legal Officer of the The University of Texas M. D. Anderson Cancer Center who has been an indispensable ally in protecting the independence of the IRB from undue political influence in good times and bad. Thank you all.

REFERENCES

1. Ott, M.B. and Yingling, G.L.; Guide to Good Clinical Practice, Tab 100, p. 7, 1999.
2. Ott, M.B. and Yingling, G.L.; Guide to Good Clinical Practice, Tab 200, p. 7, 1998.
3. Amdur, R.J. and Bankert, E.A.; in: Institutional Review Board Management and Function (Amdur, R.J. and Bankert, E.A., eds.), p. 27, 2002.
4. Cohen, J.M.; in: Institutional Review Board Management and Function (Amdur, R.J. and Bankert, E.A., eds.), p. 313, 2002.
5. Ott, M.B. and Yingling, G.L.; Guide to Good Clinical Practice, Tab 100, p. 8, 1999.
6. Bodenheimer, T.; New England Journal of Medicine 342: 1539, 2000.
7. Simone, J.; Clinical Cancer Research 5: 2281, 1998.
8. Simone, J.; Journal of Clinical Oncology 20: 4503, 2002.
9. Homer, R. Krebs, R., and Medwar, L. in: Institutional Review Board Management and Function (Amdur, R.J. and Bankert, E.A., eds.), p. 180, 2002.
10. From the Office of Research Integrity, "Introductory Workshop for Institutional Misconduct Officials", June 6, 1997.
11. Martin, J.B. and Kasper, D.L.; New England Journal of Medicine 343: 1646, 2000.
12. Thompson, D., New England Journal of Medicine 329: 573, 1993 as cited in Bekelman, J.E., Li, Y., and Gross, C.P.; Journal of the American Medical Association 289: 454, 2003.
13. Krimsky, S.; Science in the Private Interest; p. 126, 2003.
14. DeAngelis, C.D.; Journal of the American Medical Association 284: 2237, 2000.
15. Krimsky, S.; Science in the Private Interest; p. 1, 2003.
16. Krimsky, S.; Science in the Private Interest; p. 181, 2003.
17. Angell, M.; New England Journal of Medicine 342: 1516, 2000.
18. Zuger, A.; New York Times, 2/24/04.
19. Barnes, M. and Florenico, P.S.; Journal of Law, Medicine and Ethics 30: 390, 2002.
20. Coyle, S.L.; Annals of Internal Medicine 136: 396, 2002.
21. Krimsky, S.; Science in the Private Interest; p. 132-134, 2003.
22. Gelsinger, P. in: Institutional Review Board Management and Function (Amdur, R.J. and Bankert, E.A., eds.), p. xv-xxii, 2002.
23. Goldner, J.A.; Journal of Law, Medicine and Ethics 28:379, 2000.
24. Zimmerman, R.; Wall Street Journal, 9/23/02.
25. Stolberg, S.G.; New York Times, 2/6/02.
26. Hensley, S.; Wall Street Journal, 1/14/03.
27. Schlegel, D.; Houston Chronicle, 11/3/02.
28. Willman, D.; Los Angeles Times, 12/7/03.
29. Goldberg, K.B.; Cancer Letter 30:1, 2004

Chapter 15

THE CLINICAL RESEARCH PROCESS: BUILDING A SYSTEM IN HARMONY WITH ITS USERS

Greg Koski, MD, PhD

Associate Professor of Anesthesia, Senior Scientist, Institute for Health Policy, Massachusetts General Hospital, Harvard Medical School, Boston, Massachusetts, USA; Former Director, Office for Human Research Protections, U.S. Department of Health and Human Services, Washington, DC, USA

1. INTRODUCTION

An article in one of the world's pre-eminent scientific journals recently made a disturbing disclosure about the conduct of scientists and the status of our approach to human research and protection of human research participants. Among scientists at both junior and mid-career levels, a shocking number voluntarily admitted to knowingly engaging in various forms of scientific misbehavior (Martinson et al, 2005), including initiating or conducting research prior to IRB approval, misrepresenting protocols and research procedures to the IRB, disregarding the specific requirements of research protocols and other intentional actions to avoid what some see as undesirable and inappropriate interference by the IRB in their research activities. That investigators would intentionally disregard institutional requirements and federal regulations for protection of human subjects and expose themselves to the potential adverse consequences of these behaviors on their professional careers is hard to understand, and yet, the phenomenon is clearly not unusual. According to Patricia Keith-Spiegel, an ethics researcher at Simmons College in Boston, evidence suggests that some research ethics panels are alienating researchers and inadvertently promoting misbehavior be being inflexible, overly picky and insufficiently responsive to the needs and concerns of investigators and the research community (Giles, 2005). If this is indeed the case, it suggests that a more user-friendly system may be needed.

After a more than a decade of growing concern that our national 'system' for protection of human research subjects may not be up to its charge, many institutions and their IRBs have responded by tightening-up their policies and practices to ensure compliance with regulatory requirements, but in doing so, may have fallen into a pattern of what has been called "reactive hyper-protectionism", a practice that may be adversely affecting not only the behavior of investigators, but of the very progress of science. The term 'system' is best used advisedly in this context, for many would argue that few responsibilities in the conduct and oversight of human research are less systematic than protection of human subjects. Rather than being a system, a more accurate description of the current approach might be a diverse collection of well-intended groups composed of largely volunteers attempting, often with too few resources and too little guidance, to meet the challenges presented by federal regulations that require prospective approval and continuing review of human research studies.

Although IRBs operate within a framework of ethical principles that provide a foundation for the relevant regulations, and while they are subject to some degree of oversight by federal agencies, such as the Food and Drug Administration (FDA) and the Office for Human Research Protections (OHRP) of the Department of Health and Human Services (DHHS), that they are actually effective in preventing harm to research participants is presumed, not proven. That they are costly, time consuming, over-burdened and often idiosyncratic in their decision-making is widely accepted, even if the data to support these views is at least in part anecdotal. Nevertheless, experience teaches us that relationships between IRBs and investigators can often be, or become, confrontational, particularly when an IRB's decisions seem arbitrary, irrational, uninformed and obstinate in addition to being inadequately documented and communicated--which is exactly how some investigators characterize their experiences with IRBs.

To the extent that this characterization reflects current reality, one is perhaps not surprised that an investigator, even a well-trained and otherwise responsible scientist feeling misunderstood and abused by the process, may resort to a variety of tactics to circumvent or avoid the process entirely, a behavior pattern sometimes referred to as juridification by legal scholars (Gatter, 2003). Indeed, the imposition through law and regulations of a process for oversight of scientists earlier in this century may have set the stage for a confrontational environment between scientists and review boards, however justified and well-intentioned the oversight process may have been, or how strong was its justification (Koski, 2003). In truth, there have been sufficiently numerous instances of irresponsible and unethical conduct among scientists conducting human research and abuses of human research participants to justify sufficiently the creation of a process for review and oversight. The concern is not so much that we have such a process for review and oversight of human research, but rather, whether or not that process is serving either the interests of science, society or research participants.

In this volume, several respected scientists, ethicists and administrators discuss ways to promote research into the causes, prevention, diagnosis and treatment of cancer through research. This chapter considers steps that might be taken to facilitate that research by making the processes upon which it depends simpler, more uniform, more efficient and more effective—and more harmonious and "user-friendly." While there are certainly opportunities to improve the processes for making and administering grants and sponsorship of research, this chapter focuses on the critical infrastructure for doing and overseeing cancer research, particularly in the realm of clinical trials and protection of research participants. I will argue that much can be accomplished by applying a systems approach and a bit of *feng shui* to the research process.

2. WHY BUCK THE SYSTEM?

One can reasonably argue that clinical research in oncology is more sophisticated and well-developed as a process than in any other medical discipline, with HIV/AIDS and cardiology also being disciplines in which a more systematic approach is notable and productive. In these cases, cooperative clinical trials groups have been established to ensure that protocols are rigorously designed and powered to examine specific, important research questions according to priorities set by leading scientists in the field. More often than not, the protocols developed by these cooperative groups are performed at specific sites that have made a commitment to the cooperative group studies. They are, essentially, members of the club. Under this arrangement, there is an opportunity to screen specific centers as prospective performance sites on the basis of several criteria, such as availability of appropriate study subjects, investigators, facilities, resources, etc. In the case of cancer research, a major step toward a more efficient and effective process was the creation of a so-called "central institutional review board" (CIRB) to conduct a single high-level review of the science, safety and ethics of proposed research studies (Christian, 2002). This important step, taken with the leadership of the National Cancer Institute (NCI) and the Office for Human Research Protections, has still not been fully implemented, largely due to reluctance among the participating research sites to relinquish autonomy or to expose them to liability. The NCI also implemented a sophisticated electronic system for reporting and monitoring adverse events in studies conducted by its cooperative groups. Important alliances exist between research groups and advocacy groups for patients with various types of cancers, including the

American Cancer Society, one of the largest and most effective professional organizations in medicine. Why then, despite these efforts, are so few eligible caner patients actually participating in cancer trials?

There is no simple answer, but it is well known that fewer than 5% of patients eligible for participation in clinical trials choose to do so. We find ourselves in a situation where in spite of major efforts to promote research activities, few patients are inclined to volunteer to be research subjects, many practicing oncologists do not choose not to be clinical investigators, streamlined ethics review processes are underutilized and institutions frequently fail to take advantage of opportunities to reduce administrative burdens through more effective use of electronic information systems technologies, all this despite the fact that all parties would benefit from a robust clinical research endeavor. If we cannot do better in the discipline with what is ostensibly the 'best of breed' system for clinical research, it is not surprising that other disciplines are probably even less effective. Today, the vast majority of clinical trials are seriously delayed in accrual of subjects, and because clinical trials are the final common pathway for bringing new knowledge, therapies and diagnostics to fruition, we clearly face a challenge. Simply maintaining the *status quo* is not likely to result in rewarding progress--this then is the catalyst for "bucking the system". We must take a hard look at how we are conducting our activities today, identify opportunities for change and improvement, and develop a realizable plan for future success.

3. WHAT IS WRONG WITH THE SYSTEM?

The major problem with the system we have is that it is not really a system at all. A *system* is defined as a group of independent but interrelated elements comprising a *unified* whole. Beyond this core definition lies a broader context that includes an infrastructure and operational rules that provide necessary integration of the independent elements to create a true system--instrumentality that combines interrelated, interacting components designed to work as a coherent entity and a complex of methods or rules governing behavior to ensure a procedure or process for obtaining an objective.

We do have today a well established group of independent and interrelated elements engaged in the research process, many of them of very high quality, but we lack the unification, the infrastructure and operational rules to support the degree of integration and coherence necessary to create a truly effective and efficient system for conducting clinical research in oncology (or any other field for that matter). This deficiency is not due to a lack of trying, or to a lack of leadership. In large measure it is related to the culture surrounding the research enterprise, fiscal and political realities, and societal expectations. Competing interests among the parties may be contributing to our inability to be more effective and efficient.

Prior to the '60's, academic science and industry were largely independent endeavors. The ineffectiveness of university efforts, such as they were, to capitalize on their basic discoveries fostered greater interaction with industry's more experienced developmental teams to create and market products. Congress catalyzed these interactions through passage of the Bayh-Dole Act in the early '80s. Since that time, science has become more entrepreneurial, even at academic centers (Campbell et al, 2005). Some have argued that as a result, academic scientists are less willing to share their discoveries and research materials, preferring instead to seek patents that may preserve financial interests for themselves and their universities. Empirical evidence to support these views is scant, but the concern may be justified. Few in science today would argue that the climate of openness is stronger than it was two decades ago, or that entrepreneurial opportunities have less importance today than they once did. Whether driven by financial interests or the prospect of academic promotion and recognition, a scientist unwilling to share data and research materials with colleagues in search of new treatments would seem to be putting personal interest before the pursuit of knowledge, and certainly before the interests of patients and the public.

Such behaviors are contrary to what some see as the altruistic tradition of science--a tradition that may be more perception that reality-- as personal recognition has probably always been and will continue to be an important source of motivation for scientists. Few would decline the Nobel Prize, and although I have no first hand knowledge of what happens to the prize money, I doubt that most of it is given back to support research or given to charity. The current situation is perhaps not unlike the Olympic games, where a champion athlete may have once reveled in the glory of victory and a crown of olive branches, today the promise of lucrative endorsement contracts is not lost on athletes, at least in those sports highly recognized by the public. The present entrepreneurial spirit in science has led Sheldon Krimsky, a professor at Tufts University, in his book *Science in the Private Interest*, to argue that the lure of profits has corrupted the idealism and the practice of science, even fostering misconduct in its worst forms in some cases. But it is probably not all about money, as many have pointed out--noted 'gene-therapy' scientist, James Wilson, stated that he was more interested in winning the Nobel Prize than in the financial gains to be reaped from discovery of a safe and effective vector for gene-transfer in humans. In my own institution, the Massachusetts General Hospital, an institution with a long and productive tradition in biomedical research, this tension was evident during a discussion of 'institutional values' at a strategic planning retreat in the late 90's. Unable to bridge the gap between those who favored unhindered collegiality and collaboration, on the one hand, and those who were committed to a more competitive entrepreneurial approach on the other, the group finally settled upon a somewhat oxymoronic construct dubbed 'entrepreneurial teamwork' as being core to its mission.

At a time when discovery is rarely the result of a single individual's work, progress is more dependent upon collegiality and collaboration than ever. This is certainly true in clinical research for several reasons, not the least of which is the need for large numbers and diversity of patients with specific medical conditions to permit research studies to meet accrual goals in a timely manner and to ensure generalizability of study data. Although this reality has driven the formation of collaborative study groups such as those common in the discipline of oncology, and yet, these groups have failed to reach their full potential. To what extent this is the result of unwillingness to collaborate for pursuit of personal financial and academic interests is unknown, but greater willingness to engage colleagues in collaborations for the good of science, patients and society can hardly hurt. Some universities have actually tackled this thorny financial issue by creating the equivalent of faculty or alumni 'mutual funds' in which the financial rewards of the discoveries of all, or a few, can benefit all as well as the mission. It seems unlikely to me that there will be a rush to adopt such models, even with current concerns over financial conflicts of interest at the individual and institutional levels, but they may offer an alternative approach and set the stage for a renaissance of altruism and beneficence in medicine and biomedical science at a time when it is seriously needed. Here, the HIV-AIDS crisis is perhaps more visible and compelling than even the "war on cancer". In much of the world, people with cancer die without treatment because of insufficient awareness, delayed diagnosis, limited access to treatment, and insufficient resources. The HIV-AIDS crisis has demonstrated the need for a more effective system to promote public health and provide more equitable access to medical care and effective treatment more dramatically than any medical condition in recent memory. In the face of this humanitarian and health crisis, and a public outcry for social justice, some pharmaceutical companies have responded by developing programs to make their expensive drugs for treatment or prevention more readily available in developing countries, and for this they should be applauded. One can but hope that the healthcare industry and the companies whose products have contributed so much to improving treatment and life quality will continue recent trends to be more socially responsible in their conduct as we try to address the disparities that tarnish the promise of modern medicine around the world.

While investigators and sponsors of research represent one part of the enterprise, institutions and their research ethics review boards (RERBs), commonly called institutional review boards (IRBs), are also given to idiosyncratic and self-interested behaviors that may be detrimental to research progress. An example is the apparent reluctance of institutions to participate in the NCI central review process mentioned earlier. On its face, a system that can eliminate much of the wasteful and costly redundancy that is inherent in the review and oversight process would seem to be the Holy Grail for promoting more efficient cancer research. And yet, many institutions and their IRBs have declined to participate for reasons that include fears of liability and a lack of trust in a centralized review process. This said, it is inaccurate to characterize the NCI's CIRB process as just 'a central IRB', because it is in fact a distributed, tandem process that uses an central review board at one level to facilitate review at the local level, thereby allowing local sites to more effectively devote their time and resources to activities that are best done at a local level (Figure 1). This may sound good, but it has been very difficult to realize, contrary to what would seem to be common sense. Whatever the basis for this kind of behavior may be, unless it changes, the likelihood of implementing a more efficient and effective system for clinical research, whether in oncology or another discipline seems remote.

Figure 1: A 'tandem' model for facilitated cooperative review of multicenter clinical trials. Review by a central board can be accepted or rejected by local boards according to defined terms of participation, reducing redundancy and permitting local resources to be dedicated to conduct of the trial at the site.

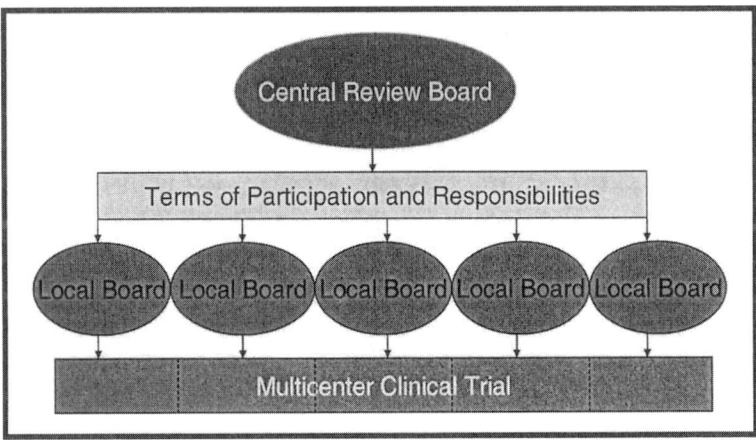

In the final analysis, we must decide what we really what to accomplish-- as individuals, as institutions, as an industry and as a society. What do we want to do and how do we hope to do it? What kind of society do we want to be? In pursuit of our research and health agendas, are we willing to forego individual interests, personal gain and recognition for a greater good, a shared good that will benefit many? Again, these are very difficult questions, but questions that are more than rhetorical. If those involved in the health-sciences enterprise can find a way to work together more collegially, to invest in a robust, shared research infrastructure and to collaborate with a spirit that 'a rising tide floats all boats', then great progress may be possible in a relatively short period, but major changes and reforms of the current 'system' are needed.

4. TOWARD A MORE USER-FRIENDLY SYSTEM

The first and most important step toward a more user-friendly clinical research system is, not surprisingly, to actually build a system--and then to have more friendly users. Consider for example another system that seems to serve society's interests quite well for the most part, for individuals, for commerce and individual countries, the air transportation safety system. I am not an expert on the airline industry by any means, despite having earned nearly a million frequent-flyer miles, but I do know that when a plane takes off for the Far East from New England, everyone involved with the flight has a common goal -- to arrive safely and on time at the destination, realizing fully that there is a very real possibility of encountering turbulence, mechanical problems, air traffic, on board illness, and a host of other challenges. The pilots and crew are generally well-trained, experienced, licensed, rested, sober, well mannered and otherwise prepared for the flight. They will fly over several countries, over vast oceans, through several time zones, over many language barriers and will do so while remaining in contact at all times with a network of global air traffic controllers monitoring their course and speed, proximity to other aircraft, adverse weather conditions, and other threats to the safety and well being of the plane, its crew and its passengers, as well as the safety and well being of the public at large that reaps the benefits of safe, convenient air travel.

In the aviation industry, we have developed a true system, one that provides safety as well as efficiency, and it works. The global system of air-traffic control centers is totally integrated so that the location of every plane in the sky is known precisely at every moment, coordinating take-offs and landings and keeping planes from colliding. As a result, air travel is the safest mode of transportation in the world. We have agreed internationally upon separation zones, and have adopted a common language for international communications. Many of the airlines even use a fully integrated reservations system to facilitate scheduling and for tracking passengers and luggage. Needless to say, this did not all happen spontaneously. It all required careful planning, training, cooperation, coordination and compromise--and major investment of resources.

The clinical research process

In the United States, the system is supported by the national Airport and Airway Trust Fund (AATF), which was created by the Airport and Airway Revenue Act of 1970:
(http://www.faa.gov/about/office_org/headquarters_offices/aep/aatf/). The AATF provides funding for the federal commitment to the nation's aviation system through several aviation-related excise taxes. Funding currently comes from collections related to passenger tickets, passenger flight segments, international arrivals/departures, cargo waybills, aviation fuels, and frequent flyer mile awards from non-airline sources like credit cards. In recent Congressional testimony by Ruth Marlin, Executive Vice President of the National Air Traffic Controllers Association (NATCA) pointed out that:

"Over thirty years ago the Airport and Airway Trust Fund was established to ensure adequate capital investment in our nation's aviation infrastructure. Since its inception, the U.S. has used the Trust Fund to make capital improvements: investing in airports; air traffic control facilities and equipment; and research and development...Through the Trust Fund, investment in our nation's aviation infrastructure has resulted in the most accessible, affordable and efficient aviation system in the world."

(http://www.house.gov/transportation/aviation/05-04-05/marlin.pdf)

If we wish to begin to move toward creating a true system for clinical research, the aviation industry may provide a useful model.

If we are to have an effective system, creation of a national trust fund to support a shared infrastructure for clinical research could be a first step. With relatively modest support from industry and government, a national research information system could be established using platform independent, web-based communications tools and databases to facilitate almost every operational component of the research process, including for example, registration of clinical trials, submission of protocols for review by RERBs, tracking and facilitating enrollment of subjects, reporting and monitoring adverse events, all while coordinating and facilitating communications among all parties to the process. Such a system could draw from already available systems such as the GeMCRIS (http://www.gemcris.od.nih.gov/) adverse event reporting system developed by the Food and Drug Administration and the Office for Biotechnology Affairs at the National Institutes of Health for monitoring high-risk gene-transfer studies. With relatively minor modifications, this system could be scaled-up and enhanced to serve the entire clinical research endeavor. Many institutions have already invested heavily, both in terms of money and intellect, to develop information systems to facilitate protocol development and IRB submission, to streamline IRB review, and to communicate with investigators in a timely manner. Many pharmaceutical and biotech companies have undoubtedly made similar investments in information systems that could have broader utility outside of an individual corporate environment. Certainly this is the case for electronic data-capture systems for clinical trials, but there has been little cooperation or standardization across the industry. The result is the proliferation of proprietary systems with limited capabilities to interact with other systems, even if doing so could be advantageous to the industry as a whole by increasing productivity and reducing expenses. A best-of-breed assessment by an appropriately appointed steering committee could identify those components that would best serve the needs of the research community and incorporate them into a national system that would provide the backbone of a national clinical research system.

Perhaps the most glaring and crucial example of an opportunity to reduce redundancy and costs while improving efficiency and effectiveness is the process for review and oversight by RERBs (IRBs). Although the actual number of IRBs in operation today is unknown, estimates are generally in the 4,000 to 5,000 range. The existing "one institution, one review board" model was created by federal regulations promulgated three decades ago. Many, including the National Bioethics Advisory Commission and the Institute of Medicine have noted the inefficiency and redundancy of the existing process, while investigators and sponsors often regard the process as a serious and frustrating impediment to research initiation. While the original desire for local input into the approval process remains, the approach to research then and now is dramatically different. Today, large-scale multicenter research studies are the norm, and in general are preferable to smaller, often underpowered studies done at individual sites, but the IRB process is ill suited to support the collaborative multicenter approach. Initiation of even a straightforward cancer trial comparing two established treatments today could require review and approval by several hundred RERBs, with several hundred variations of a model consent form, and hundreds of sets of duplicate files, all at enormous cost. If this level of local authority and redundancy could be shown to provide a measurable increase in the protections accorded the research participants, its continuation could be justified. Few would argue this to be the case.

Concern regarding the capabilities and effectiveness of local review boards is widespread, as is concern over their inefficiency and costs. These concerns exist both here in the United States and internationally, particularly in Europe, where they have been addressed in the European Union's Directive on Clinical Trials (available at http://europa.eu.int/smartapi/cgi/sga_doc?smartapi!celexapi!prod!CELEXnumdoc&lg=EN&numdoc=32001L0020&model=guichett). By requiring a single ethical opinion from each participating member state regarding a given protocol within a specified time-frame, the Directive has catalyzed a shift toward more centralized or cooperative review mechanisms and movement away from the inefficient and often idiosyncratic institution-based model of review. The United Kingdom adopted a system of regional review boards a few years ago, an approach recently modified in light of the

EU Directive, and regional review boards have been proposed for the U.S., where a few fledgling efforts in collaborative review are also underway (Koski et al, 2005). These efforts arise not from government mandates, but from institutions that envision opportunities to cut costs and improve effectiveness. For its part, the U.S. government facilitates such efforts through the streamlined and flexible Federalwide assurance process first introduced five years ago and formally in 2004. It is still too early to know whether collaborative review models, implemented either regionally or nationally, will provide the anticipated improvements in operational efficiency or cost reduction. It is clear, however, that relatively few institutions in the U.S. as yet seem willing to adopt these models, so some action by the federal government to promote them may be in order, especially for a well established research-based discipline like oncology. Overcoming this reluctance is a necessary step toward creating a more efficient system. Incentives, in the form of financial support and reduced regulatory and administrative burdens, might be effective in this regard.

The reluctance of individual sites or institutions to participate in collaborative research and review processes may be diminished by accreditation processes developed over the last few years and now taking hold both in the U.S. and abroad. In the wake of high-profile clinical research tragedies in the U.S. in recent years, and recognition that government regulatory agencies lack sufficient resources to effectively oversee review boards and investigators, private sector approaches to validate competencies, or at least, process capabilities, are gaining broader acceptance. Of these, certification of individual members of clinical research teams (for more information, visit the Association of Clinical Research Professionals at http://www.acrpnet.org) and accreditation of human subjects protection programs (see the Association for Accreditation of Human Research Protection Programs at http://www.aahrpp.org) are best developed and most widely recognized, and accreditation of research performance sites is just beginning. As confidence in these accreditation and certification programs grows, so will their value to the research enterprise and to the public. An institution with an accredited human research protection program is likely to be more willing to enter into a cooperative, reciprocal review process with another institution because the level of trust is enhanced through an objective, independent accreditation process. With less concern over potential liability, institutions will be more willing to work together on common protocols. Growth is site accreditation and professional certification of individual members of research teams will similarly help to build confidence and foster collaboration. The resources made available through reduced redundancy can then be applied locally to further strengthen the local research infrastructure.

5. A FIELD OF DREAMS?

No one would be surprised that a sweeping proposal for a national research system engenders great skepticism. Many will likely argue that such a system would be too expensive, that it would be too complicated, that it would be insensitive to local considerations important to the ethical review and conduct of the research, among a host of other objections. However, it is generally easier to give into skepticism that to venture forth into new territory--real progress is unlikely to occur until both the research community and the public accept that the present system is largely unworkable. If, however, we have indeed reached the point that responsible investigators are being driven by frustration to breaking the law and engaging in other forms of scientific and ethical misconduct in order to see their work move forward, then recognition of the need for a better approach cannot be far behind.

Oncology is well positioned to be the prototype for a national clinical research system. Many of the essential components are already available and with some modification, a truly effective system for cancer research is feasible within five years. The basic design would draw upon the current initiatives of the National Cancer Institute, the Office for Human Research Protections, the National Institutes of Health and other organizations, but would also include pharmaceutical companies and industry organizations, as well as public health and patient advocacy groups that share interests in realizing such a system. In its 2006 budget, the NCI requested over $170 M to develop a systems approach to oncology research, its program encompassing most of the components mentioned here and then some, but largely lacking the critical participation of industry in the process (Table 1).

Table 1: NCI Integrated Clinical Trials System Budget Increase Request for Fiscal Year 2006

Strengthening scientific prioritization & coordination, $116.00 M

Flexible collaborations
State-of-the-science & other planning meetings
Standardization, coordination, & tracking of trials
Centralized IRB & administrative support
Increased use of imaging
Staffing & training
New approaches & prototypes for networks

Speeding novel agent development & biomarker validation, $28.00 M

Trials employing novel validation principles
Identification of surrogate endpoints & biomarkers
Laboratory-based correlative studies

Expanding the goals of clinical trials, $24.00 M

Increased access for minority & underserved populations
Symptom management studies
Patient tracking & record keeping
Studies of long-term effects of treatment
Use of quality- of- life & economic endpoints

Management & Support 2.85 M

Total $170.85 M

6. CONCLUSION

In the war against cancer, industry must be a part of the "coalition of the willing", and that poses an enormous set of challenges (Bodenheimer, 2000). Most specifically, the industry must be willing to invest in the shared infrastructure rather than to expect the public, through taxpayer dollars, to bear the full cost of a system that provides enormous benefits to the industry and its shareholders. In part, industry support must come in the form of monies paid into a joint public-private trust fund to support the system, as in the aviation industry. Beyond that, the industry must also be willing to enter into a process of evidence-based development and treatment in which companies address priorities set by teams of independent clinician scientists operating with transparency and public oversight. This will undoubtedly be unsettling to companies that have generally, and understandably, given their proprietary interests top priority. In such a system, clinical trials would be developed objectively according to what the best available data indicate is likely to be the most effective therapeutic approach, and competing therapies would be tested head-to-head. Under such a system, companies will be rewarded solely on the basis of the effectiveness of their products, rather than on the effectiveness of their marketing strategies. It will be necessary to ensure that the process does not stifle the spirit of discovery and entrepreneurialism that has driven the industry for so long, but the emphasis must be shifted to fulfilling the mission, not the money coffers--which brings us back to 'entrepreneurial teamwork'--perhaps the construct is not so oxymoronic after all.

Under such a system, investigators and sponsors attitudes toward RERBs must also change, and vice versa. The ethics review and approval process must be accepted as part of the critical mission infrastructure, not merely as an administrative process, and the resources to support it must flow accordingly. A system of truly expert central and/or regional review boards, all of which are of course fully accredited, working in tandem with local boards to ensure that all studies are not only properly and efficiently reviewed according to the highest ethical and scientific standards, but are also conducted with the safety and well being of the subjects and the integrity of the science as the foremost priorities. With well-trained, committed individuals properly supported by sufficient funds and a robust information system, these goals are readily achievable. Paperwork and administrative processing times can be markedly reduced, trials initiated and conducted much more efficiently, and the overall cost-savings can be re-invested in the research process. Investigators must accept their responsibility to be fully trained to design and conduct the research and should demonstrate their commitment by completing rigorous training programs and seeking certification through a rigorous examination process. Finally, the public must be willing to accept its role in the research process. Cancer is still a leading killer, and while great progress has been made, much remains to be accomplished. We do not know who among us will become a victim of cancer, but when and if we do, we will all want to be survivors. Toward realizing this hope, and this goal, we all have a responsibility to be part of the process, to learn more about research, and like the three generations of citizens in Framingham, Massachusetts who have allowed us to benefit from their participation in the long-running Framingham Heart Study sponsored by the National Heart Lung and Blood Institute, we all need to consider participating actively in cancer research from which we all can benefit.

The important initiatives that the NCI has proposed in its 2006 strategic plan and budget set the stage for an even more aggressive and far-reaching effort to create a comprehensive system for clinical research in oncology. If we can muster the vision, the will and the resources to make such a system work for cancer research, it could serve as a prototype for a new model for clinical research across the board, one that is less fraught with the competing and conflicting interests that plague clinical research today, one that is less driven by the quest for profits rather than the quest for cures and better lives. Many will simply dismiss such an approach as sheer folly, but others will see it as both a challenge and an opportunity. There are obviously many details that need to be defined and huge compromises that would be required just to get started, and even if we are successful, the question remains, "If will build it, will they come?" In the final analysis, there is really only one way to find out.

Given the current state of the process and the pressing needs and hopes of society, we can ill afford to wait.

In the meantime, we can begin on a less grand scale to implement and expand efforts to improve upon what we have today. Opportunities for simplification of our regulatory scheme, such as harmonizing regulatory requirements and consolidating oversight agencies to make it easier to understand and meet our responsibilities is long overdue and would be welcomed by the entire research community, whether based in academia or industry, in the public or private sector. Investigators and sponsors could improve their lot by better appreciating the very difficult task confronting research ethics review boards. If investigators and sponsors accepted fully their responsibilities for protecting the interests of research participants and gave those responsibilities the same consideration and effort they give their scientific interests, their interactions with the RERB/IRB would be considerably less confrontational, more collaborative and more efficient. In reality, the bar is not set very high. If every research protocol were to include a thoughtful presentation and discussion of the ethical issues implicit in the study and specifically how those issues have been addressed to protect the interests and safety of the subjects, most proposals would slide with far greater easy through what seem to be the sticky wickets of the review process. Many companies recognized long ago that a good relationship with the FDA is an extremely valuable asset, well worth cultivating--mindful investigators and sponsors are well advised to similarly cultivate their relationships with their ethics review boards. And if the review boards are able to focus more on real issues of science, ethics and safety, as opposed to 'word smithing' consent forms, are able to exercise the flexibility of judgment granted in their guiding regulations, and communicate their concerns more logically, directly and explicitly to investigators in a timely manner, our process would operate more smoothly and efficiently. Of course, they must be given the resources necessary to do so.

Those who engage in research studies of other human beings are granted enormous privilege, and with that privilege comes enormous responsibility. In the end, clinical research is truly a team effort, and all members of the team have a common interest in the fruits of this labor. Done well, it warrants the respect and trust of all, but even hard-earned respect and well-deserved trust is fragile and easily squandered with but a few irresponsible actions by those who fail to understand and meet their responsibilities. Facing and meeting those responsibilities head on is our challenge--if we are to continue to bring the great promise of science and technology to all, we must not fail.

REFERENCES

1. Bodenheimer, T. Uneasy Alliance--Clinical Investigators and the Pharmaceutical Industry. N. Eng. J. Med., 2000; 342: 1539-1544. Available online at http://content.nejm.org/cgi/content/full/342/20/1539
2. Campbell, E., Koski, G., Zinner, D., and Blumenthal, D. Managing the Triple Helix in the Life Sciences. Issues in Science and Technology, Winter, 2005; 1: 32-39. National Academies Press, Washington, DC. Available online at http://www.issues.org/21.2/campbell.html.
3. Christian, M., Goldberg, J., Killen, J., Abrams, J., McCabe, M., Mauer, J., and Wittes, R. A central institutional review board for multi-institutional trials. N. Eng. J. Med. 2002; 346: 1405-1408. Available online at http://content.nejm.org/cgi/content/full/346/18/1405
4. Gatter, R. Walking the Talk of Trust in Human Subjects Research: the Challenge of Regulating Financial Conflicts of Interest. Emory Law Journal, 2003; 52: 327-402.
5. Giles, J. Researchers break the rules in frustration at review boards. Nature, 2005; 438:136-137. Available online at http://www.nature.com/nature/journal/v438/n7065/full/438136b.html
6. Koski, G. Research, Regulations and Responsibility: Confronting the Compliance Myth. Emory Law Journal, 2003; 52: 403-416
7. Koski, G., Aungst, J., Kupersmith, J., Getz, K., and Rimoin, D. Enhancing Safety and Efficiency in Clinical Research: Cooperative Research Ethics Review Boards—A Win-Win Solution? IRB: Ethics & Human Research, 2005; 27: 1-7. Available online at http://www.medscape.com/viewarticle/505154_print.
8. Martinson, B., Anderson, M., and de Vries, R. Scientists behaving badly. Nature, 2005; 435: 737-738. Available online at http://www.nature.com/nature/journal/v435/n7043/full/435737a.html

Chapter 16

CANCER RESEARCH AND CLINICAL TRIAL IN ACTION: AN IMPORTANT EXERCISE BEFORE YOU EMBARK ON YOUR STUDY

Larry Carbone, DVM, PhD[1], Scott H. Kurtzman, MD[2] and Stanley P.L. Leong, MD[3]
[1]*Department of Vetinary Medicine, UCSF Medical Center, San Francisco, CA, USA;* [2]*Department of Surgery, University of Connecticut, Farmington, CT & Waterbury Hospital, Waterbury, CT;* [3]*Department of Surgery, University of California, San Francisco, CA, USA*

1. INTRODUCTION

Before the FDA will approve a Phase I study of a potential cancer chemotherapeutic agent, animal studies using at least two animal species generally must be submitted. But animal studies themselves require considerable planning to meet scientific, ethical and regulatory commitments.

These commitments are herein reviewed in a question and answer format.

Q. Must all cancer studies in animals be performed using FDA's Good Laboratory Practices as their standard?

A. Data to be presented to the FDA in support of an Investigational New Drug (IND) application usually must follow GLP standards. Initial, exploratory studies may employ less stringent standards of quality control and of tissue and records archiving.

Q. Which animal studies require prior approval of the Institutional Animal Care and Use Committee?

A. As a general rule, all vertebrate animal work, must be approved by the institution's animal care and use committee prior to obtaining animals or proceeding with the experiment. Pilot studies, though they use few animals, carry the potential for a great deal of animal pain or distress, and so even small pilot projects must be approved before they are begun.

Q. What regulations require Institutional Animal Care and Use Committees? Are there exceptions?

A. In the United States, two main bodies of regulation require IACUCs. The Animal Welfare Act (7 U.S.C. §§ 2131 – 59; Title 9 Code of Federal Regulations) requires committee reviews for research using the animal species that law covers (currently, all mammals except laboratory-bred mice and rats), regardless of the source of funding for the research. Likewise, the Public Health Service (PHS) Policy on Humane Care and Use of Laboratory Animals requires committee review for projects at all PHS-conducted and PHS-funded projects. This policy applies to all vertebrate animals (i.e., fish, amphibians, reptiles, birds and mammals).

Work that uses only laboratory-bred mice or rats, frogs, or other species not covered by the Animal Welfare Act, and that is not funded by the Public Health Service or its divisions (such as the National Institutes of Health) potentially may not require the approval of an Institutional Animal Care and Use Committee. However, in many states, there are state regulations that may apply.[1]

Q. What principles guide Institutional Animal Care and Use Committee deliberations?

A. IACUCs have responsibility for oversight of the use of animals in experiments, as well as for their procurement, housing, health and veterinary care. IACUCs focus on efforts to minimize any potential pain or distress that research projects might cause the animals. This includes assuring that animals used for research are healthy, that efforts are made to reduce their numbers to the minimum required for sound scientific data, that anesthetics and analgesics are used when appropriate and that experimental endpoints are set such that animals are removed from study (usually by euthanasia) before significant adverse effects on health and well-being develop.[2]

Perhaps because institutions own and house their animal subjects, and because animals cannot opt out of a project in progress as human subjects can IACUCs have a longer history of post-approval compliance monitoring than human subjects Institutional Review Boards have had. Initial protocol approval is an early step in the IACUC's oversight animal studies.

Q. What alternatives are there for animal cancer studies?

A. Following Russell and Burch's *Principles of Humane Experimental Technique*[3], investigators consider three types of alternatives:

1) *Replacement alternatives* refers to replacing vertebrate animals entirely, with cell or organ culture systems, microbiological models, invertebrate animals (such as *Drosophila* fruit flies), or computer models. Examples include production of monoclonal antibodies in tissue culture rather than in mouse ascites fluid, or using cell membrane extracts (liposomes) to investigator membrane transport phenomena *in vitro*.

2) *Reduction alternatives* refers to careful statistical methods that allow for smaller numbers of subjects to yield statistically valid data. Examples may include use of historical controls (when valid), or employing assays that can analyze small samples derived from single animals over multiple time-points, rather than many animals sampled once.

3) *Refinement alternatives* refers to the myriad ways of changing experimental design to minimize pain and distress. In addition to anesthesia and analgesia, refinements can include setting humane endpoints, training animals to cooperate with experimental technique, using telemetry devices for less invasive physiological monitoring, and improved imaging techniques.

Q. When might animals on cancer studies experience pain?

A. Surgery is always a potential source of pain if animals are not appropriately anesthetized, or not fully treated with post-surgical analgesics. Common surgeries performed in cancer research may include embryo transfer for development of transgenic rodent strains and implantation of subcutaneous osmotic pumps for delivery of test medications. Specific studies call for specific experimental techniques. Studies of brain cancers, for example, may involve intracerebral inoculation of tumor cells into rodents' brains or ventricles, which may require surgical exposure of the surface of the skull, and drilling through the bone. Placement in a stereotactic head restrainer itself is a likely source of pain.

Some cancers are probably directly painful to the animals, once induced. Subcutaneous tumors may be quite tolerable, until the overlying skin ulcerates; this is a standard criterion for euthanasia in many studies. Metastasis of experimental tumors, especially to bone, has the potential to cause significant pain.

Q. How can animal pain be recognized?

A. The United States government *Principles for the Utilization and Care of Vertebrate Animals Used in Testing, Research, and Training* state that "unless the contrary is established, investigators should consider that procedures that cause pain or distress in human beings may cause pain and distress in other animals."[4] This is often the starting point in deciding whether animals are likely to be in pain related to an experimental protocol or not.

Beyond this "critical anthropomorphism," diagnosing animal pain, especially chronic pain, can be very difficult. Pain diagnosis will depend on the species of animal, the experimental manipulations, and the type of pain expected. Animals in pain may limp or refuse to move; on the other hand, they may be nervous and excitable. They may stop grooming themselves, or decrease their food or water intake.

For group-housed nocturnal animals (i.e., for most mice and rats), individual behaviors are difficult to assess and loss of weight or loss of body condition can be important objective indicators of pain or distress.[5]

Q. How can animal pain be managed?

A. The first step in animal pain management is prevention. To the extent possible, researchers should avoid procedures that could cause pain. After that, most acutely painful procedures should be performed under anesthesia, with appropriate post-procedural analgesia.

Treatment of animal pain by pharmacologic means is similar to human pain treatment. Multimodal analgesia involves using medications of several different classes. For example, a surgery may include pretreatment with ketamine, local infiltration of bupivicaine and lidocaine at the incision site, and maintenance on an inhalant anesthetic. Post-surgical pain management might then include further use of local analgesic, a systemic opioid such as fentanyl or buprenorphine, as well as a non-steroidal anti-inflammatory drug such as meloxicam or carprofen.[6-8]

Researchers should remember that many disease processes, not just surgical procedures, can lead to animal pain. Dental disease, some metastatic cancers, arthritis and other illnesses can cause chronic pain in animals just as in people.

Non-pharmacologic adjuncts to pain management can include immobilizing an injured limb, hot or cool compresses, additional deep bedding for animals who have difficulty ambulating. Softened food and food placed in easy reach may reduce the pain of moving to acquire or to chew food.

Q. How can animal distress be recognized and treated?

A. Not all animal distress or illness involves pain; nonetheless, it is still a serious animal welfare concern that must be addressed. Russell and Burch identified a typology of "inhumanity" (i.e., pain and distress) in the animal laboratory, noting that some distress is inherent to some experiments ("direct inhumanity"), and some is extrinsic ("contingent inhumanity").[3]

As a general rule, any induction of disease should be considered a possible source of pain and/or distress. In cancer studies, this would potentially include the induction of tumors, though early stage benign tumors may cause no distress or illness. Once a tumor has metastasized to vital organ, has grown to a size that interferes with ambulation, feeding or other activities, or has caused skin ulceration, it should be considered a painful and distressing condition, and treated appropriately.

Additional sources of potential distress that are not necessarily painful include food and water deprivation, use of paralytic agents, some behavioral testing, or maintenance in cold environments. The need to employ these conditions must be carefully justified to the IACUC.

"Contingent inhumanity" includes husbandry and housing conditions that are distressful, but are not a required part of an experiment. Laboratory animals inhabit a social world that includes conspecifics, whether in their home cage or just within the room, as well as humans; social isolation and inter-animal aggression are both potential sources of distress for animals. Animals that are timid can be acclimated and trained to cooperate with research and husbandry procedures. Environmental conditions such as temperature and lighting and lack of a hiding opportunity can cause animal distress and can be fixed in the animals' favor without compromising the study.

Given the variety of causes and types of animal distress, recognizing it can be difficult. Careful observation of behavior, as well as monitoring physical signs (weight loss in particular) are the most useful approaches to diagnosing distress in individual animal subjects.[9, 10] Stereotypical behaviors may indicate distressing housing conditions that have persisted over time.[11] Most often, the likelihood of distress must be inferred from knowledge of species biology and normal behavior, and assessment of the animals' housing environment.

Q. What advice is there for getting a protocol approved by the Institutional Animal Care and Use Committee in a timely fashion?

A. It should be obvious that completely answering all of the questions on the IACUC's application form is prerequisite to timely review and approval of an animal-use protocol. Given the IACUC's wide-ranging oversight of animal use, animal housing, personnel qualifications, veterinary care and (human) occupational health, an investigator may need to address a range of questions satisfactorily to obtain approval.

The key to an acceptable and well-written animal protocol is for the scientist to try to envision and identify, from initial acquisition (or breeding) until final disposition (usually euthanasia), all steps that pose threats to animal welfare and to develop plans to prevent, treat, or justify the pain and distress. The best-written animal protocols briefly enumerate these, whether they are animal identification methods, surgical procedures, induction of disease states, methods of tissue collection, restraint, and answer these questions for each one:

- What is the degree of pain and/or distress likely to accompany this procedure?
- How is this pain/distress likely to manifest?
- How will it be monitored and on what timetable?
- Can the pain or distress be treated without invalidating the data being collected?
- If it can be treated, what anesthetics, analgesics and tranquilizers will be used, under what circumstances, and at what dose and frequency?
- Can endpoints be set to terminate pain or distress before they become severe?
- Has a literature search for alternatives been conducted that targets each potentially painful or distressful procedure as keywords?

If any of these questions are left unaddressed for any potentially painful or distressful procedure, the IACUC will not find itself able to approve the protocol.

2. AN EXERCISE

. . . or How to get your protocol approved by your Institutional Animal Care and Use Committee:
You've cloned a protein subunit of an ion channel. You believe it may have a role in inter-cellular communication during tumor formation. Eventually, you hope that you can develop a drug that will block the abnormal function of this ion channel in some human cancers.

2.1 Step 1: Antibodies

To determine how the subunits might combine to form an ion channel, you'll need to generate some monoclonal antibodies.

Q: Do I even need IACUC approval for this?

A: Some antibodies are commercially available; to buy these from a supplier, you do not need IACUC review and approval. If you are generating your own, you will need live mice, and you will need approval.

Q: What will the IACUC review if I decide I must make my own antibodies?

A: Making monoclonal antibodies begins by immunizing an animal to elicit a polyclonal population of antibody-producing lymphocytes. These will then be fused with myeloma cells to produce a hybridoma. The hybridoma secrets the monoclonal antibodies. There are two stages that may require live animals: the initial production of polyclonal lymphocytes, and the propagation of antibody-producing hybridoma cells.

Q: Must I consider alternatives? How do I do that?

A: You must consider alternatives to procedures that may cause more than minor or momentary pain or distress to the animals.

Start by considering which procedures those might be. In this project, for the initial polyclonal immunization, you will need to inject adjuvants, and they can cause painful inflammation. You will need to collect blood samples in the mice. You will need to euthanize them and collect their spleens. Later, once you've generated a hybridoma that produces the monoclonal antibody that you want, you may consider injecting the hybridoma cells into a mouse's abdomen; they will secrete monoclonal antibodies into the peritoneal cavity which will swell with ascites fluid full of antibodies. First though, you must 'prime' the abdomen with an inflammatory agent such as pristane to elicit the macrophages that will nourish the hybridoma cells, but which can produce painful inflammation. The abdominal distention may also be painful, and if it interferes with the mouse's ability to walk, it will cause distress.

Having identified the procedures that may cause pain or distress, think of three types of alternatives – replacement, reduction, refinement – and start doing your literature search.

Q: Are replacement alternatives possible?

A: Monoclonal antibody production is one of the great success stories in replacing live animal use with *in vitro* technologies. In most cases, most hybridoma lines will produce good yields of good quality antibody in tissue culture flasks. Your IACUC will require very strong justification before allowing you to produce monoclonals in mouse ascites fluids. For the initial polyclonal immunization, you will almost certainly need to immunize live mice.

Q: What about reduction?

A: You will need to explain to your IACUC how you chose the number of mice you plan to immunize. Five mice per antigen is fairly standard. If your antigen is not highly immunogenic (say, it's not a complex protein, or it's so similar to a mouse's endogenous proteins that they may not recognize it as foreign), you may need more.

Q: What refinements must I consider?

A: The standard for decades has been to use Freund's complete and incomplete adjuvants for antibody production. There are now less inflammatory proprietary commercial adjuvants that may work with your antigen. You certainly must be careful about how many times you inject Freund's complete adjuvant – more than once, and you'll elicit profound inflammation and peritonitis. What route will you use for blood collection? Collection from tail or lateral saphenous veins may be gentler on the animals than retro-orbital collection. You may need to use anesthesia, depending on the blood collection route you choose. You must monitor your mice for signs of peritonitis and have a plan (usually, humane euthanasia) if they start to look ill or lose weight or body condition. Finally, you must choose a euthanasia method that is consistent with the American Veterinary Medical Association Panel on Euthanasia recommendations.[12]

Q: How do I search for these alternatives?

A: Electronic database searches are often the first step. In the eyes of government regulators and many IACUCs, they are seen as crucial. The federal government's Animal Welfare Information Center maintain a staff and a website that are helpful in learning how to conduct literature searches targeted to finding information about animal alternatives. They also produce bibliographies on common topics. The search must be narrowed down, using keywords such as *alternatives, in vitro, blood collection* to be useful.

Unfortunately, database searching is better at reviewing the literature to assure non-duplication of existing work than it is at finding alternatives, especially refinement alternatives. Often the best sources of information on alternatives are your campus laboratory animal professionals (for common procedures) and scientists who have published work using methods similar to those you'll be needing.

2.2 Step 2: Investigating how the ion channel functions.

Experimental design for this step requires expressing the channel in frog oocyte cell membranes. Currently, the only way to obtain frog eggs is from frogs.

Q: Does my IACUC review use of frog oocytes?

A: Technically, oocytes are not vertebrate animals and they are not covered by animal welfare regulations. If a colleague offered to share her frog oocytes with you, there is no government requirement that you undergo IACUC review. However, if you are using live frogs to obtain the oocytes, you will need IACUC approval.

Q: What will the IACUC review if I decide I must use frogs as a source of oocytes?

A: Most projects using frog oocytes require early stage oocytes that are surgically removed from the female, rather than passed naturally through the cloaca. Any surgery is a potential source of distress, and strategies for anesthesia, sterile procedure, and after care must be reviewed.

Q: Must I consider alternatives?

A: Absolutely. You must explain to your IACUC why you require surgical collection of early-stage oocytes rather than harvesting later-stage oocytes that the female has passed (possibly in response to hormone injections). You must justify the numbers of frogs you will use. Because the frogs themselves are not units of statistical comparison in this project, numbers are justified based on the need for oocyte membranes, how many you can get from a single surgery, and how many surgeries you will perform on each frog. Finally, you must consider refinements by researching the most up-to-date information on frog anesthesia and post-operative analgesia. The latter question is in flux at the time of this publication, with minimal research data to date describing a really good post-operative analgesic for frogs.[13]

Q: What special review does vertebrate animal surgery require?

A: Regardless of the species, aseptic technique is required.[14] (p. 62) Though oocyte collection is a major surgery (in that it penetrates a major body cavity), it may be performed on the laboratory bench in a clean area. Sterile instruments, proper skin disinfection, and use of sterile surgical gloves are the standard of care.

The IACUC must review the qualifications and training of individuals who will perform surgery and anesthesia on a case-by-case basis. Specific degrees or certifications are not required.

The IACUC and attending veterinarian must review plans for anesthesia and post-operative care. Immersion anesthesia (such as tricaine methanesulfonate, or MS-222) is the most common anesthetic for *Xenopus* frogs. Use of hypothermia as part of the anesthetic regimen is common, but controversial.

As a general principle, multiple major survival surgeries on individual animals are discouraged.[14] (p. 12) However, an exemption to this principle exists on many campuses for frog oocyte collection; at the time of this publication, for example, the NIH intramural animal care and use program, allows up to five survival frog laparotomies per frog, plus a sixth non-survival surgery.[15]

2.3 Step 3: Developing transgenic mice with inducible genes for the ion channel

Transgenic and "knock-out" mice are extremely useful for studying the effects of individual genes and their products. At this stage of the project, you're ready to modify the genetic make-up of mice such that constitutive expression of the gene in question has been "knocked out" but an oxytetracylcine-inducible version of the gene has been inserted.

Q. What special welfare concerns does production of genetically modified rodents entail?

A. The creation of new strains of transgenic rodents raises concern for the manipulations of the animals (including surgery of both the males and females), the need to monitor new phenotypes for adverse outcomes, animal identification methods, and biosafety issues.

Cancer research and clinical trial in action

Rodent surgery requires that the PI address the same issues raised by frog surgery, including aseptic technique, safe and effective anesthesia, and effective post-operative care, including use of post-operative analgesics. Laparotomy for vasectomy and for embryo-transfer are both major survival surgical procedures. It is now standard practice in many laboratories to treat potential post-operative pain for 12-24 hours or longer with opioids (typically, buprenorphine) and/or non-steroidal anti-inflammatory drugs. Embryonic loss does not appear to be a problem and fear of embryonic loss is not a justification for withholding analgesics.[16]

Genetic manipulation can result in a range of desired and undesired genotypes and phenotypes. Animals must be carefully monitored throughout their development for evidence of adverse phenotypes. Systematic weight and growth measurements, behavioral tests, and other clinical observations are required to assure that the new transgenic line does not carry animal welfare problems.

Methods of genotyping and identifying transgenic rodents must be considered. Common practice allows tail-tip sampling of animals up to 3 weeks of age (before significant tail vertebra ossification has occurred); tail biopsy beyond that age certainly calls for anesthesia. Identification of baby mice is also challenging. Removing toes is banned in some countries. If considered, it must be done at an early age (5 – 10 days old), preferably under inhalant anesthesia.

Biosafety issues arise if human genes are being inserted into mice, or if viral vectors are used to introduce the genes. These practices are reviewed by a biosafety committee or biosafety officer.

Step 4: Preclinical safety and efficacy testing using animals.

Ultimately, potential therapeutic interventions will go to human clinical trials, but rarely without preliminary safety and efficacy testing in animal models.

Q. Do I need Food and Drug Administration approval to begin safety and efficacy trials of cancer chemotherapeutics in animals?

A. No. An FDA-approved Investigational New Drug (IND) Application is required before Phase I human studies are begun. Animal data are usually required for this application, and so must be largely completed before filing this application.

Q. What animal welfare regulations does the FDA impose?

A. Animal welfare does not figure prominently in FDA's oversight of animal use, and is not mentioned in the FDA's regulation of preclinical trials.[17]

Q. What other animal-use regulations does the FDA impose?

A. The FDA's oversight of animal use focuses on assuring the quality of the data generated in animal studies. FDA regulations include standards for animal identification, for avoiding accidental exposure to test substances, and assurance that food, water, bedding and pest control materials do not compromise the study in any way. Animals should be free of health problems that could complicate a study, and potentially infected animals must be isolated, if necessary, to control contagion.

Data that will be used to support IND applications must be accompanied by strict quality control and compliance with Good Laboratory Practices. This quality control, with associated internal audits and internal quality assurance units, is generally much stricter than that required for preliminary scientific studies that precede the FDA-related studies.

2.4 Clinical Studies

Vaccine study of human malignant melanoma

Overview:

Visceral metastases from malignant melanoma is invariably a fatal circumstance for which there is no effective treatment. Using harvested lymph nodes you would like to develop a vaccine. The purpose of the study is to test whether or not the vaccine can prevent the development of visceral metastases.

2.5 An Exercise

Q: What is your hypothesis?

A: A vaccine can be prepared from melanoma resection that will prevent the development of visceral metastases.

Q: What is your study design?

A: Portions of melanoma obtained either from biopsies or from operative specimens will be processed and prepared as single cells to be frozen in liquid nitrogen. Patients will be randomized to receive vaccine or a placebo. Patients will be followed for development of metastases. In addition, periodic blood samples will be taken to look for evidence of immunity. Genetic analysis of the tumors will be carried out to see if markers can identify patients who are likely to respond to the vaccination procedure.

Q. What do you have to submit to your IRB?

A: Most IRB's will require submission of a brief application in addition to the full protocol. In this application, you need to convey top the IRB the purpose of the research. Most IRB's distribute the main application to all the members, but only distribute the complete protocol to one or two members who serve as the primary reviewers. A clue to how they handle applications is how many copies are requested. Often the requirement will be for a large number of copies of the IRB application, but only two or three copies of the full scientific protocol. The reason that this is important is that not all of the committee members will have an oncology or even a scientific background. Federal regulations[18] require that some committee members represent the public, and some are from a non-scientific background. Since you only get one chance to make a first impression, it is imperative that the abstract be easy to understand.

Q: What is your scientific rationale?

A: The IRB is primarily interested in deciding whether or not it is ethical to subject humans to the research you are proposing. The application must convince them that you are asking a valid question and that the experiment proposed has a reasonable likelihood of answering the question. You should not have to convince them that you are doing Nobel laureate work. In my opinion, it also not their function to decide what kind of research is carried out at your institution. The hospital or department chair might not want you doing a particular protocol, but that is not a human subject protection issue. While the scientific aspects of the project are important, and care should be taken to ensure that valid data can be obtained, the IRB should not be criticizing specific methodology such as the concentration of glutamate that you have selected for your culture medium. However, if the reviewer feels that your scientific background is so poor that you are not qualified to do the research and perhaps don't even understand the question the project may be rejected. In addition, if the reviewers determine that the research design is so flawed that there is no possibility of obtaining meaningful data then the IRB can rule that it is not ethical to subject the patients to even the slightest risk and will turn down the protocol.

Q: What is your subject selection?

A: There are a number of important issues to be addressed with respect to subject selection. First, is the group of subjects selected to the research appropriate? Is that population available to the investigators. Second, you must address how the number of patients was determined. It is very important to enlist the help of a statistician to do a careful and thoughtful power analysis. These analyses are always subject to some speculation. For example, it is often difficult to determine what the response rate will be to a treatment. The protocol must address this and the assumptions should be based on some scientific principles or previous similar experience. Another important issue is who the subjects are. The IRB will carefully scrutinize whether the group of subjects selected is being chosen for the convenience of the investigator only. Projects that would not be approved would be ones where a vulnerable population such as the underserved are preferentially used. In the past, this group had been used because they were often uneducated and not facile in working their way through the healthcare system. They are more vulnerable to coercion, especially financial coercion.

On the other hand, underserved populations can also not be excluded from research if there is a reasonable likelihood that benefit could accrue as a result of participation. Similarly, particular ethnic groups need to be included in numbers proportional to the local population. The potential risks and benefits of the research should be equitably distributed. For example, if a particular ethnic group or gender is excluded from the research, then if the treatment is found to be effective, they will be deprived of the benefit since they were not included. This has occurred with children, pre-menopausal (fertile) women, African- Americans and others.

The research plan must therefore include a plan to recruit and retain a diverse population if that is appropriate. It is the PI responsibility to convey this information to the IRB in a manner that will allow them to make a rational decision.

Q: What are the safety concerns?

A: In this section, you will need to assure the IRB members that all precautions have been taken to minimize the risks to the patient. The IRB understands that there is a variable amount of risk inherent in almost any protocol. It is not necessary to convince the committee that you have eliminated all the risks but rather that you have identified the risks and have taken appropriate precautions to protect the subjects.

In a study involving biologic materials such as this vaccine trial for example, you will need to provide evidence of good laboratory practices e.g., sterility, non-pyrogenicity, prevention of viral transfer etc. The researchers involved in the project must be properly qualified to perform the tasks required of them. While non-physicians can certainly be principal investigators in human research, they can not be allowed to perform procedures or prescribe medications. Most IRB's will accept that once precautions have been minimized as best possible, that an informed adult should be allowed to decide whether or not he or she would like to participate and accept the risks that remain.

Q: How will the subjects be recruited?

A: In this section of the application you will need to describe how patients will be identified and invited to participate in the research. This is often an area of confusion among investigators, and IRB's . As a guiding principle, only clinicians participating in the care of patients are entitled to know anything about a patient. This includes knowledge that a particular individual has a disease and might therefore be eligible to participate in the project. Accordingly, it is appropriate for a member of the health care team to identify subjects and seek their permission to participate. The clinicians may also ask their patients if the research team who might not be known to them can contact them regarding the clinical trial. If you are going to take this latter approach remember to find out the restrictions the patients might impose on the nature of the contact. Keep in mind that some patients might choose not tell family members or others they live with about their diagnosis. A poorly planned phone call answered by a young child might be devastating.

It is permissible to advertise the study. Again as a general rule though, anytime the research team contacts the public with information regarding research, this is considered the beginning of the informed consent process and is subject to IRB jurisdiction and approval. However, communication between health care providers is not considered in this way and is permissible. For example, you can feel free to discuss your protocol on the telephone with other clinicians who might be referral sources or you can present the protocol at professional conferences. If you plan to discuss this with a lay audience this should receive IRB approval so that it is clear that the information presented is unbiased, not coercive and presented in a way that can be understood by potential patients. The same rule applies to media advertising.

Q: How do you construct your informed consent?

A: IRB's consider informed consent a process, not simply a document. As stated earlier, the informed consent process begins at the very introduction of the protocol. In this section of the application, you must explain to the committee how you will help the potential subject understand the nature and purpose of the research, what the possible risks and benefits are to them, what it might cost them, how they can withdraw as well as the many other issues discussed in previous chapters. The IRB will be concerned with issues such as when and how the patient is made aware of the protocol. Patients are especially vulnerable to coercion when they are told bad news and when they are alone. For many projects, it will be important to specify that the information regarding the experiment will be presented at a separate time from when consent is obtained. It is often highly desirable to present the patient with an information sheet as well as the informed consent document and then allow them time to go home and review the material with family members, a primary care physician or other resources such as the internet. The IRB will be suspicious of a process where the subject is asked to give consent at the same visit when a cancer diagnosis or staging change has been given. Subjects also need to be told that they can withdraw from the research. Often there are risks to withdrawing for which they need to be made aware. In this study that involves vaccination there is not likely to be a risk to withdrawing, but if the protocol utilizes immunosuppression then there might be times when it would be dangerous for the patients to withdraw.

Q: What are the issues regarding compensation and costs?

A: IRB's and investigators alike struggle with issues regarding compensation and expenses. A guiding principle is that third party payors should not be expected to bear the cost of research. Subjects should be allowed to make a decision as to whether or not they are willing to bear the costs of experimental treatments. Any costs that are associated with the normal routine care are allowed. The use of medications, treatments or examinations that would not normally be utilized in the care of patients with this medical problem must be accounted for. Sometimes the issues are not entirely clear. For example in a study of a vaccine treatment, is a periodic CT scan routine or part of the study. Clearly the investigators need to know if their treatment is effective. The question that needs to be addressed is whether or not the CT would have normally have been obtained if the patient was not on the study. Many times insurance carriers are willing to cover such costs, but it is not their responsibility and if they deny cover, the patient is required to cover the costs. The IRB will therefore require a careful analysis of the protocol with these issues in mind. Compensation of subjects is an equally controversial issue. There are three basic reasons why patients may be compensated: 1) to cover costs associated with participation; 2) as an inducement to participate or 3) to compensate them for tolerating discomfort or inconvenience. While all three are valid reasons, the latter is the most problematic. The danger is not that the compensation is inadequate but rather that the compensation is so high so as to be coercive. This threshold will vary with the discomfort and risk as perceived by the IRB. The standard compensation for a blood draw will be lower than for a bone marrow biopsy or excision of a vaccination site. It is permissible not to compensate subjects at all. If the patients are willing to participate because they feel a moral obligation to be of help then they are free to make that decision. However, the same compensation should be made available to all subjects.

Q: How do you compare your protocol to standard treatment?

A: Most studies are designed to compare a new treatment to what is considered to be standard treatment. Often this an elusive term. Is a relatively ineffective treatment that is commonly used the proper comparison group to a novel treatment or is the proper comparator no treatment? This is more relevant question when an effective regimen is accepted by the medical community.
In this section of the application, the IRB will be expecting you to explain why it is acceptable to allow subjects to receive treatment in the experimental arm. You must tell the committee why it is morally acceptable to deny the patients what is considered standard care for their disease. The task is relatively easier if the patients will be randomized to standard treatment alone or standard treatment plus the experimental arm. The underlying principle here is that patients should not be denied effective treatment for the sake of the experiment.

Q: How will the experiment be monitored and ended?

A: The IRB will expect that there is independent oversight of the experiment. For minimal risk studies such as blood drawing only, minimal supervision is needed. For studies that represent higher risk often a Data Safety Monitoring Board (DSMB) is needed. It is imperative that you detail the stopping rules for the IRB. Stopping rules must cover most contingencies. It is unethical to continue the experiment when 1) there is no longer any possibility that there can be a positive result; 2) the study goal has been met and the addition of additional subjects could not possibly change the outcome or 3) the rate of complications exceeds the tolerance described in the protocol. Again depending on the risks involved in the study these study end points should be monitored by a group that includes a statistician that has no vested interest in the outcome of the experiment. A mechanism for such monitoring must be described including a protocol for ending the study. In this section you must also describe what will be done with PHI once the study is completed.

Q: What are the issues regarding confidentiality?

A: Protection of the patient's privacy is an extremely sensitive issue for the IRB. In this portion of the application you must tell the IRB how you will prevent the release of PHI. The rigor with which study records must be guarded is a function of the type of material that is retained. If the study information is completely stripped of protected health information (PHI), i.e., there is no way for anyone to ever match a record to a particular individual then there is less risk. If on the other hand the records are either directly identified or are linked to a separately held code sheet then appropriate cautions will be expected. The mechanisms might be a locked cabinet or a password protected or encrypted computer file. Whichever way this is done, it must be detailed for the IRB and included in the informed consent. At my institution we once suspended an investigator when we repeatedly found his office door unlocked or guarded and the research files easily available to unexpected visitors to the office.

REFERENCES

1. Animal Welfare Institute. Animals and their legal rights, animal welfare institute; 1990.
2. Carbone L. *What Animals Want: Expertise and advocacy in laboratory animal welfare policy.* New York: Oxford; 2004.
3. Russell WMS, Burch RL. *The Principles of Humane Experimental Technique.* London: Methuen & Co. Ltd.; 1959.
4. United States Interagency Research Animal Committee. *Principles for the Utilization and Care of Vertebrate Animals Used in Testing, Research, and Training.* In: Federal Register, May 20, 1985; 1985:20864-5.
5. Ullman-Cullere MH, Foltz CJ. Body condition scoring: A rapid and accurate method for assessing health status in mice. *Laboratory Animal Science* 1999;49(3):319-23.

6. Flecknell PA. *Laboratory Animal Anesthesia: Second edition, A practical introduction for research workers and technicians.* London: Academic Press; 1996.
7. Kohn DF, Wixson SK, White WJ, Benson GJ, eds. *Anesthesia and Analgesia in Laboratory Animals.* San Diego: Academic Press; 1997.
8. Panel on the Recognition and Alleviation of Animal Pain and Distress. Panel Report on the Colloquium on Recognition and Alleviation of Animal Pain and Distress. *JAVMA* 1987;191(10):1186-91.
9. Moberg GP, Mench JA, eds. *The Biology of Animal Stress: Basic principles and implications for animal welfare.* Wallingford, UK ; New York, NY: CABI Pub.; 2000.
10. Dallman MF, Akana SF, Bell ME, et al. Warning! Nearby construction can profoundly affect your experiments. Endocrine 1999;11(2):111-3.
11. Garner JP, Mason GJ. Evidence for a relationship between cage stereotypes and behavioural disinhibition in laboratory rodents. Behav Brain Res 2002;136(1):83-92.
12. Beaver BV, Reed W, Leary S, et al. 2000 Report of the AVMA Panel on Euthanasia. J Am Vet Med Assoc 2001;218(5):669-96.
13. Green SL. Postoperative analgesics in South African Clawed frogs (Xenopus laevis) after surgical harvest of oocytes. Comp Med 2003;53(3):244-7.
14. Institute of Laboratory Animal Resources. *Guide for the Care and Use of Laboratory Animals.* Washington DC: National Academy Press; 1996.
15. Oocyte Harvesting in *Xenopus laevis* (ARAC Guidelines). 2004. (Accessed December 9, 2004)
16. BVAAWF/FRAME/RSPCA/UFAW Joint Working Group on Refinement. Refinement and reduction in production of genetically modified mice. *Laboratory Animals* 2003;37 Suppl 1:S1-S49.
17. Food and Drug Administration DoHaHS. Good Laboratory Practice for Nonclinical Laboratory Studies (21 CFR 58.90). In. Washington, D. C.: Office of the Federal Register; 2001 (revised).
18. *Code of Federal Regulations.* 2001.

INDEX

Academic environment, 161
Access. *See also* Fair Access to Clinical Trials Act
   INDs and, 88–91
   in international studies, 26–27
Accreditation, 285
Accrual
   community outreach and, 140
   patient advocates and, 135
ACoS. *See* American College of Surgeons
Adult solid tumors, 116–17
AIS. *See* Audit Information System
American College of Surgeons (ACoS), 210
American College of Surgeons Oncology Group, 195
Animal studies, 291–302
   alternatives to, 293
   approval of, 196, 292
   distress in, 295
   FDA and, 291
   pain in, 293–95
   process of, 297–302
   regulations governing, 292
Animal Welfare Act, 292
Anonymizing, 204–6
Approvals
   of animal studies, 292, 296
   CoC and, 214
   FDA and, 54, 106–7
Association for Accreditation of Human Research Protection Programs, 285
Association of American Medical Colleges, 226–27
Association of Clinical Research Professionals, 285
Audit(s), 179–96
   assessment of, 190–94
      communication of, 191–92
      institutional response to, 192–93
      rating criteria in, 191*t*
      scientific misconduct and, 193–94
   clinical trials infrastructure and, 257–58
   components of, 185–86
      consent form reviews and, 187–88
      IRB documentation reviews and, 187–88
      patient record reviews and, 189–90
   CTEP and, 32–33
   CTMB and
      rating system of, 187
      responsibilities of, 181–83
   federal requirements for, 181–83
   goals for, 180–81
   impact of, 194–96
   NCI policy and, 179
   pharmacy reviews and, 188–89
   preparations for, 183–87
      institutional, 186–87
      on-site team selection and, 185
      protocol and patient selections and, 184–85
      scheduling and, 184
   of principle investigators, 164–65, 169–70
   quality assurance and, 179–80, 257–58
Audit Information System (AIS)
   assessment reports and, 192
   audit scheduling and, 184

Bayh-Dole Act
   conflicts of interest and, 226
   industry and, 251
   scientific misconduct and, 279
Beecher, Henry, 12
Belmont Report
   ethical principles of, 13–15, 223
   history of, 12
   industry and, 250
   international studies and, 25–27
Beneficence, 14–15, 223
Best Pharmaceuticals for Children Act, 96–98
Biologics, 57–60
Biostatisticians, 245–46
Business associate agreements, 212–13

Cancer and Leukemia Group B, 194
Cancer Center Support Grants, 248
Cancer prevention, 118–19

Cancer Therapy Evaluation Program
(CTEP), 32–38
 annual accrual of, 46f, 47f
 audit requirements and, 181
 clinical trials and, 37–38, 47f, 48f
 cooperative groups and, 112
 CTMB responsibilities and, 181–83
 drug development program of, 34–37
 letters of intent and, 45f, 46f
 quality assurance and, 32–33
 review types in, 44f
 structure of, 42f
 trials sponsored by, 43f, 49f
Cancer Trials Support Unit (CTSU)
 accrual summary for, 48f
 audits and, 181
 development of, 39–40
 protocol history of, 49f
CCOP. *See* Community Clinical Oncology
 Program
Cellular products, 72–73
Centers for Medicare and Medicaid
 Services, 221
Childhood cancer, 116
Clinical hold
 grounds for, 76–77
 INDs and, 62
 mechanics of, 77–79
Clinical practice
 clinical trials infrastructure and, 241–43
 principle investigators and, 176f
 regulation of, 242
Clinical Research Associate, 245
Clinical research process. *See* Research
 process
Clinical trials infrastructure. *See*
 Infrastructure
Clinical Trials Monitoring Branch (CTMB)
 AIS and, 184
 audits and, 265
  assessment reports and, 192
  guidelines for, 181–85
  rating system for, 187
  requirements for, 187–90
 data reporting to, 236–37
Clinicaltrials.gov, 88
CoC. *See* Commission on Cancer
Code of Federal Regulations, 12
Collaboration, 280
Combined modality therapy, 117–18
Commission on Cancer (CoC)
 approvals and, 214
 conferences and, 214–15
 follow-up and, 215–16
 goals of, 210–11
 HIPAA and, 212–13
 Privacy Rule and, 210
 quality improvement activities of, 213–14
 surveys and, 215
Common Rule
 history of, 12
 impact of, 204–6
 Privacy Rule and, 203–6
Community Clinical Oncology Program
 (CCOP)
 audits and, 181
 cooperative groups and, 113–15
Compensation. *See also* Conflicts of interest
 human research process and, 306–7
 phase I studies and, 18–19
Competition, 280
Compliance
 recommendations for, 228
 support systems for, 222
Conferences
 CoC-sponsored, 214–15
 NBCCF-sponsored, 147–48
 ORI-sponsored, 237
Confidentiality, 268
Conflicts of interest
 Bayh-Dole Act and, 226
 databases for, 265
 Gelsinger, Jesse, case and, 225–26, 271
 guidelines on, 226–27
 in multicenter clinical trials, 5–6
 policies for, 272
 Science in the Private Interest (Krimsky)
  and, 269
 stages of, 269–70
Consent forms
 audits of, 187–88
 language of, 16
 non-therapeutic trials and, 17–18
 phase I studies and, 18–19
 phase II and III studies and, 19–20
 reviews of, 187–88
 therapeutic misconception and, 7
 translation of, 16
Contract research organizations, 3
Contracts, 5, 232
Cooperative groups, 111–25
 activities of, 115–21
  cancer prevention and, 118–19
  cancer treatment and, 116–18
  correlative science and, 119

Index

economic outcomes research and, 120–21
quality of life and, 120
standards setting and, 115
challenges for, 122–23
clinical trial development and, 125*t*
CTEP and, 34, 37
future directions of, 123–24
list of, 47*f*
NCI and, 111–12, 124*t*
processes for, 112–15
strengths of, 121–22
structure of, 112–13
Correlative science, 119
CTEP. *See* Cancer Therapy Evaluation Program
CTMB. *See* Clinical Trials Monitoring Branch
CTSU. *See* Cancer Trials Support Unit

Data
management of, 36–37
sequestration of, 268
Data managers, 245
Data Safety and Monitoring Plan, 248–49
Databases
clinical trials infrastructure and, 262–63
Privacy rule and, 202–3
Decedent research, 202
Declaration of Helsinki, human research and, 2
Department of Defense Breast Cancer Research Program, 150–51
Department of Health and Human Services
ORI and, 232
OSI and, 231–32
Privacy Rule and, 200
Detachment, 159
Directive on Clinical Trials, 284–85
Docu-Mart, 38
Drug Development Group, 45*f*

Electronic medical record, 209
Entrepreneurialism, 279–80
Ethics, 219–28. *See also* Conflicts of interest; Scientific misconduct
compliance support systems and, 222
conflicts of interest and, 225–27
physician-as-researcher and, 224
principle investigators and, 163–64
principles of, 13–15, 222–23
regulatory environment and, 220–21
therapeutic misconception and, 224–25

Ethics and Regulation of Clinical Research (Levine), 222
European Organization for Research and Treatment of Cancer, 195

Fair Access to Clinical Trials Act, 151
Falsification, fabrication, and plagiarism (FFP)
definition of, 266
examples of, 233–35
Fast Track designation, 102–3
FDA. *See* Food and Drug Administration
Federal-Wide Assurance document (FWA), 247–48
Food and Drug Administration (FDA), 51–109. *See also* Investigational New Drug
animal studies and, 291
approvals and, 54, 106–7
authority of, 51–53
biologics and, 57–60
clinical trials infrastructure and, 249–50
Fast Track designation and, 102–3
Food, Drug and Cosmetic Act and, 56
GCP and, 242
history of, 55–57
laws enforced by, 52*t*
marketing applications and, 103–9
accelerated approval of, 106–7
priority review of, 107–8
product labels and, 105–6
regulations of, 103–5
supplemental claims and, 108–9
meetings with, 98–101, 99*t*
organization of, 54
orphan drugs and, 95–96
pediatric programs and, 96–98
Privacy Rule and, 199–200
products regulated by, 53*t*
regulatory environment and, 220–21
special protocol assessments and, 101–2
sponsors and, 60–61
therapeutic development process and, 61*f*
Food, Drug and Cosmetic Act
FDA history and, 55
IND regulations and, 61–64
Fossel, Eric, 234
Fraud, 166
Funding
CTEP and, 36
principle investigators and, 168–69
from private-sector sources, 270

FWA. *See* Federal-Wide Assurance document

GCP. *See* Good Clinical Practice
Gelsinger, Jesse, 2–3, 225–26, 271
GeMCRIS, 283
Gene therapy, 73–74
Gene transfer products, 58
Good Clinical Practice (GCP)
  human subjects research and, 242
  Investigator's Agreement in, 244
Guide for Grants and Contracts (NIH), 232

Hanneken, Vicki, 234
Health Insurance Portability and Accountability Act (HIPAA)
  business associate agreements and, 212–13
  CoC and, 212–13
  electronic medical record standardization and, 209
  Privacy Rule of, 199–207
    anonymizing and, 204–6
    authorization and, 201
    Common Rule and, 203–6
    databases and, 202–3
    decedent research and, 202
    impact of, 204–6
    PHI and, 200–201
    Privacy Board and, 201
    regulations relating to, 199–200
    research review and, 201–2
  regulatory environment and, 221
Herman, Terence, 235
HIPAA. *See* Health Insurance Portability and Accountability Act
Honesty, 159
Human research. *See also* Research process
  clinical practice and, 242
  ethical guidelines for, 12
  funding of, 3
  historical background of, 2–4
  planning exercise for, 302–8
    compensation and, 306–7
    completion and, 307–8
    confidentiality and, 308
    expenses and, 306–7
    hypothesis in, 301
    informed consent and, 306
    IRBs and, 303
    monitoring and, 307–8
    protocols and, 307
    recruitment and, 305–6
    safety and, 304–5

  scientific rationale and, 303–4
  subject selection for, 21–22, 304
Human subjects
  biostatistics and, 246
  definition of, 241
  protections of, 3–4

IND. *See* Investigational New Drug
Industry
  Bayh-Dole Act and, 251
  Belmont Report and, 250
  clinical trials infrastructure and, 250–52
  funding by, 270
  intellectual property and, 251
  systems approach to research and, 287
Informed consent. *See also* Consent forms
  human research process and, 306
  INDs and, 62
  in international studies, 25–27
  IRBs and, 15–17
  patient advocates and, 135
  of prisoners, 23–25
  quality of, 6
  scientific review and, 253
Infrastructure, 241–73
  clinical practice v. clinical research and, 241–43
  conflicts of interest and, 269–73
  information systems and, 261–65
    clinical research databases and, 262–63
    conflicts of interest databases and, 265
    protocol authoring and, 263–64
    web sites and, 264
  institutions in
    culture of, 252–53
    FDA and, 249–50
    IRBs and, 255–57
    NCI and, 248–49
    OHRP and, 247–48
  personnel in
    clinical research associates and, 245
    investigators and, 243–44
    pharmacists and, 246
    research administration officers and, 246–47
    research nurses and, 244–45
  quality assurance and, 257–61
    audits for, 257–58
    monitoring for, 258–59
    ombudsman offices and, 261
    training for, 259–61
  scientific misconduct and, 266–69
    FFP and, 266

Index

investigations into, 268–69
ORI and, 266–67
scientific review in, 253–55
Inhumanity, 295
Initial treatment audits, 184
Institutional Animal Care and Use
  Committee
  approval from, 292, 296
  responsibility of, 292–93
Institutional Review Board (IRB), 11–29
  clinical trials infrastructure and, 255–57
  document audits and, 187–88
  ethical principles and, 14–15
  FWA and, 247–48
  history of, 2–3, 12–13
  human subject protection and, 3–4
  informed consent and, 15–17
  non-therapeutic trials and, 17–18
  phase I studies and, 18–19
  Privacy Rule and, 200
  research process problems and, 280–81
  risk assessment and, 20–21
  special situations and
    international studies and, 25–27
    prisoners and, 23–25
    terminal patients and, 27
  subject selection and, 21–22
  systems approach to research and, 288
  tissue banking and, 28–29
Intellectual property, 251
International Conference on Harmonization, 57
International studies, 25–27
Investigational New Drug (IND), 61–88
  access to, 88–91
    Clinicaltrials.gov, 88
    regulatory mechanisms of, 88
  annual reports and, 87
  applications for, 71–75
    amendments to, 80–83
    cellular products and, 72–73
    gene therapy and, 73–74
    toxicology reports and, 71–72
  charging for, 92
  clinical hold and, 76–79
  clinical trials infrastructure and, 249–50
  consultation and, 68–69
  CTEP and, 34
  expedited safety reports and, 85t
  Fast Track and, 100–1
  filing of, 69–71
  import and export of, 91–92
  investigator responsibilities and, 83–87

legal basis of, 61–65
  clinical hold and, 62–64
  data requirements and, 62
  distribution and, 63
  informed consent and, 62
  pediatric plan and, 62
  record keeping and, 63
  risk and, 63
  scientific justification and, 61
regulations of, 64–66
requirements for, 66–70
  administration routes and, 68
  Guidance Document for, 68
  marketed products and, 66
  promotion and, 67
  review process for, 75–76
  shipping of, 79–80
IRB. *See* Institutional Review Board

Juridification, 276
Justice, 15, 223

Krimsky, Sheldon, 269–70

Legal issues, 219–28
  compliance support systems and, 222
  conflicts of interest and, 225–27
  general principles and, 222–23
  physician-as-researcher and, 224
  regulatory environment and, 220–21
  therapeutic misconception and, 224–25
Levine, Robert J., 222
Limited data set, 213

Monitoring, 258–59
Multicenter clinical trials
  conflicts of interest in, 5–6
  facilitated cooperative review of, 281
  informed consent in, 6–7
  oversight of, 4–5
  systems approach to research with, 284

National Breast Cancer Coalition, 150–51
National Breast Cancer Coalition Fund
  (NBCCF), 143–56
  clinical trial initiatives of, 144–45
  education and
    advocacy training conferences and, 147–48
    Project LEAD® and, 146–47
    published materials for, 148–49
  mission of, 143
  patient advocate perspective of, 144

public policy and, 150–51
scientific collaboration and, 152–55
National Cancer Database, 211–12
National Cancer Institute (NCI), 31–49. *See also* Cancer Therapy Evaluation Program
  audit policy of, 179
  budget of, 286–87
  clinical trials infrastructure and, 248–49
  compliance support systems and, 222
  Cooperative Group Program of, 111–12
  cooperative groups sponsored by, 124*t*
  CTSU and, 39–40, 48*f,* 49*f*
  divisions of, 31–32
  Drug Development Group and, 45*f*
  future directions of, 40–41
  multicenter clinical trials and, 4
  ORI findings and, 233
National Commission for the Protection of Subjects of Biomedical and Behavioral Research, 12
National Institute of Health (NIH)
  compliance support systems and, 222
  Guide for Grants and Contracts by, 232
  ORI and, 232
  OSI and, 231–32
  regulatory environment and, 221
National Research Act, 12
NBCCF. *See* National Breast Cancer Coalition Fund
NCI. *See* National Cancer Institute
NIH. *See* National Institute of Health
Non-therapeutic trials, 17–18

Objective response, 7
Off-cycle audits, 184
Office of Human Research Protections (OHRP)
  clinical trials infrastructure and, 247
  FWA and, 247–48
  history of, 13
  Privacy Rule and, 200
  regulatory environment and, 220
Office of Protection from Research Risks. *See* Office of Human Research Protections
Office of Protocol Research (OPR), 254
Office of Research Integrity (ORI), 231–39
  background of, 231–32
  clinical trials infrastructure and, 266–67
  conferences sponsored by, 237
  scientific misconduct and
    cases of, 233–35, 238*t*–239*t*
    causes of, 236
Office of Scientific Integrity (OSI), 231–32
OHRP. *See* Office of Human Research Protections
Ombudsman offices, 261
OPR. *See* Office of Protocol Research
Oral consent, 26
ORI. *See* Office of Research Integrity
Orphan Drug Act
  FDA history and, 57
  orphan designation and, 95–96
Orphan drugs, 95–96
OSI. *See* Office of Scientific Integrity

Pain, 293–95
Palliative care, 120
Patient advocates, 131–41. *See also* National Breast Cancer Coalition
  accrual and, 135
  community outreach and, 139–41
  function of, 133–34
  grants for, 134–35
  history of, 131–32
  independent projects by, 136
  informed consent and, 135
  NBCCF training conferences for, 147–48
  partnerships with, 136–39
  study development and, 135–36
  training of, 132–33
PDOL. *See* Protocol Document On-Line
Pediatric programs, 96–98
Pediatric Research Equity Act, 98
Personal identifiers, 206
Pharmacies
  audit rating criteria for, 191*t*
  audits of, 188–89
Pharmacists, 246
Phase I studies, 18–19
Phase II studies, 19–20
Phase III studies, 19–20
PHI. *See* Protected health information
Philpot, Thomas, 234–35
Physician-as-researcher, 224
Placebo arms, 24
Poisson, Roger, 233–34
Principle investigators, 157–77
  audits and, 164–65, 169–70
  challenges to
    academic environment and, 161
    collegial, 160
    individual, 159
    institutional, 161–63
  characteristics of, 173*t*

Index

clinical practice v. clinical research and, 176*f*
clinical research methods of, 175*f*
ethical issues and, 163–64
funding issues and, 168–69
GCP and, 244
legal issues and, 167–68
modus operandi of, 174*t*
obligations of, 157–58, 172*t*
regulatory issues and, 164–67
rules for, 174*t*
Prisoners, 23–25
Privacy Board, 201
Privacy Rule, 199–207
anonymizing and, 204–6
authorization and, 201
CoC and, 210
Common Rule and, 203–6
databases and, 202–3
decedent research and, 202
HIPAA and, 199
impact of, 204–6
PHI and, 200–201
Privacy Board and, 201
regulations relating to, 199–200
research review and, 201–2
Project LEAD®, 146–47
Protected health information (PHI)
anonymizing and, 204–6
definition of, 200–201
personal identifiers and, 206
Protocol authoring, 263–64
Protocol Document On-Line (PDOL), 254
Public Health Service Policy on Humane Care and Use of Laboratory Animals, 292

Quality assurance, 257–61
audits for, 257–58
CTEP and, 32–33
monitoring for, 258–59
ombudsman offices and, 261
training for, 259–61
Quality assurance audits. *See* Audits
Quality of life, 120

Regulatory issues
principle investigators and, 164–67
systems approach to research and, 289
Reputation, 268
Research administration office, 246–47
Research ethics review board. *See* Institutional Review Board

Research nurses, 244–45
Research process, 275–89
problems with, 277–82
collaboration v. competition and, 280
entrepreneurialism and, 279–80
IRBs and, 280–81
regulatory requirements and, 289
researcher alienation and, 275–76
systems approach to, 277, 282–85
accreditation and, 285
GeMCRIS and, 283
local v. central review and, 284–85
multicenter trials and, 284
national trust fund for, 283
NCI budget and, 286–87
Respect for persons, 14, 223
Risk
INDs and, 64
IRBs and, 20–21
therapeutic misconception and, 224–25

Science in the Private Interest (Krimsky), 269
Scientific misconduct
audits and, 193–94
Bayh-Dole Act and, 279
cases of, 233–35, 238*t*–239*t*
causes of
ethics panels and, 275–76
overwork, 236
definition of, 193
FFP and, 266
investigations into, 268–69
ORI and, 266–67
Scientific review
informed consent and, 253
OPR and, 254
PDOL and, 254
protocol for, 253–55
Somatic cell therapy, 58, 72–73
Southwestern Oncology Group (SWOG), 194
Special protocol assessments, 101–2
Sponsors
FDA interaction with, 60–61
IND filing and, 69–71
responsibilities of, 173*t*
Surveys, 215
Survivorship, 120
SWOG. *See* Southwestern Oncology Group
Systems approach, 277, 282–87

Tanner, Vivian, 235

Terminal patients, 27
Therapeutic development, 60*f*
Therapeutic misconception
　informed consent and, 6–7
　risk and, 224–25
Tissue banking, 27–29
　federal regulations and, 28–29
　ownership and, 18
Toxicology reports, 73–74
Training
　clinical trials infrastructure and, 259–61
　for patient advocates, 132–33, 147–48
Transgenic mice, 300–301
Translation, 16
Treatment, 116–18
Tuskegee study
　human research and, 2
　subjection selection for, 21

Web sites, 264
Whistle-blowers, 160

Printed in the United States